MW01143212

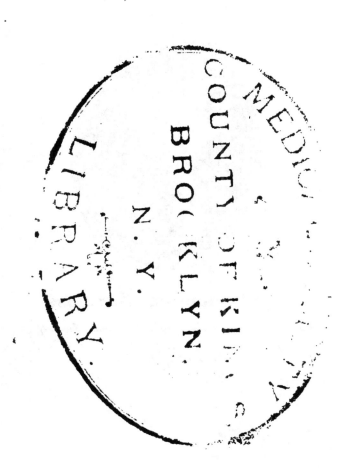

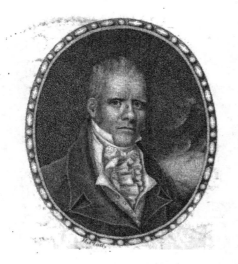

SAMl. THOMSON — BOTANIST.

His System and practice originating with himself

Born Feby 9th 1769.

NEW
GUIDE TO HEALTH;

OR,

BOTANIC FAMILY PHYSICIAN.

CONTAINING

A COMPLETE SYSTEM OF PRACTICE,

On a Plan entirely New;

WITH A DESCRIPTION OF THE VEGETABLES MADE USE OF, AND DIRECTIONS FOR PREPARING AND ADMINISTERING THEM, TO CURE DISEASE.

TO WHICH IS PREFIXED,

A NARRATIVE

OF THE

LIFE & MEDICAL DISCOVERIES

OF THE AUTHOR.

Third Edition.

BY SAMUEL THOMSON.

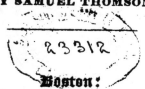
Boston:
Printed for the Author, and Sold by him at No. 4, Clark Street;
and by the Agent, Office of the Investigator,
Merchants' Hall.
1832.
J. Howe, Printer, Merchants Row.

District of Massachusetts....to wit:

DISTRICT CLERK'S OFFICE.

BE IT REMEMBERED, That on the thirtieth day of November, A. D. 1822, in the forty-seventh year of the Independence of the United States, of America, SAMUEL THOMSON, of the said District, has deposited in this Office the Title of a Book, the right whereof he claims as Author and Proprietor, in the words following, to wit:

"New Guide to Health; or, Botanic Family Physician. Containing a complete System of Practice, on a plan entirely new; with a description of the vegetables made use of, and directions for preparing and administering them to cure disease. To which is prefixed, a Narrative of the Life and Medical Discoveries of the author. By Samuel Thomson."

In conformity to the Act of the Congress of the United States, entitled, "An Act for the Encouragement of Learning, by securing the Copies of Maps, Charts and Books, to the Authors and Proprietors of such Copies, during the times therein mentioned:" and also to An Act entitled "An Act Supplementary to an Act, entitled, An Act for the Encouragement of Learning, by securing the Copies of Maps, Charts, and Books to the Authors and Proprietors of such Copies during the times therein mentioned; and extending the benefits thereof to the Arts of Designing, Engraving and Etching Historical and other Prints."

JNO. W. DAVIS,
Clerk of the District of Massachusetts.

ADVERTISEMENT.

TO THE PUBLIC.

The preparing the following work for the. press, has been a task of much difficulty and labour, for to comprise in a short compass, and to convey a correct understanding of the subject, from such a mass of materials as I have been enabled to collect, by thirty years practice, is a business of no small magnitude. The plan that has been adopted I thought the best to give a correct knowledge of my system of practice; and am confident that the descriptions and directions are sufficiently explained to be understood by all those who take an interest in this important subject. Much more might have been written; but the main object has been to confine it to the practice, and nothing more is stated of the theory, than what was necessary to give a general knowledge of the system. If any errors should be discovered, it is hoped that they will be viewed with candour; for in first publishing a work, such things are to be expected; but much care has been taken that there should be no error, which would cause any mistake in the practice, or preparing the medicine.

Many persons are practising by my system, who are in the habit of pretending that they have made great improvements, and in some instances it is well known that poisonous drugs have been made use of under the name of my medicine, which has counteracted its operation, and thereby tended to destroy the confidence of the public in my system of practice, this has never been authorized by me.   The public are therefore cautioned against such conduct, and all those who are well disposed towards my system, are desired to lend their aid in exposing all such dishonest practices, in order that justice may be done.   Those who possess this work, may, by examining it, be able to detect any improper deviations therefrom; and they are assured that any practice which is not conformable to the directions given, and does not agree with the principles herein laid down, is unauthorized by me.

PREFACE.

Written by a Friend.

There is no subject in which the great family of mankind have a deeper interest, than that of medicine; to lessen the sum of human suffering by alleviating pain, and removing those diseases that all are subject to, is a duty of the greatest importance of any undertaking that man can engage in. Health is the greatest blessing that can be enjoyed in this life; and to be deprived of it, takes away all our pleasures and comforts, and makes every thing in this world appear a dreary waste. This will readily be admitted by every one; but in what manner disorder can best be removed or prevented, is a subject that has engaged the attention of many wise men, who have existed in different ages, from the earliest times to the present day, without, as we humbly conceive, very much benefitting mankind by their labours. Their inquiries, it would seem, have been directed to the investigation of visionary theories, of the form and curious construction of the body and members, upon mechanical principles; to the neglect of what is of the greatest importance, a correct and useful practice by a direct application to the cause of disease. This is like pursuing a shadow, and losing sight of the substance; for there are certain causes and effects in the works of creation, that are beyond the comprehension of man, and the general principles of animated nature are as correctly known by the whole human family as by the most wise and learned.

In the different ages of the world, the medical faculty have been very prolific in forming systems of the theory and practice of medicine. One man builds up a system

1*

for another that comes after him, to pull down, who erects one of his own, which is followed for a time, and is then supplanted by another. They have gone on in this way, almost every age producing a new system, to the present time ; each one pronounces the other to be wrong, they certainly cannot all be right, and the most natural conclusion is, that they are all wrong; for no good has resulted from all they have done, but on the contrary, it has tended to produce much confusion and doubt, in the minds of all who seek to gain a correct knowledge of the subject. The best evidence of this, is the bad success that has attended the regular faculty in all their practice, for they do not pretend to a knowledge of a certain remedy for any case of disease ; and it is readily admitted by the most distinguished men in the profession, that there is no art or science, so little understood and miserably conducted, as that of medicine.

The way to become a fashionable doctor at the present day, is to spend three or four years in what they call reading physic, when they receive a degree and a diploma from some medical society. This time is spent in learning the Latin names of the different preparations of medicine, according to the plan adopted by the faculty, as also of the different parts of the human body, with the names, colours and symptoms of all kinds of disease, divided and subdivided into as many classes and forms as language can be found to express; and sufficient knowledge of the nature of medicine to know how much poison can be given without causing immediate death. With these qualifications and a little self-importance, they commence their medical career, as ignorant of what is really useful in curing disease, as though they had been shut up in a cloister all the time. Their heads are filled with the theory, but all that is most important in the removal of disorder, they have to learn by practice, which can never be learned in any other way. Those patients who are so unfortunate as to come under their care, become subjects for them to learn upon, and have to suffer from their experiments. After pursuing this course for many years, they begin to learn that their practice has been wrong ; and it is a fact well known, that all our old and most experienced physicians, who have become distinguished in the profession, make use of but very little medicine; prescribing principally simples, with directions how they may cure themselves; the greater part of their patients, are such as have been run down, and had their constitutions destroyed by the improper treatment they have received from the young and inexperienced part of the faculty.

This picture may be considered by some as highly coloured; but if prejudice is laid aside, and viewed with candour, it will be found not to be far from the truth. There are no doubt many exceptions among the practising physicians; but their manner of treating disease by bleeding and blistering, and administering mercury, arsenic, nitre, antimony, opium, &c. is directly opposed to nature, and cannot be justified by any principles founded on natural causes and effects. Another serious difficulty exists, which is, that the people are kept ignorant of every thing of importance in medicine, by its being kept in a dead language, for which there can be no good reason given. Dr. Buchan has made some very good remarks on this subject, to show the impropriety of such a practice, and gives it as his opinion, that if physicians would write their prescriptions in the language of our own country, and lay medicine more open to the people, much good would result from it. In the new Pharmacopocia, got up lately by the medical societies in this country, an entire new arrangement is made, and new names adopted, which is to be revised every ten years; this will completely keep the people in ignorance of the medicine they use, when prescribed by the faculty.

There can be not the least doubt but there is medicine enough grows in our country, to answer all the purposes necessary in curing every disease incident to the climate, if the people had a knowledge of it; but the doctors have so much influence in society, and manage their affairs with so much art, for their own profit and praise, that the common people are kept back from a knowledge of what is of the utmost importance for them to know. If any man undertakes to pursue a practice differing from what is sanctioned by the regular faculty, let him show ever so much ingenuity in his discoveries, or be ever so successful in curing disease, he is hunted down like a wild beast; and a hue and cry raised against him from one end of the country to the other. There must be some reason for all this, more than an aim to the public good ; for the people are certainly capable of judging for themselves, whether what is done for them, removes their complaint, or increases it. It is not unreasonable, we think, to conclude, that it arises from a fear, that the craft is in danger.

Nothing could more fully exemplify the above opinion than the treatment which Dr. Thomson has received from the medical faculty, during the whole of his practice. He has been persecuted and pursued with all the malice of demons, for no other cause that can be imagined, than because of his extraordinary success in curing disease, which has tended to enlighten the people, and do away their blind confidence in the infallibility of doctors. This opposition has not been from the people at large, for all who have been attended by him, and those who have had a correct knowledge of his system of practice, are not only well satisfied, but are thoroughly convinced of its superiority over the practice of the doctors ; and some of the faculty who have examined the subject, allow the discovery to be original and ingenius, and that the principles upon which it is founded, are correct. If the physicians generally had, instead of trying to destroy him and his practice, inquired into and made themselves acquainted with his improvements, and treated him with that courtesy due to every ingenius man, who devotes himself to the advancement of the arts and sciences, they would have received much useful information on one of the most important branches of the medical art, that is, of the medicinal virtues of the vegetables of this country, with the best method of preparing and administering them to cure disease ; but they seem to consider every thing relating to the subject as a sort of holy ground, on which no one has a right to tread, but the regularly initiated.

Dr. Thomson began his practice as it were from accident, with no other view than an honest endeavour to be useful to his fellow creatures; and had nothing to guide him but his own experience. He not having had an education, has received no advantages from reading books, which left his mind unshackled by the visionary theories and opinions of others; his whole studies have been in the great book of nature, and his conclusions have all been drawn from that unerring guide; by this he was enabled to form correct opinions of the fitness of things. His first inquiry was to know of what all animal bodies were formed, and then to ascertain what caused disease. After being satisfied on this head, the next thing was to find what medicine was the best calculated to remove disease and restore health. For this he looked into the vegetable kingdom, where he found a large field for contemplation, and for the exercise of his inquiring mind. Here, by an invention of his own, that of ascertaining the qualities and power of vegetables by their taste, he was enabled at all times to find something to answer the desired purpose; his apothecary's shop was the woods and the fields.

In his practice, it has always been his first object to learn the course pointed out by nature, and has followed by administering those things best calculated to aid her in restoring health. This is unquestionably the only correct course that can be pursued with any chance of success, for all the good that can be expected by giving medicine, is to assist nature to remove the disease. The success with which his practice has been attended, has astonished all who witnessed it, and has led the people to wonder how a man without learning could perform what could not be done by the learned doctors; this is not strange, for people most generally form their opinions by what is fashionable, without examining into the nature of things. A man can be great without the advantages of an education; but learning can never make a wise man of a fool; the practice of physic requires a knowledge that cannot be got by reading books, it must be obtained by actual observation and experience.

It is very common with the doctors, to call all those who practise, and have not been regularly educated to the profession, quacks, and empirics. The definition of the word quack, is an ignorant pretender; and those who are entitled to this appellation, are best known by the knowledge they possess in their profession, and the success with which they pursue it; and there may be probably more ignorant pretenders found among those who have received a diploma, than in any other class. An empiric is one who is governed in his practice by his own experimental knowledge; and Dr. Thomson can have no reasonable objection to be honoured by this title, for there is nothing valuable in the whole range of the medical science, but what has been derived from this source. In ancient times the man who could discover any thing that proved to be useful in curing disease, was entitled to honourable notice, and a reward for his ingenuity, without regarding whether he was learned or unlearned. In this way the faculty have obtained all their knowledge of vegetable medicine, and if they had confined themseves to this, it would have been much better for the people, than to make use of those poisonous minerals, which have been the production of the learned, and is the only addition they have been able to make to the Materia Medica.

In the following work, Dr. Thompson has endeavoured to embody in a small compass, and to convey to the public, in as plain and simple terms as he was capable, a correct knowledge of his system of practice, with his manner of treating disease, together with a description of all the vegetable productions of our own country that he has found to be useful in curing disorder, and the best manner of preparing and administering them. It will be found of the greatest importance to the people; being the result of thirty years constant practice, in attending on all kinds of disease common in this country. It offers to the public an opportunity to make themselves sufficiently acquainted with the subject, to enable every one who avails himself of it to become his own physician, with a trifling expense.

To introduce a new system of medical practice, and to make an entire change of the public opinion on so important a subject, is an undertaking of too great magnitude to be effected without much difficulty, let its superiority over all others be ever so great; for whoever undertakes it, must expect to have to contend against the interest of a large class of the community, and the prejudices of the whole. That Dr. Thomson has been able to effect so much, is more surprising, than that he has not done more, for he has laboured under many difficulties, besides being opposed by a powerful combination, whose interest it is to keep the people back from adopting his practice. He has been obliged to satisfy the people of what is for their interest, as well as for their peace and happiness, against their own inclinations; and has pursued his own plan with wonderful perseverance, and with an honest and determined zeal, to do what he thought to be his duty. He seems to have had in view more the public good than his own interest, for his whole plan has been to give information to the people, as well as to relieve them from disease; and to put it in their power to cure themselves and families in all cases of sickness, without being under the necessity of employing a doctor. In pursuing this object, he has spent the best part of his days, and has received but very small compensation for all his labours; the pecuniary benefit that he has realised for his practice and rights sold, would be no temptation to any one to undergo the hundredth part of what he has suffered from persecution.

Notwithstanding all the difficulties Dr. Thomson has met with, and all the opposition he has had to contend against, his system is made use of by the people generally, in many places, and it is fast spreading in all parts of the United States. Wherever the people become acquainted with it they universally adopt it, and consider it of the greatest value; so much so, that there are hundreds who would not be deprived of the information they have received, for any sum of money whatever. In several towns, large societies have been formed of those who have purchased the rights, and who obligate themselves to assist each other in cases of sickness; where this has been the case, great benefit has been derived and the success of the practice has been complete. This seems to be the best plan for introducing a correct knowledge of the system and practice among the people, and putting it in their power to derive the most advantage from its use ; and if a few of those men who have the most influence in society, would examine into the subject with impartiality, they would readily be convinced of its superior usefulness, and by taking an interest in diffusing a knowledge of the practice among the people, they would confer a greater benefit on mankind, than by any charitable act they could perform.

There has been one great obstacle in the way of a general extension of a knowledge of the practice, for the want of some means to convey correct information how to prepare and administer the medicine, with the best manner of treatment in curing disease ; and also to prevent all who adopt this system of practice, from being imposed upon by those who pretend to make use of it without a proper knowledge of the subject; for there are quacks under this system as well as others. This is obviated by the following work, in which it is thought will be found sufficient explanations and directions to enable any one who pays strict attention to them, to make use of the practice with safety and success.

NARRATIVE

LIFE, &c. OF SAMUEL THOMSON.

THERE is, nothing, perhaps, more unpleasant than to write one's own life; for in doing it we are obliged to pass over again, as it were, many scenes, which we might wish to have forgotten, and relate many particulars, which, though they may seem very important to ourselves, yet would be very uninteresting to the reader. It is not my intention to attempt to write a history of my life, nor would it be in my power to do it if I had such a wish; but as I have been the greater part of my life engaged in one of the most important pursuits, and which is of more consequence to the great human family, than any other that could be undertaken by man; that of alleviating human misery, by curing all cases of disease by the most simple, safe, and certain method of practice, I think the public will be interested to know something of me, and the reason of my having taken upon myself so important a calling, without being regularly educated to the profession, which is thought by the world to be indispensably necessary; but I shall take the liberty to disagree a little with them in this particular; for, although learning may be a great advantage in acquiring a profession, yet that alone will never make a great man, where there is no natural gift.

By giving a short sketch of the early part of my existence, and relating those accidental circumstances that have occurred during my life, and which were principally the cause of my engaging in the healing art, will enable the public to judge more correctly, whether I

2

have taken that course, in fulfilling my duty in this life, which the God of nature hath pointed out for me. In doing this, I shall endeavour to give a plain and simple narrative of facts as they took place, and relate only those particulars of my life, with such of the cases that have come under my care, as will best convey to the reader, the most correct information of my system of practice in curing disease.

I was born February 9, 1769, in the town of Alstead, county of Cheshire, and State of New Hampshire. My father, John Thomson, was born in Northbridge, county of Worcester, and State of Massachusetts; he was twenty-five years old when I was born. My mother's name was Hannah Cobb; she was born in Medway, Mass. and was four years older than my father. I had one sister older than myself, and three brothers and one sister younger, who are all living except my second brother, who died in his fourteenth year. My oldest sister married Samuel Hills, and lives in Surry, New Hampshire, and my two brothers live in Jericho, Vermont. My youngest sister married Waters Mather, and lives in the State of Ohio.

That country was a wilderness when I was born; my father had began there about a year before, at which time there was no house within three miles one way, and about one the other; there were no roads, and they had to go by marked trees. The snow was very deep when they moved there, and my mother had to travel over a mile on snow shoes through the woods to get to their habitation. My parents were poor, having nothing to begin the world with; but had to depend upon their labour for support. My father had bought a piece of wild land on credit, and had to pay for it by his labour in what he could make off the land, which caused us great hardships and deprivations for a long time.

As soon as I began to form any correct ideas of things, my mind was much irritated by the impressions made on it by my parents, who, no doubt with very good intentions, filled my young head with all kinds of hob-goblin and witch-stories, which made a very deep impression on my mind, and which were not entirely eradicated for many years. I mention this as a caution to parents, not to tell their children any thing but the truth; for young children naturally believe whatever their parents tell them, and when they frighten them with such stories, for the purpose of making them behave well, it will most generally have a very bad effect; for when they arrive at years of discretion, and find that all those stories are falsehoods, they will naturally form very unfavourable opinions of their parents, whose duty it is to set them better examples.

My father and mother were of the Baptist persuasion, and were very strict in their religious duties. They attended meeting every Sabbath, and my father prayed night and morning in his family. One day they went to meeting, and left me and my sister at home alone, and told us that if we were wicked they should send the bear or the knocker to carry us off. While they were absent I was at play, when we heard a hard knocking on the outside of the house, which frightened us very much, and when they came home I told them what had happened; but instead of letting us know what it was, they told us it was the knocker they had told us of, and that or the bear would always come, if we were wicked, and did not mind and do as they told us. It was several years after that my reason taught me that this knocker, as they called it, was a wood-pecker that came on the end of the house. Parents ought to be careful to impress on the minds of young children, correct ideas of things, and not mislead their understandings by telling them falsehoods; for it will be of the greatest importance as respects their future conduct and pursuits in life.

When I was between three and four years old, my father took me out with him to work. The first business I was set to do was to drive the cows to pasture, and watch the geese, with other small chores, which occupation kept me all day in the fields. I was very curious to know the names of all the herbs which I saw growing, and what they were good for; and, to satisfy my curiosity was constantly making inquiries of the persons I happened to be with, for that purpose. All the information I thus obtained, or by my own observation, I carefully laid up in my memory, and never forgot. There was an old lady by the name of Benton lived near us,

who used to attend our family when there was any sickness.   At that time there was no such thing as a Doctor
known among us, there not being any within ten miles.
The whole of her practice was with roots and herbs, applied to the patient, or given in hot drinks, to produce
sweating ; which always answered the purpose.   When
one thing did not produce the desired effect, she would
try something else, till they were relieved.   By her
attention to the family, and the benefits they received
from her skill, we became very much attached to her ;
and when she used to go out to collect roots and herbs,
she would take me with her, and learn me their names,
with what they were good for ; and I used to be very
curious in my inquiries, and in tasting every thing that
I found.   The information I thus obtained at this early
age, was afterwards of great use to me.

Sometime in the summer, after I was four years old,
being out in the fields in search of the cows, I discovered a plant which had a singular branch and pods, that
I had never before seen, and I had the curiosity to pick
some of the pods and chew them ; the taste and operation produced was so remarkable, that I never forgot it.
I afterwards used to induce other boys to chew it, merely
by way of sport, to see them vomit.   I tried this herb
in this way for nearly twenty years, without knowing
any thing of its medical virtues.   This plant is what I
have called the Emetic Herb, and is the most important
article I make use of in my practice.   It is very common
in most parts of this country, and may be prepared and
used in almost any manner.   It is a certain counter poison, having never been known to fail to counteract the
effects of the most deadly poison, even when taken
in large quantities for self-destruction.   There is no
danger to be apprehended from its use, as it is perfectly harmless in its operation; even when a large
quantity is taken ; it operates as an emetic, cleanses
the stomach from all improper aliment, promotes an internal heat, which is immediately felt at the extremities, and produces perspiration.   The exclusive right
of using this plant for medical purposes is secured to
me by patent, and my right to the discovery has never
been disputed ; though the Doctors have done every

thing they could to destroy the credit of it, by false statements, representing it to be a deadly poison, and at the same time they knew to the contrary, for they have made use of it themselves for several years, and have tried to defraud me of the discovery. I feel perfectly convinced from near thirty years experience of its medical properties, that the discovery is of incalculable importance, and if properly understood by the people will be more useful in curing the diseases incident to this climate, than the drugs and medicines sold by all the apothecaries in the country.

At five years of age my father put me to hard work, and was very strict, using the greatest severity towards me. I used to suffer very much from pains in my hips and back, being lame from my birth, and the hard work made me so stiff, that in the morning it was with difficulty I could walk. My father's severity towards me made me very unhappy; for I was constantly in fear lest he should call and I should not hear him, in which case, he used to punish me very severely. I continued in this situation till I was eight years old, when my brothers began to be some help, which took part of the burthen off from me. We suffered great hardships and lived very poorly; but we always had something to eat, and were contented, for we knew of nothing better; a dish of bean-porridge and some potatoes, were our constant fare, and this was better than many others had. The greatest part of this winter we had to live in the barn. In July my father had got a part of the roof of a new house covered, and we moved into it; which was more comfortable than the barn. About this time my mother was taken sick, and was carried to Mrs. Benton's for her to take care of, where she remained for several weeks, during which time, by using such means as this old lady prescribed, she recovered. At this time I had never been to school, or had any chance whatever to learn to read. My father kept me constantly at work all week days, and on Sunday I had to go a considerable distance on foot to meeting, and the rest of the day was kept on my feet in hearing him read the catechism, creed and prayers, so that I had little time to rest on that day.

2*

The winter I was eight years old, I was very sick with the canker-rash; but was attended by the widow Benton, who cured me by making use of such medicine as our country afforded, and I was in a short time able to be about.   After I had got well, my mind was more attentive to the use of roots and herbs as medicine, than ever.   I had at that time a very good knowledge of the principal roots and herbs to be found in that part of the country, with their names and medical uses; and the neighbours were in the habit of getting me to go with them to show them such roots and herbs as the doctors ordered to be made use of in sickness, for syrups, &c. and by way of sport they used to call me doctor.   While in the field at work I used often to find the herb, which I tasted when four years old, and gave it to those who worked with me, to see them spit-and often vomit; but I never observed any bad effect produced by it, which simple experiments eventually led me to observe the value of it in disease.

When I was about ten years old, there was a school a little more than a mile from my father's, where I had the opportunity of attending for one month.   The weather was cold and the going bad, which caused me to make very slow progress in my learning; but the chance we considered a great privilege, for the country was new and people poor, and the opportunity for children to get learning very small.   I took a great dislike to working on a farm, and never could be reconciled to it.; for nothing could strike me with greater dread than to hear the name of a plough, or any other thing used on a farm mentioned.   This I have always attributed to the hardships I underwent, and the severity which my father used constantly to exercise towards me from the time I was five to ten years old.   At that time, I used to think that if I ever had any land I would not plough it; and if my father's treatment of me was the effect of his religion, I never wished to have any. This was when he was under the strongest influence of the baptist persuasion, and used to be very zealous in his religious duties, praying night and morning, and sometimes three times a day.   He was a man of violent and quick temper, and when in his fits of passion, my mother used frequently to remind him of certain parts of his prayer; such as this, which I never forgot: " May we live soberly, righteously, and godly, in the present evil world." She was a woman much respected in the town where we lived.

About the time I was fourteen years old, my father left the baptist persuasion and embraced that of universal salvation ; By grace are ye saved, through faith not of yourselves, it is the gift of God. If he ever experienced a change of heart for the better, it was at this time ; his love to God and man was great, and I had great reason to rejoice, for he was like another man in his house. He continued to enjoy the same belief, with much comfort to the time of his death, which took place in August, 1820, aged 76. My mother remained many years in the full belief of the salvation of all men, and continued so till her death.

Sometime during the year that I was sixteen years old, I heard my parents say, that as my mind was so much taken up with roots and herbs, they thought it best to send me to live with a Doctor Fuller, of Westmoreland, who was called a root doctor. This pleased me very much, and in some measure raised my ambition; but I was soon after disappointed in my hopes, for they said I had not learning enough, and they did not know how to spare me from my work, which depressed my spirits, and was very discouraging to me. I now gave up all hopes of going to any other business, and tried to reconcile myself to spend my days in working on a farm, which made me very unhappy. I had little learning, and was awkward and ignorant of the world, as my father had never given me any chance to go into company, to learn how to behave, which caused me great uneasiness.

In the year 1788, when I was in my nineteenth year, my father purchased a piece of land on Onion river, in the state of Vermont, and on the 12th day of October, he started from Alstead, and took me with him, to go to work on the land and clear up some of it to build a house on, as it was all covered with wood. In about

four days after our arrival, we were enabled to clear a
small spot and to build us a camp to live in ; we had to
do our own cooking and washing; our fare was poor,
and we had to work very hard ; but we got along tolera-
bly well till the 2d of December, when I had the misfortune to cut my ancle very badly, which accident prevented me from doing any labour for a long time, and
almost deprived me of life.   The wound was a very bad
one, as it split the joint and laid the bone entirely bare,
so as to lose the juices of my ancle joint to such a degree as to reduce my strength very much.   My father
sent for a Doctor Cole, of Jericho, who ordered sweet
apple-tree bark to be boiled, and the wound to be washed with it, which caused great pain, and made it much
worse, so that in eight days my strength was almost exhausted ; the flesh on my leg and thigh was mostly gone,
and my life was despaired of ; the doctor said he could
do no more for me ; my father was greatly alarmed about
me, and said that if Dr. Kitteridge, of Walpole, could
be sent for, he thought he might help me ; but I told
him it would be in vain to send for him, for I could
not live so long as it would take to go after him,
without some immediate assistance.   He said he did not
know what to do ; I told him that there was one thing I
had thought of which I wished to have tried, if it could
be obtained, that I thought would help me.   He anxious-
ly inquired what it was, and I told him if he could find
some comfrey root, I would try a plaster made of that
and turpentine.   He immediately went to an old place
that was settled before the war, and had the good luck
to find some ; a plaster was prepared by my directions and applied to my ancle, the side opposite to the
wound, and had the desired effect ; the juices stopped
running in about six hours, and I was very much
relieved ; though the pain continued to be very severe
and the inflammation was great ; the juices settled
between the skin and bone, and caused a suppura-
tion, which broke in about three weeks ; during which
time I did not have three nights sleep, nor did I eat any
thing.   This accidental remedy was found through
necessity, and was the first time the mother of invention held forth her hand to me.   The success

which attended this experiment, and the natural turn of my mind to those things, I think was a principal cause of my continuing to practise the healing art to this time.

Our stock of provisions being now exhausted, and my wound somewhat better, my father was very anxious to return to Alstead. He asked me if I thought I could bear the journey, if he should place me on a bed laid in a sled. I answered that I was willing to try. He immediately went to work and fixed a sled, and put me in it on a straw bed; and on the first day of January, 1789, we began our journey. There was very little snow, and the road rough, which caused the sled to jolt very much, and my sufferings were great. It was very doubtful with my father, and likewise with me, whether I should live to perform the journey; but we proceeded on, however, without any thing important happening, except wearing out the runners of our sled, and having to make new ones, and accomplished twenty miles the first day. At a place where we stopped all night, there was a woman whose situation appeared to me so much worse than my own, that I felt much encouraged. She had been sick with a fever, and the doctor had given so much poisonous medicine, to break the fever, as he called it, she was left in a most miserable situation. Her side and shoulder were in a putrid state, and in full as bad a condition as my ancle. My father in dressing my wound had drawn a string through between the heel-cord and bone, and another between that and the skin; so that two thirds of the way round my ancle was hollow.

At a place where we stopped on the third night, a circumstance had occurred which, from its novelty, I think worth mentioning. A young woman who lived in the family had discovered a strong inclination to sleep more than what is common; and had expressed a wish that they would let her sleep enough once. She went to bed on Sunday night, and did not wake again till Tuesday morning, having slept thirty-six hours. On awaking, she had no idea of having slept more than one night; but began to make preparation for washing, as was the custom on Mondays, till she was informed that they had washed the day before. Her health was good and she never after that required more sleep than other persons.

When we got on to the high land there was considerable snow, and we got along much more comfortably. I had to be carried in on the bed and laid by the fire, every night during the journey. The people generally, where we stopped, treated me with kindness, and showed much pity for me in my distressed situation; but they all thought that I should not live to get through the journey. The doctors had advised to have my leg cut off, as the only means of saving my life, and all those who saw me during our journey, expressed the same opinion; and I think it would have been done had I given my consent; but I positively refused to agree to it, so the plan was given up. I preferred to take my chance with my leg on, to having it taken off; which resolution I have never repented of, to this day.

On arriving in Walpole, my father proceeded immediately to the house of the famous Dr. Kitteridge, to have him dress my wound, and get his opinion of my situation; he not being at home, and it being nearly dark, we concluded to put up for the night, and I was carried in on my bed and laid by the fire. The doctor soon came home, and on entering the room where I was, cried out in a very rough manner, who have you here! His wife answered, a sick man. The devil, replied he, I want no sick man here. I was much terrified by his coarse manner of speaking, and thought if he was so rough in his conversation, what will he be when he comes to dress my wound; but I was happily disappointed, for he took off the dressing with great care, and handled me very tenderly. On seeing the strings that were in the wound, he exclaimed, what the devil are these halters here for? My father told him they were put in to keep the sore open. He said he thought the sore open enough now, for it is all rotten. Being anxious to know his opinion of me, my father asked him what he thought of my situation. What do I think? said he, why I think he will die; and then looking very pleasantly at me, said, though I think young man, you will get well first. In the morning he

dressed my ancle again, and gave me some salve to use
in future; and my father asked him for his bill, which
was, I think, for our keeping and his attending me,
about fifty cents. A great contrast between this and
what is charged at the present time by our regular physicians; for they will hardly look at a person without
making them pay two or three dollars. I have been
more particular in describing this interview with Dr.
Kitteridge, on account of his extraordinary skill in
surgery, and the great name he acquired, and justly
deserved, among the people throughout the country.
His system of practice was peculiarly his own, and all
the medicines he used were prepared by himself, from
the roots and herbs of our own country. He was a
very eccentric character, and uncouth in his manners;
but he possessed a good heart, and a benevolent disposition. He was governed in his practice by that
great plan which is dictated by nature; and the uncommon success he met with is evidence enough to
satisfy any reasonable mind, of the superiority of it
over what is the practice of those who become doctors
by reading only, with their poisons and their instruments
of torture.

We left Walpole, and arrived at our home about noon,
and my mother, brothers and sisters, were much re-
joiced to see me, though grieved at my distressed situation; and never was any one more in need of the tender care of friends than I was at this time. My mother
proved to me the old saying, that a friend in need is a
friend indeed. My case was considered doubtful for
some time. I was from the first of December to the
first of March unable to walk; but by good nursing and
constant care, I was enabled in the spring to attend to
the business at home, so that my father left me in charge
of the farm, and went with my brother to Onion river,
again to work on his land.

On the 9th of February, 1790, I was twenty-one years
of age, and my father gave me a deed of one half of
his farm in Alstead, consisting of one hundred and
twenty-five acres; and I carried it on for three years,
and he had the liberty to take such stock as he pleased.
He then made preparations and removed to Onion river,

and left my mother and sister in my care. Soon after I took a bad cold, which threw me into a slow fever. In the month of March we all had the meazles, and my mother had what the doctors called the black kind, and was so bad that her life was despaired of. The disease turned in and seated on her lungs, and she never recovered her health. Several doctors attended her without doing her any good. Her cough was very severe and her mouth was sore, and she was greatly distressed. I attended upon her under the direction of the doctors, and took the cough, and had much the same symptoms. She continued to grow worse daily; the doctors gave her over, and gave her disease the name of galloping consumption, which I thought was a very appropriate name; for they are the riders, and their whip is mercury, opium and vitriol, and they galloped her out of the world in about nine weeks. She died on the 13th day of May, 1790.

I was at this time very low with the same disorder that my mother died with, and the doctor often importuned me to take some of his medicine; but I declined it, thinking I had rather die a natural death. He tried to frighten me by telling me it was the last chance of getting help, and he thought he could cure me; but I told him I had observed the effect his medicine had on my mother, for she constantly grew worse under the operation of it, and I had no desire to risk it on myself. I have always been of the opinion, that if I had followed his advice, I should have been galloped out of the world the same as my mother was; and I have never repented of my refusal to this day.

After my mother died, I undertook to doctor myself, and made some syrups of such things as I had the knowledge of, which relieved my cough; and with the warm weather, I so far recovered my health, as to be able to work some time in June. Being without women's help, I was obliged to hire such as I could get, which proved a disadvantage to my interest, and I thought it would be best to find some person who would take an interest in saving my property. On the 7th day of July, 1790, I was married to Susan Allen. We were both young, and had great hardships to encounter; but we got along very well, and both enjoyed good health until our first child was born, which was on the fourth day of July following. My wife was taken ill on Saturday, and sent for help; she lingered along till Sunday night, when she became very bad; her situation was dangerous, and she was in hand constantly the whole night, until sunrise the next morning, when she was delivered; but her senses were gone. During the whole night it was one continued struggle of forcing nature, which produced so great an injury to the nervous system, as to cause strong convulsion fits in about an hour after her delivery. The witnessing of this horrid scene of human butchery, was one great cause of my paying attention to midwifery, and my practice has since been very successful in it.

Her fits continued and grew worse; there were six doctors attended her that day, and a seventh was sent for; but she grew worse under their care; for one would give her medicine, and another said that he did wrong; another would bleed her, and the other would say he had done wrong, and so on through the whole. I heard one of them say that his experience in this case was worth fifty dollars. I found that they were trying their practice by experiments; and was so dissatisfied with their conduct, that at night I told them what I thought; and that I had heard them accusing each other of doing wrong; but I was convinced that they had all told the truth, for they had all done wrong. They all gave her over to die, and I dismissed them, having seen enough of their conduct to convince me that they were doing more hurt than good.

After they were gone, I sent for Dr. Watts and Dr. Fuller, who were called root doctors. They attended her through the night, and in the morning about the same hour that they began, the fits left her. She had in the whole, eighteen of the most shocking convulsion fits that had been ever seen by any one present. The spasms were so violent that it jarred the whole house. After the fits had left her, she was entirely senseless, and was raving distracted for three days; and then became perfectly stupid, and lay in that situation for three days; she then laughed three days, and then cried three

3

days; after which she seemed to awake like a person
from sleep, and had no knowledge of what had passed,
or that she had been sick, or had a child.   These two
doctors continued to attend her, and used all the means
in their power to strengthen the nervous system.   She
gained very slowly, and it was a long time before she
got about; but she never got entirely over it.   This
sickness put me back in my business very much, and
the expense was above two hundred dollars.

In about a month after my wife had recovered from
her sickness, she was attacked with the cholic, which
required all my attention, and that of the two doctors
who attended her before ; but all our exertions appeared to be in vain, for the disease had its regular
course for several days and then left her.   These attacks continued once a month, or oftener, and it was so
much trouble to go for the doctor so often, as I had to
during these turns, that I let a young man who studied
with Dr. Watts, have a house on my farm, so as to have
him handy ; but I soon found that by having a doctor
so near, there was plenty of business for him; for there
was not a month in the year but what I had somebody sick in my family.   If a child was attacked with
any trifling complaint, the doctor was sent for, and they
were sure to have a long sickness; so he paid his rent
and keeping very easy.   This doctor lived on my farm
seven years, during which time I had a very good
knowledge of all the medicine he made use of, and his
manner of curing disease, which has been of great use
to me, in finding out the use, or rather the abuse and
imposition of a family doctor, as the family is of no use
to the doctor, unless they are sick, and it is for his profit,
if not sick, to make them so.   During the first of his
practice, he used chiefly roots and herbs, and his success was very great in curing canker and old complaints; but he afterwards got into the fashionable mode
of treating his patients, by giving them apothecary's
drugs; which made him more popular with the faculty,
and less useful to his fellow creatures.

My mind was bent on learning the medical properties of such vegetables as I met with, and was constantly in the habit of tasting every thing of the kind I saw;

and having a retentive memory I have always recollected the taste and use of all that were ever shown me by others, and likewise of all that I discovered myself. This practice of tasing of herbs and roots has been of great advantage to me, as I have always been able to ascertain what is useful for any particular disease, by that means. I was often told that I should poison myself by tasting every thing I saw; but I thought I ought to have as much knowledge as a beast, for they possess an instinct to discover what is good for food, and what is necessary for medicine. I had but very little knowledge of disease at this time; but had a great inclination to learn whatever I had an opportunity; and my own experience, which is the best school, had often called my attention to the subject.

The herb which I had discovered when four years old, I had often met with; but it had never occurred to me that it was of any value as medicine, until about this time, when mowing in the field with a number of men one day, I cut a sprig of it, and gave to the man next to me, who eat it; when we had got to the end of the piece, which was about six rods, he said that he believed what I had given him would kill him, for he never felt so in his life. I looked at him and saw that he was in a most profuse perspiration, being as wet all over as he could be; he trembled very much, and there was no more colour in him than a corpse. I told him to go to the spring and drink some water; he attempted to go, and got as far as the wall, but was unable to get over it, and laid down on the ground and vomited several times. He said he thought he threw off his stomach two quarts. I then helped him into the house, and in about two hours he ate a very hearty dinner, and in the afternoon was able to do a good half day's labour. He afterwards told me that he never had any thing do him so much good in his life; his appetite was remarkably good, and he felt better than he had for a long time. This circumstance gave me the first idea of the medical virtues of this valuable plant, which I have since found by twenty years experience, in which time I have made use of it in every disease I have met with, to great advantage, that it is a discovery of the greatest importance.

In March, 1794, my second daughter was born; and my wife had no medical assistance except what I could do for her, with the advice of the doctor who lived on my farm.　After this she was never again afflicted with the cholic.　In the course of this year the lease of my father's half of the farm expired, and we made a division of the stock.　My half was five yearlings and half a colt; this, with half the farm, containing about one hundred and twenty-five acres, was all the property I possessed, and I was mostly clear of debt.　Soon after, I purchased of my father the other half of the farm, for which I gave six hundred and thirty-six dollars, payable in stock, one half in two years, and the other in four. In order to meet these payments, I purchased calves and colts; but it proved hard for me, as they brought, when the payments became due, but little more than the first cost, after having to keep them two years; I offered them to my father for what the hay they ate the last year would have sold for, but he would not agree to it. I settled with him, however, and paid him according to contract.　I afterwards purchased of a neighbour a small piece of land, which incommoded me by keeping the sun from my house part of the forenoon; for which I agreed to pay him seventy-three dollars and thirty-three cents, in three years, with interest.　This turned out a troublesome affair for me, for when I came to pay the interest the second year, the note was more than when first given, having been altered; and I refused to pay any thing.　When the note became due, I would pay no more than what it was given for, and it was sued and my cattle and horses were attached.　It went through a course of law and cost us both a great deal of expense and trouble; but I finally beat him; he lost his note and I recovered damage for his taking my cattle and horses.　This was the first time I had any thing to do with the law, and in the whole it cost me about one hundred dollars; but it was a good lesson, and has been worth to me the expense.

When my second daughter was about two years old she was taken sick, and had what is called the canker-rash.　Dr. Bliss, who lived on my farm, was sent for, and he said she had that disorder as bad as any one he ever saw. He tried his utmost skill to prevent putrefaction, which he feared would take place; but after using every exertion in his power, without doing her any good, he said he could do no more, she must die. She was senseless and the canker was to be seen in her mouth, nose, and ears, and one of her eyes was covered with it and closed; the other began to swell and turn purple also. I asked the doctor if he could not keep the canker out of this eye; but he said it would be of no use, for she could not live. I told him that if he could do no more, I would try what I could do myself. I found that if the canker could not be stopped immediately, she would be blind with both eyes. She was so distressed for breath that she would spring straight up on end in struggling to breathe. I sat myself in a chair, and held her in my lap, and put a blanket round us both; then my wife held a hot spider or shovel between my feet, and I poured on vinegar to raise a steam, and kept it as hot as I found she could bear, changing them as soon as they became cold; and by following this plan for about twenty minutes, she became comfortable and breathed easy. I kept a cloth wet with cold water on her eyes, changing it often, as it grew warm. I followed this plan, steaming her every two hours, for about a week, when she began to gain. Her eyes came open, and the one that was the worst, was completely covered with canker, and was as white as paper. I used a wash of rosemary to take off the canker; and when the scale came off, the sight came out with it; and it entirely perished. The other eye was saved, to the astonishment of all who saw her, particularly the doctor, who used frequently to call to see how she did. He said she was saved entirely by the plan I had pursued, and the great care and attention paid to her. She entirely recovered from the disease, with the exception of the loss of one eye, and has enjoyed good health to this time. This was the first of my finding out the plan of steaming and using cold water. After this I found by experience that by putting a hot stone into a thing of hot water, leaving it partly out of the water, and then pouring vinegar on the stone, was an improvement. Care should be taken not to raise the heat too fast; and I used to put a cloth wet with cold

3*

water on the stomach, at the same time giving hot medicine to raise the heat inside; and when they had been steamed in this manner as long as I thought they could bear it, then rub them all over with a cloth wet with spirit, vinegar, or cold water, change their clothes and bed clothes, and then let them go to bed.

A short time before this daughter was sick, my oldest son was born, and was very weakly in consequence of his mother's having previous to his birth, what is called a three months' fever, which experience gave me a pretty good knowledge of the practice of the doctors in prolonging a disease; for I never could reconcile myself to the idea, that a doctor could be of any use, if the fever must have its course, and nature had to perform the cure, at the same time the doctor gets his pay and the credit of it. If the patients' constitution is so strong as to enable them to struggle against the operation of the medicine and the disorder, they will recover; but if not, they run down in what the doctors call a galloping consumption. The doctor proceeded in this way with my wife, until I was satisfied of his plan, when I interfered and dismissed him. As soon as she left off taking his medicine, she began gradually to gain her health, and soon got about.

· When this son was about six weeks old, he was attacked with the croup, or rattles. He was taken a little before sunset with a hoarseness, was very much clogged with phlegm, and breathed with so much difficulty, that he could be heard all over the house. I sent for the doctor, and he attended him till about ten o'clock at night without doing him any good, and then went away, saying that he would not live till morning. After he was gone, I was again obliged to call on the mother of invention, and try what I could do myself. I searched the house for some rattle-snake's oil, and was so fortunate as to find about three or four drops, which I immediately gave him, and it loosened the phlegm, and he soon began to breathe easy; by close attention through the night, the child was quite comfortable in the morning. The doctor came in the next day and expressed great astonishment on finding the child alive: and was anxious to know by what means he had been relieved from so desperate a situation. On my informing him, he seemed well pleased with the information; and observed that he was willing to allow, that the greatest knowledge that doctors ever obtained was either by accident or through necessity. So the discovery of a cure for this desperate disease by necessity, was of great use both to me and the doctor; notwithstanding, however, the information he gained of me, instead of giving me credit for it, he charged me for his useless visit.

I was in the habit at this time of gathering and preserving in the proper season, all kinds of medical herbs and roots that I was acquainted with, in order to be able at all times to prevent as well as to cure disease; for I found by experience, that one ounce of prevention was better than a pound of cure. Only the simple article of mayweed, when a person has taken a bad cold, by taking a strong cup of the tea when going to bed, will prevent more disease in one night, with one cent's expense, than would be cured by the doctor in one month, and one hundred dollars expense in their charges, apothecaries' drugs, and nurses.

I had not the most distant idea at this time of ever engaging in the practice of medicine, more than to assist my own family; and little did I think what those severe trials and sufferings I experienced in the cases that have been mentioned, and which I was drove to by necessity, were to bring about. It seemed as a judgment upon me, that either myself or family, or some one living with me, were sick most of the time the doctor lived on my farm, which was about seven years. Since I have had more experience, and become better acquainted with the subject, I am satisfied in my own mind of the cause. Whenever any of the family took a cold, the doctor was sent for, who would always either bleed or give physic. Taking away the blood reduces the heat, and gives power to the cold they had taken, which increases the disorder, and the coldness of the stomach causes canker; the physic drives all the determining powers from the surface inwardly, and scatters the canker through the stomach and bowels, which holds the cold inside, and drives the heat on the outside. The consequence is, that perspiration ceases, because

internal heat is the sole cause of this important evacua-
tion; and a settled fever takes place, which will continue as long as the cold keeps the upper hand. My
experience has taught me that by giving hot medicine,
the internal heat was increased, and by applying the
steam externally, the natural perspiration was restored;
and by giving medicine to clear the stomach and bowels
from canker, till the cold is driven out and the heat returns, which is the turn of the fever, they will recover
the digestive powers, so that food will keep the heat
where it naturally belongs, which is the fuel that continues the fire or life of man.

After the doctor, who lived on my farm, moved away,
I had very little sickness in my family. On the birth
of my second son, which was about two years from
the birth of the first son, we had no occasion for a
doctor; my wife did well, and the child was much more
healthy than the others had been; and I have never
employed a doctor since; for I had found from sad
experience, that they made much more sickness than
they cured. Whenever any of my family were sick, I
had no difficulty in restoring them to health by such
means as were within my own knowledge. As fast as
my children arrived at years of discretion, I instructed them how to relieve themselves, and they have all
enjoyed good health ever since. If parents would adopt
the same plan, and depend more upon themselves, and
less upon the doctors, they would avoid much sickness
in their families, as well as save the expense attending the employment of one of the regular physicians,
whenever any trifling sickness occurs, whose extravagant charges is a grievous and heavy burthen upon the
people. I shall endeavour to instruct them all in my
power, by giving a plain and clear view of the experience I have had, that they may benefit by it. If they
do not, the fault will not be mine, for I shall have done
my duty. I am certain of the fact, that there is medicine enough in the country within the reach of every
one, to cure all the disease incident to it, if timely and
properly administered.

At the birth of our third son, my wife was again given
over by the midwife. Soon after the child was born,

she was taken with ague fits and cramp in the stomach; she was in great pain, and we were much alarmed at her situation. I proposed giving her some medicines, but the midwife was much opposed to it; she said she wished to have a doctor, and the sooner the better. I immediately sent for one, and tried to persuade her to give something which I thought would relieve my wife until the doctor could come; but she objected to it, saying that her case was a very difficult one, and would not allow to be trifled with; she said she was sensible of the dangerous situation my wife was in, for not one out of twenty lived through it, and probably she would not be alive in twenty-four hours from that time. We were thus kept in suspense until the man returned and the doctor could not be found, and there was no other within six miles. I then came to the determination of hearing to no one's advise any longer, but to pursue my own plan. I told my wife, that as the midwife said she could not live more than twenty-four hours, her life could not be cut short more than that time, therefore there would be no hazard in trying what I could do to relieve her. I gave her some warm medicine to raise the inward heat, and then applied the steam, which was very much opposed by the midwife; but I persisted in it according to the best of my judgment, and relieved her in about one hour, after she had laid in that situation above four hours, without any thing being done. The midwife expressed a great deal of astonishment at the success I had met with, and said that I had saved her life, for she was certain that without the means I had used, she could not have lived. She continued to do well and soon recovered. This makes the fifth time I had applied to the mother of invention for assistance, and in all of them was completely successful.

These things began to be taken some notice of about this time, and caused much conversation in the neighbourhood. My assistance was called for by some of the neighbours, and I attended several cases with good success. I had previous to this time, paid some attention to the farrier business, and had been useful in that line. This, however, gave occasion for the ignorant and credulous to ridicule me and laugh at those whom I attend-

ed; but these things had little weight with me, for I
had no other object in view but to be serviceable to
my fellow creatures, and I was too firmly fixed in my
determination to pursue that course, which I considered was pointed out as my duty, by the experience
and many hard trials I had suffered, to be deterred by
the foolish remarks of the envious or malicious part of
society.

The last sickness of my wife, I think took place in
the year 1799, and about two years after she had another
son and did well, making five sons that she had in succession; she afterwards had another daughter, which
was the last, making eight children in the whole that
she was the mother of; five sons and three daughters.
I mention these particulars in order that the reader may
the better understand many things that took place in
my family, which will give some idea of the experience
and trouble I had to encounter in bringing up so large
a family, especially with the many trials I had to go
through in the various cases of sickness and troubles,
which are naturally attendant on all families, and of
which I had a very large share.   The knowledge and
experience, however, which I gained by these trying
scenes I have reason to be satisfied with, as it has proved
to be a blessing, not only to me, but many hundreds who
have been relieved from sickness and distress through
my means ; and I hope and trust that it will eventually
be the cause of throwing off the veil of ignorance from
the eyes of the good people of this country, and do away
the blind confidence they are so much in the habit of
placing in those who call themselves physicians, who
fare sumptuously every day ; living in splendour and
magnificence, supported by the impositions they practise upon a deluded and credulous people; for they have
much more regard for their own interest than they
have for the health and happiness of those who are
so unfortunate as to have any thing to do with them.
If this was the worst side of the picture, it might be
borne with more patience; but their practice is altogether experimental, to try the effect of their poisons upon
the constitutions of their patients, and if they happen
to give more than nature can bear, they either die or

become miserable invalids the rest of their lives, and
their friends console themselves with the idea that it
is the will of God, and it is their duty to submit; the
doctor gets well paid for his services and that is an end
of the tragedy. It may be thought by some that this is
a highly coloured picture, and that I am uncharitable
to apply it to all who practise as physicians; but the
truth of the statements, as respects what are called regular physicians, or those who get diplomas from the
medical society, will not be doubted by any who are
acquainted with the subject, and will throw aside prejudice and reflect seriously upon it—those whom the coat
fits I am willing should wear it. There are, however,
many physicians within my knowledge, who do not follow the fashionable mode of practice of the day, but
are governed by their own judgments, and make use of
the vegetable medicine of our own country, with the
mode of treatment most consistent with nature; and
what is the conduct of those who have undertaken to
dictate to the people how and by whom they shall be attended when sick, towards them? Why, means that
would disgrace the lowest dregs of society, that savages
would not be guilty of, are resorted to for the purpose of
injuring them, and destroying their credit with the public.
I have had a pretty large share of this kind of treatment
from the faculty, the particulars of which, and the sufferings I have undergone, will be given in detail in the
course of this narrative.

Sometime in the month of November, 1802, my children had the measles, and some of them had them very
bad. The want of knowing how to treat them gave me
a great deal of trouble, much more than it would at the
present time, for experience has taught me that they
are very easy to manage. One of the children took the
disease and gave it to the rest, and I think we had four
down with them at the same time. My third son had
the disorder very bad; they would not come out, but
turned in, and he became stupid. The canker was
much in the throat and mouth, and the rosemary would
have no effect. Putrid symptoms made their appearance, and I was under the necessity of inventing something for that, and for the canker. I used the steam of

vinegar to guard against putrefaction, and gold thread, or yellow root, with red oak acorns pounded and steeped together, for the canker. These had the desired effect; and by close attention he soon got better. The second son was then taken down pretty much in the same manner, and I pursued the same mode of treatment, with similar success; but the disease had so effected his lungs, that I feared it would leave him in a consumption, as was the case with my mother. He could not speak loud for three weeks. I could get nothing that would help him for some time, till at last I gave him several portions of the emetic herb, which relieved him and he soon got well. During this sickness we suffered much from fatigue and want of sleep; for neither my wife nor myself had our clothes off for twelve nights. This was a good fortnight's school to me, in which I learned the nature of the measles; and found it to be canker and putrefaction. This experience enabled me to relieve many others in this disease, and likewise in the canker-rash; in these two disorders, and the small pox, I found a looking-glass, in which we may see the nature of every other disease. I had the small pox in the year 1798, and examined its symptoms with all the skill I was capable of, to ascertain the nature of the disease; and found that it was the highest stage of canker and putrefaction that the human system was capable of receiving; the measles the next, and the canker-rash the third; and other disorders partake more or less of the same, which I am satisfied is a key to the whole; for by knowing how to cure this, is a general rule to know how to cure all other cases; as the same means that will put out a large fire will put out a candle.

Soon after my family had got well of the measles, I was sent for to see a woman by the name of Redding, in the neighbourhood. She had been for many years afflicted with the cholic, and could get no relief from the doctors. I attended her and found the disorder was caused by canker, and pursued the plan that my former experience had taught me, which relieved her from the pain, and so far removed the cause that she never had another attack of the disease. In this case the cure was so simply and easily performed, that it became a subject of ridicule, for when she was asked about it, she was ashamed to say that I cured her. The popular practice of the physicians had so much influence on the minds of the people, that they thought nothing could be right but what was done by them. I attended in this family for several years, and always answered the desired purpose ; but my practice was so simple, that it was not worthy of notice, and being dissatisfied with the treatment I received, I refused to do any thing more for them. After this they employed the more fashionable practitioners, who were ready enough to make the most of a job, and they had sickness and expense enough to satisfy them, for one of the sons was soon after taken sick and was given over by the doctor, who left him to die; but after he left off giving him medicine he got well of himself, and the doctor not only had the credit of it, but for this job and one other similar his charges amounted to over one hundred dollars. This satisfied me of the foolishness of the people, whose prejudices are always in favour of any thing that is fashionable, or that is done by those who profess great learning ; and prefer long sickness and great expense, if done in this way, to a simple and natural relief, with a trifling expense.

Soon after this, I was called on to attend a Mrs. Wetherbee, in the neighbourhood, who had the same disorder. She had been afflicted with the colick for several years having periodical turns of it about once a month ; had been under the care of a number of doctors who had used all their skill without affording her any relief, excepting a temporary one by stupifying her with opium and giving physic, which kept her along till nature could wear it off, when she would get a little better for a few days, and then have another turn. After hearing of my curing Mrs. Redding, they sent for me ; I gave her my medicine to remove the canker, and steamed her, which gave relief in one hour. She had a very large family to attend to, having thirteen children, and before she had recovered her strength she exposed herself and had another turn ; I attended again and relieved her in the same manner as before; but she could not wait till she gained her strength, and exposed.

4

herself again as before, took cold and had another turn.
Her husband said I only relieved her for the time, but
did not remove the cause, and being dissatisfied with
what I had done, he sent for a doctor to remove the
cause; who carried her through a course of physic, and
reduced her so low, that she lingered along for eight
weeks, being unable to do any thing the whole time;
they then decided that she had the consumption, and
gave her over to die. After the doctors had left her in
this situation as incurable, she applied again to me; but
I declined doing any thing for her, as I knew her case
was much more difficult than it was before she applied
to the doctor, and if I should fail in curing her, the
blame would all be laid to me, or if she got well I should
get no credit by it; for which reason I felt very unwilling to do any thing for her. After finishing my forenoon's work, on going home to dinner, I found her at
my house, waiting for me, and she insisted so much upon
my undertaking to cure her, and seemed to have so
much faith in my being able to do it, that I at last told
her, if she would come to my house and stay with my
wife, who was sick at the time, I would do the best I
could to cure her. She readily consented, and staid but
three days with us; during which time I pursued my
usual plan of treatment, giving her things to remove
the canker, and steaming to produce a natural perspiration; at the end of the three days she went home,
taking with her some medicine, with directions what to
do for herself, and in a short time entirely recovered her
health. In less than a year after, she had another child,
which was a conclusion of her having children or the
colick, and she ever after enjoyed as good health as any
woman in the neighbourhood; but this cure was done
in so unfashionable a way, that they were hardly willing
to acknowledge it, and they would not apply to me for
relief when any of their family were sick, till they had
failed in getting it in any other way.

In about a year after the above case, one of this
family, a young man about sixteen years old, was attacked with a fever; the doctor was sent for, who followed the fashionable course of practice, and reduced
him with mercury and other poisons, so that he linger-

ed along for three or four months, constantly growing worse, till the doctor said it was a rheumatic fever, and afterwards that he was in a decline. He had taken so much mercury that it had settled in his back and hips, and was so stiff that he could not bring his hands lower than his knees. By this time the doctor had given him over as incurable, and he was considered a fit subject for me to undertake with. They applied to me, and I agreed to take him home to my house, and do the best I could to cure him. It was a difficult task, for I had in the first place to bring him back to the same situation he was in when he had the fever, and to destroy the effects of the poison and regulate the system by steaming, to produce a natural perspiration; by pursuing this plan, and giving such things as I could get to restore the digestive powers, in two months he was completely restored to health; for which I received but five dollars, and this was more grudgingly paid than if they had given a doctor fifty, without doing any good at all.

In the spring of the year 1805, I was sent for to go to Woodstock, in Vermont, to attend a young woman, who was considered in a decline, and the doctors could not help her. I found her very low, not being able to set up but very little. I staid and attended her about a week, and then left her, with medicines and directions what to do, and returned home. In about a month, I went again to see her, and found her much better, so that she was able to ride to her father's, which was above twenty miles. All this time I had not formed an idea that I possessed any knowledge of disorder or of medicine, more than what I had learned by accident; and all the cases I had attended were from necessity; but the success I had met with, and the extraordinary cures I had performed, made much talk, and were heard of for fifty miles around.

I began to be sent for by the people of this part of the country so much, that I found it impossible to attend to my farm and family as I ought; for the cases I had attended, I had received very little or nothing, not enough to compensate me for my time; and I found it to be my duty to give up practice altogether, or to make a business of it. I consulted with my wife and asked the advice of my friends, what was best for me to do; they all agreed, that as it seemed to be the natural turn of my mind, if I thought myself capable of such an important undertaking, it would be best to let my own judgment govern me, and to do as I thought best. I maturely weighed the matter in my mind, and viewed it as the greatest trust that any one could engage in. I considered my want of learning and my ignorance of mankind, which almost discouraged me from the undertaking; yet I had a strong inclination for the practice, of which it seemed impossible to divest my mind; and I had always had a very strong aversion to working on a farm, as every thing of the kind appeared to me to be a burthen; the reason of which I could not account for, as I had carried on the business to good advantage, and had as good a farm as any in the neighbourhood. I finally concluded to make use of that gift which I thought nature, or the God of nature had implanted in me; and if I possessed such a gift, I had no need of learning, for no one can learn that gift. I thought of what St. Paul says in his epistle to the Corinthians, concerning the different gifts by the same spirit; one had the gift of prophecy; another, the gift of healing, another, the working of miracles. I am satisfied in my own mind, that every man is made and capacitated for some particular pursuit in life, in which, if he engages, he will be more useful than he would if he happens to be so unfortunate as to follow a calling or profession, that was not congenial to his disposition. This is a very important consideration for parents, not to make their sons learn trades or professions which are contrary to their inclinations and the natural turn of their minds; for it is certain if they do, they never can be useful or happy in following them.

I am convinced myself that I possess a gift in healing the sick, because of the extraordinary success I have met with, and the protection and support I have been afforded against the attacks of all my enemies. Whether I should have been more useful had it been my lot to have had an education, and learned the profession in the fashionable way, is impossible for me to say with certainty; probably I should have been deemed more honourable in the world; but honour obtained by learning, without a natural gift, or capacity, can never, in my opinion, make a man very useful to his fellow creatures. I wish my readers to understand me, that I do not mean to convey the idea, that learning is not necessary and essential in obtaining a proper knowledge of any profession or art; but that going to college will make a wise man of a fool, is what I am ready to deny; or that a man cannot be useful and even great in a profession, or in the arts and sciences, without a classical education, is what I think no one will have the hardihood to attempt to support, as it is contrary to reason and common sense.   We have many examples of some of the greatest philosophers, physicians, and divines the world ever knew, who were entirely self-taught ; and who have done more honour, and been greater ornaments to society, than a million of those who have nothing to recommend them but having their heads crammed with learning, without sense enough to apply it to any great or useful purpose.

Among the practising physicians, I have found, and I believe it to be a well known fact, that those who are really great in the profession and have had the most experience, condemn as much as I do, the fashionable mode of practice of the present day, and use very little medical poisons, confining themselves in their treatment of patients to simples principally, and the use of such things as will promote digestion and aid nature ; and many of them disapprove of bleeding altogether. Those of this description, with whom I have had an opportunity to converse, have treated me with all due attention and civility; have heard me with pleasure, and been ready to allow me credit for my experience, and the discoveries I have made in curing disease.   The opposition and abuse that I have met with, have been uniformly from those to whom I think I can with propriety, give the name of quacks, or ignorant pretenders; as all their merit consists in their self-importance and arrogant behaviour towards all those who have not had the advantages of learning, and a degree at college. This class compose a large proportion of the medical faculty throughout our country; they have learned just enough to know how to deceive the people, and keep them in ignorance, by covering their doings under an

4*

unknown language to their patients.   There can be no
good reason given why all the technical terms in medical
works are kept in a dead language, except it be to deceive and keep the world ignorant of their doings, that
they may the better impose upon the credulity of the
people; for if they were to be written in our own language, every body would understand them, and judge for
themselves; and their poisonous drugs would be thrown
into the fire before their patients would take them.   The
ill-treatment that I have received from them, has been
mostly where I have exposed their ignorance by curing
those they had given over to die; in which cases they
have shown their malice by circulating all kinds of false
and ridiculous reports of me and my practice, in order
to destroy my credit with the people; and I am sorry to
say that I have found many too ready to join with them,
even among those who have been relieved by me from
pain and sickness.   Such ingratitude I can account for
in no other way, than by the readiness with which the
people follow whatever is fashionable, without reflecting
whether it be right or wrong.

After I had come to the determination to make a
business of the medical practice, I found it necessary to
fix upon some system or plan for my future goverment
in the treatment of disease; for what I had done had
been as it were from accident, and the necessity arising
out of the particular cases that came under my care,
without any fixed plan; in which I had been governed
by my judgment and the advantages I had received from
experience.   I deemed it necessary, not only as my own
guide, but that whatever discoveries I should make in
my practice, they might be so adapted to my plan that
my whole system might be easily taught to others, and
preserved for the benefit of the world.   I had no other
assistance than my own observations and the natural
reflections of my own mind, unaided by learning or the
opinions of others.   I took nature for my guide, and
experience as my instructer; and after seriously considering every part of the subject, I came to certain
conclusions concerning disease and the whole animal
economy, which more than thirty years experience has
perfectly satisfied me is the only correct theory.   My

practice has invariably been conformable to the general principles upon which my system is founded, and in no instance have I had reason to doubt the correctness of its application to cure all cases of disease when properly attended to; for that all disease is the effect of one general cause, and may be removed by one general remedy, is the foundation upon which I have erected my fabric, and which I shall endeavour to explain in as clear and concise a manner as I am capable, with a hope that it may be understood by my readers, and that they may be convinced of its correctness.

I found, after maturely considering the subject, that all animal bodies are formed of the four elements, earth, air, fire, and water. Earth and water constitute the solids, and air and fire, or heat, are the cause of life and motion. That cold, or lessening the power of heat, is the cause of all disease; that to restore heat to its natural state was the only way by which health could be produced; and that after restoring the natural heat, by clearing the system of all obstructions and causing a natural perspiration, the stomach would digest the food taken into it, by which means the whole body is nourished and invigourated, and heat or nature is enabled to hold its supremacy; that the constitutions of all mankind being essentially the same, and differing only in the different temperament of the same materials of which they are composed; it appeared clearly to my mind, that all disease proceeded from one general cause, and might be cured by one general remedy; that a state of perfect health arises from a due balance or temperature of the four elements; but if it is by any means destroyed, the body is more or less disordered. And when this is the case, there is always an actual diminution or absence of the element of fire, or heat; and in proportion to this diminution or absence, the body is affected by its opposite, which is cold. And I found that all disorders which the human family were afflicted with, however various the symptoms, and different the names by which they are called, arise directly from obstructed perspiration, which is always caused by cold, or want of heat; for if there is a natural heat, it is imposible but that there must be a natural perspiration.

Having fixed upon these general principles, as the only solid foundation upon which a correct and true understanding of the subject can be founded, my next business was to ascertain what kinds of medicine and treatment would best answer the purpose in conformity to this universal plan of curing disease; for it must, I think, be certain and self-evident to every one, that whatever will increase the internal heat, remove all obstructions of the system, restore the digestive powers of the stomach, and produce a natural perspiration, is universally applicable in all cases of disease, and therefore may be considered as a general remedy.

The first and most important consideration was to find a medicine that would establish a natural internal heat, so as to give nature its proper command. My emetic herb, (No. 1,) I found would effectually cleanse the stomach, and would very effectually aid in raising the heat and promoting perspiration; but would not hold it long enough to effect the desired object, so but that the cold would return again and assume its power. It was like a fire made of shavings; a strong heat for a short time, and then all go out. After much experience, and trying every thing within my knowledge, to gain this important point, I fixed upon the medicine which I have called No. 2, in my patent, for that purpose; and after using it for many years, I am perfectly convinced that it is the best thing that can be made use of to hold the heat in the stomach until the system can be cleared of obstructions, so as to produce a natural digestion of the food, which will nourish the body, establish perspiration and restore the health of the patient. I found it to be perfectly safe in all cases; and never knew any bad effects from administering it.

My next grand object was to get something that would clear the stomach and bowels from canker, which are more or less effected by it in all cases of disease to which the human family are subject. Canker and putrefaction are caused by cold, or want of heat; for whenever any part of the body is so affected by cold as to overpower the natural heat, putrefaction commences, and if not checked by medicine, or if the natural constitution is not strong enough to overcome its progress it will communicate to the blood, when death will end the contest between heat and cold, by deciding in favour of the latter. I have made use of a great many articles, which are useful in removing canker; but my preparation called No. 3, is the best for that purpose, that has come to my knowledge; though many other things may be made use of to good effect, all of which I shall give particular description of in my general directions hereafter.

Having endeavoured to convey to my readers in a brief manner a correct idea of the general principles upon which I formed my system of practice, I shall now give some account of the success I met with in the various cases that came under my care, and the difficulties and opposition that I have had to encounter in maintaining it till this time, against all my enemies.

My general plan of treatment has been in all cases of disease, to cleanse the stomach by giving No. 1, and produce as great an internal heat as I could, by giving No. 2, and when necessary, made use of steaming, in which I have always found great benefit, especially in fevers; after this, I gave No. 3, to clear off the canker; and in all cases where patients had not previously become so far reduced as to have nothing to build upon, I have been successful in restoring them to health. I found that fever was a disturbed state of the heat, or more properly, that it was caused by the efforts which nature makes to throw off disease, and therefore ought to be aided in its cause, and treated as a friend; and not as an enemy, as is the practice of the physicians. In all cases of disease, I have found that there is more or less fever, according to the state of the system; but that all fevers proceed from the same cause, differing only in the symptoms; and may be managed and brought to a crisis with much less trouble than is generally considered practicable, by increasing the internal heat, till the cold is driven out, which is the cause of it. Thus keeping the fountain above the stream, and every thing will take its natural course.

During the year 1805, a very alarming disease prevailed in Alstead and Walpole, which was considered the yellow fever, and was fatal to many who were attacked by it. -I was called on, and attended with very great success, not losing one patient that I attended; at the same time nearly one half of those who had regular physicians, died. This disease prevailed for about forty days, during which time, I was not at home but eight nights. I was obliged to be nurse as well as doctor, and do every thing myself, for the people had no knowledge of my mode of practice, and I could not depend upon what any person did, except what was under my own immediate inspection. I pursued the same general plan that I had before adopted; but the experience I had from this practice, suggested to me many improvements, which I had not before thought of, as respects the manner of treatment of patients to effect the objects I aimed at in curing the disease, which was to produce a natural perspiration. I found great benefit in steaming in the manner that I had discovered and practised with my little daughter; but I found by experience, that by putting a hot stone into a spider or iron bason, and then wetting the top of the stone with vinegar, was an important improvement; and with this simple method, with a little medicine of my own preparing, answered a much better purpose; than all the bleeding and poisonous physic of the doctors. While I was attending those who were sick, and they found that my mode of treatment relieved them from their distress, they were very ready to flatter and give great credit for my practice; but after I had worn myself out in their service, they began to think that it was not done in a fashionable way; and the doctors made use of every means in their power to ridicule me and my practice, for the purpose of maintaining their own credit with the people. This kind of treatment was a new thing to me, as I did not at that time so well understand the craft, as I have since, from hard earned experience. The word quackery, when used by the doctor against me, was a very important charm to prejudice the people against my practice; but I would ask all the candid and reflecting part of the people, the following questions, and I will leave them to their consciences to give an answer; which is the greatest quack, the one who

relieves them from their sickness by the most simple
and safe means, without any pretentions to infallibility
or skill, more than what nature and experience has
taught him? or the one who, instead of curing the disease, increases it by administering poisonous medicine,
which only tend to prolong the distress of the patient,
till either the strength of his natural constitution, or
death relieves him?

I was called upon to attend a man by the name of
Fairbanks, who lived in Walpole; he was taken with
bleeding at the lungs. I found him in a very bad condition; the family judged that he had lost nearly six
quarts of blood in twenty-four hours. He was in despair and had taken leave of his family, as they considered there was no hopes of his living. The doctor
was with him when I first entered the house; but he
fled at my approach. Both his legs were corded by
the doctor, and the first thing I did was to strip off the
cords from his legs; and then gave medicine to get as
great an internal heat as I possibly could produce; got
him to sweat profusely; then gave him medicine to
clear the canker; and in four days he was so well as to
be able to go out and attend to his business.

Sometime in October, 1805, I attended a Mrs. Goodell,
of Walpole; she had been confined and had taken
cold. The most noted doctors in the town had attended
her through what they called a fever, and she was then
pronounced by them to be in a decline. After three
months practice upon her, they had got her into so desperate a situation, that they gave her over, and said that
her case was so putrid and ulcerated that it was utterly
incurable. She had in addition to the rest of her difficulties, a cancer on her back. In this desperate situation, it was thought by her friends that she was a proper
subject for me to undertake with. I, with a great deal
of reluctance, undertook with her at her earnest solici-
tation and that of her husband; but met with much
greater success than I expected. In four weeks she
was able to be about the house and do some work.

In the same year I was sent for to attend a woman
who had been in a dropsical way for a number of
years. The disease had of late gained with rapid

progress.   Her husband had previously conversed with
me upon the subject and said that he had applied to Dr.
Sparahawk, and others, and they had agreed to make
a trial of mercury.   I told him that it would not answer
the purpose; he said he was afraid of it himself; but
the doctors said there was no other possible way.   The
doctor tried his mercurial treatment for several days,
which very nearly proved fatal; for I was sent for in
great haste, with a request that I would attend as soon
as possible, as they expected she would not live through
the day.   I found her situation very distressing; she
said it appeared to her that she was full of scalding water.   She began to turn purple in spots, and it was
expected that mortification had taken place.   In the
first place I gave her about a gill of checkerberry and
hemlock, distilled, which allayed the heat immediately.   This answered the purpose, till I could clear her
stomach, and by the greatest exertions, and close attention through the day, I was enabled to relieve her.   I
attended her for about a week, and she was so far recovered as to enjoy comfortable health for twelve years.

Notwithstanding this desperate case was cured, to the
astonishment of all who witnessed it, the doctors had so
much influence over the people, and made so many
false statements about it, that I got no credit for the
cure.   This woman's brother had said that her husband
wanted to kill her or he would not have sent for me.
Such kind of ingratitude was discouraging to me; but it
did not prevent me from persevering in my duty.

A short time after the above case happened, that
woman's brother, who made the speech about me, was
taken very sick, with what was called the yellow fever,
and sent for me.   I attended him and asked him if he
wanted to die.   He said no; why do you ask that?   I
told him, that I should suppose from the speech he made
about my being sent for to his sister, that he did, or he
would not have sent for me, if he believed his own
words.   He said he thought differently now.   I attended
him through the day with my new practice.   To sweat
him I took hemlock boughs, and put a hot stone in the
middle of a large bunch of them, wrapping the whole
in a cloth and poured on hot water till I raised a lively

steam, and then put one at his feet and another near his body. I gave him medicine to raise the inward heat, and for the canker; after attending him through the day, I went home; and on calling to see him the next morning, found his fever had turned, and he was quite comfortable, so that he was soon about his business.

I was about this time sent for to see a child in Surry, a neighbouring town, which was taken very sick, and was entirely stupid. I told the father of the child that it had the canker, and made use of my common mode of practice for that difficulty. Being sent for to go to Walpole to see two young men who had been taken the day before with the prevailing fever, I left the child, with directions how to proceed with it. I then started for Walpole, and found the two young men violently attacked with the fever. They had a brother who had been attended by the doctor for above four weeks for the same disease, and was then just able to sit up. It was thought by all, the two that were attacked last, were as violently taken as the other was; and they expressed a strong wish, that they might be cured without so long a run as their brother had. I was as anxious as they were to have a short job, and exerted all my powers to relieve them, which I was enabled to do that night, and left them in the morning quite comfortable, so that they were soon able to attend to their work. The brother who had the doctor, was unable to do any thing for several months. The doctor was paid a heavy bill for his visits; but my cure was done so quick, that it was thought not to be worthy of their notice, and I never received a cent from them for my trouble. On returning to the child that I had left the day before, I found that the doctor had been there and told them that I did not know what was the matter with the child; and had persuaded them to give him the care of it. He filled it with mercury and run it down; after having given as much mercury inside as nature could move, and the bowels grew silent, he then rubbed mercurial ointment on the bowels as long as it had any effect; after which he agreed that the child had the canker very badly; but he still persisted in the same course till the child wasted away and died, in about two months after it

5

was first taken sick.   After the child was dead, its parents were willing to allow that I understood the disorder best.   The doctor got twenty-five dollars for killing the child by inches, and I got nothing.

In the spring of 1805, a Mrs. Richardson was brought to my house.   She was brought in her bed from Westford, Vermont, about 180 miles, and was attended by a son and daughter, the one 21 and the other 18 years of age.   The mother had lain in her bed most part of the time for ten years.   All the doctors in that part of the country had been applied to without any advantage ; and they had spent nearly all their property.   I undertook with her more from a charitable feeling for the young man and woman, than from any expectation of a cure.   Their conduct towards their helpless mother, was the greatest example of affection of children to a parent that I ever witnessed.   The young man stated to me that his mother had been a year together without opening her eyes ; that when she could open them, they thought her almost well.   She was perfectly helpless, not being able to do the least thing ; not even to brush off a fly, any more than an infant.   She had laid so long that her knee joints had become stiff.

I began with her by cleansing her stomach, and promoting perspiration ; after which, I used to try to give her some exercise.   The first trial I made was to put her bed into a wheelbarrow and lay her on it : when I would run her out, till she appeared to be weary ; sometimes I would make a mistep and fall, pretending that I had hurt me ; in order to try to get her to move herself by frightening her.   After exercising her in this way for a few days, I put her in a wagon, sitting on a bed, and drove her about in that manner ; and when her joints became more limber, I sat her on the seat of the wagon.   She insisted that she should fall off, for she said she could not use her feet ; but the driver would sometimes drive on ground that was sideling, and rather than turn over, she would start her foot unexpectedly.   After exercising her in this way sometime, I put her on a horse behind her son ; she at first insisted that she should fall off ; but when I told her she was at liberty to fall, if she chose, she would

not, choosing rather to exert herself to hold on. When
she had rode a few times in this way, I put her on the
horse alone, and after a few trials she would ride very
well, so that in the course of two months she would
ride four miles out and back every day. She used to
be tired after riding, and would lay down and not move
for six hours. I continued to give her medicine to keep
up perspiration, and restore the digestive powers, and
to strengthen the nervous system. I attended her in
this way for three months, and then went with her and
her son and daughter to Manchester; she rode upwards
of thirty miles in a day, and stood the journey very well.
I never received any pay for all my trouble and expense
of keeping them for three months, except what the two
young people did more than take care of their mother;
but I accomplished what I undertook, and relieved these
two unfortunate orphans from their burthen; which was
more satisfaction to me than to have received a large
sum of money, without doing any good. I saw this
woman three years after at the wedding of her son,
and she was quite comfortable, and has enjoyed a tolerable degree of health to this time, being able to wait
on herself.

On my return from Manchester, I stopped at Walpole,
and it being on the Sabbath, I attended meeting. In
the afternoon during service, a young woman was taken
in a fit and carried out of the meeting-house. I went
out to see her and found that she had been subject to
fits for some time. She was much bloated, and very
large, weighing about three hundred. A few days after,
her friends brought her to my house, and were very
urgent that I should undertake to help her; but I told
them I was satisfied that it would be a very difficult undertaking, and I did not feel willing to engage in it;
but they were so urgent, I agreed to do what I could
for her. Every time she took medicine, when I first
began with her, she would have a strong convulsion
fit; but I soon got her to sweat freely, and her fits were
at an end. By persevering in my usual plan of treatment, I got a natural perspiration, and her other evacuations became regular; she was considerably reduced
in size, and I have never heard of her having any fits

since.   The cause of her fits was taking sudden cold,
and all perspiration and the greater part of other evacuations ceased, leaving the water in her body.

In the fall of 1805, I was sent for to go to Rich-
mond, to see the family of Elder Bowles, who were all
sick with the dyssentary ; and Mrs. Bowles had a
cancer on her breast.   I relieved them of their disorders by my usual mode of practice; and gave the woman
medicine for the cancer, which relieved her.   I had
occasion to visit her again, and the tumour was about
the size of an egg ; but by following my prescriptions,
it was dissolved without causing any pain, and she has
been well for twelve years.   I then practised in different parts of Royalston and Warwick, and my practising in these places, was the way that my mode of
sweating for the spotted fever, came to be known and
practised by the physicians in Petersham.   I had discovered the benefit of steaming by trying it upon my
daughter two years before, and had been constantly
practising it ever since ; but the doctors, though they
condemned me and my practice, were willing to introduce it and take the credit to themselves as an important discovery.

After returning home, I was sent for to attend a
woman in the neighbourhood, who had been under the
care of a celebrated doctor, for a cancer in her breast.
He had tortured her with his caustics, till her breast
was burnt through to the bone ; and by its corrosive nature, had caused the cords to draw up into knots ; he
had likewise burnt her leg to the cords.   She had been
under his care eleven weeks; until she was much
wasted away, and her strength nearly gone.   In this
situation the doctor was willing to get her off his hands,
and wished me to take charge of her.   After some
hesitation, I consented, and attended her three weeks,
in which time I healed up her sores, and cleared her of
the humour so effectually, that she has ever since enjoyed good health.

While attending upon this case, another woman was
brought to me from Hillsborough, who had a cancer
on the back of her neck.   I dissolved the tumour, and
cured her by applying my cancer balsam, and the com-

mon course of medicine, in three weeks, without any pain ; and she has ever since enjoyed good health.

About this time I was called on to attend a woman in the town where I lived. She was an old maid, and had lately been married to a widower, who was very fond of her. She had been much disordered for many years, and was very spleeny ; she had been under the care of several doctors without receiving any benefit. I visited her several times and gave general satisfaction ; so much so that she allowed that I had done her more good than all the others that had attended her. A short time after I had done visiting her, the old man came out one morning to my house at sunrise, and I being about six miles from home, he came with all speed where I was, and said he wished me to come to his house as soon as possible, for his wife was very sick. I told him to return, and I would be there as soon as he could. I soon after sat out, and we both arrived there about the same time ; and I was very much astonished to find his wife about her work. I was asked into another room by the old man and his wife, and he said she had something to say to me. She then said that " if I could not attend her without giving her love powder, she did not wish me to attend her at all." I was very much astonished at her speech, and asked what she meant. She said that ever since she had taken my medicine she had felt so curiously, that she did not know what to make of it. The old man affirmed to the same, and he thought that I had given her love powder, and did not know what the event might be.

This foolish whim of the old man and his wife, caused a great bluster, and was food for those idle minds, who seem to take delight in slandering their neighbours ; and was made a great handle of by the doctors, who spread all kinds of ridiculous stories about me during my absence in the summer of 1806. In the autumn, when I had returned home, I found that a certain doctor of Alstead, had circulated some very foolish and slanderous reports about me and the old woman, and had given to them so much importance, that many people believed them. I found that I could prove his assertions, and sued him for defamation ; supposing that by appealing

5*

to the laws of my country I could get redress; but I was disappointed in my expectations, for I was persuaded to leave the case to a reference, and he had raised such a strong prejudice in the minds of the people against me, that they were more ready to favour a man whom they considered great and learned, because he had been to college, than to do justice to me; so they gave the case against me, and I had to pay the cost. After this, I refused to attend those people who had assisted in injuring me, and gave them up to their fashionable doctor. A curse seemed to follow them and his practice; for the spotted fever prevailed in this place soon after, and the doctor took charge of those who had sided with him against me, and if he had been a butcher and used the knife, there would not have been more destruction among them. Two men who swore falsely in his favour, and by whose means he got his cause, were among his first victims; and of the whole that he attended, about nine tenths died. He lost upwards of sixty patients in the town of Alstead in a short time.

I attended the funeral of a young man, one of his patients, who was sick but twenty-four hours, and but twelve under the operation of his medicine. He was as black as a blackberry, and swelled so as to be difficult to screw down the lid of the coffin; when I went into the room where the corpse was, the doctor followed me, and gave directions to have the coffin secured so as to prevent the corpse being seen; and then began to insult me, to attract the attention of the people. He said to me, I understand, sir, that you have a patent to cure such disorders as that, pointing to the corpse. I said no, and at the same time intimated what I thought of him. He put on an air of great importance, and said to me, what can you know about medicine? You have no learning; you cannot parse one sentence in grammar. I told him I never knew that grammar was made use of as medicine; but if a portion of grammar is so much like the operation of ratsbane, as appears on this corpse, I should never wish to know the use of it. This unexpected application of the meaning of what he said, displeased the medical gentleman very much; and finding that many of the people present had the same opinion that I had, it irritated him so much, that he threatened to horsewhip me; but I told him that he might do what he pleased to me, provided he did not poison me with his grammar. He did not attempt to carry his threat into execution, so I have escaped his whip and his poison; but the people were justly punished for their ingratitude and folly, in preferring death and misery, because it was done more fashionably, to a mode of practice by which they might relieve themselves in a simple and safe manner.

I have been more particular in relating these circumstances, in order to show my reasons for refusing to practice so near home; for I had been in constant practice among them for four or five years, and had been very successful, not having lost one patient during the whole time. My house had been constantly filled with patients from all parts of the country, for which I had received very little pay; myself and family were worn out with nursing and attending upon them; so that I was compelled in a measure, to leave home to free myself and family from so heavy a burthen. Besides, I felt it more a duty to assist the people in those parts where I had been treated with more friendship, and had received more assistance through my troubles, than what I had experienced from those whom I had reason to consider as under the greatest obligations to me.

In the spring of the year 1806, I came to a determination to go to New York, for the purpose of ascertaining the nature of the yellow fever, having been impressed with the idea, that this disease was similar to that which had been prevalent in different parts of the country, only differing in causes which were local. I made arrangements with a man to take charge of my farm, and on the 26th of June started for Boston, where I took passage for New York, and sailed on the third of July. In passing through the Sound, I was very sensibly affected by the cold chills I experienced in consequence of the sea air; having never been on the salt water before, this was new to me; although the weather was very hot on the land, I suffered with the cold. We arrived at New York in eight days; and the weather was extremely hot when I landed; this sudden change

produced a powerful effect on my feelings; the cause
of which I was satisfied in my own mind, was in consequence of the cold I had experienced on the water,
having reduced the natural heat of the body; thus,
coming into a very warm atmosphere, the external and
internal heat were upon nearly an equal scale, and when
there is an exact balance, so as to stop the determining
powers to the surface, mortification immediately takes
place, and death follows. This is the cause why the
fever is so fatal to those who go from the northward into
a warm climate.

On my arrival, I looked round to find a place to board,
and took up my lodgings with a Mr. Kavanagh, an
Irishman, and a Roman Catholic. After spending some
time in viewing the city, I applied to the Mayor of the
city, and to the Board of Health, to ascertain whether I
could have an opportunity to try the effect of my medicine and system of practice on the prevailing fever.
They told me that I could; but that I could get no pay
for it by law. I went to see Dr. Miller, who was then
President of the board of health, and had some conversation with him upon the subject. He told me
the same as the Mayor had, and inquired of me in what
manner I expected to give relief; I told him my plan
was to cause perspiration. He said if I could cause
them to sweat, he thought there was a good chance to
effect a cure.

After spending several days in New York, I went
to West Chester Creek to procure some medicine. I
thought that I was going to have the yellow fever, for
I felt all the symptoms, as I thought, of that disease;
my strength was nearly gone, my eyes were yellow,
and a noise in my head; my tongue was black, and
what passed my bowels was like tar. I was among
strangers, and had little money; I went to the house of
a Quaker woman, and asked her to let me stay with her
that day; she gave her consent. Had but little medicine with me, and could find nothing that I could relish
but salt and vinegar; I used about half a pint of salt,
and double that quantity of vinegar, which gave me
relief, and I gained so much strength, that the next day
I was able to return to the city of New York. On my

arrival there, I was so weak that it was with the greatest
difficulty I could walk to my boarding house, which
was about forty rods from the place where we landed. I immediately took Nos. 2 and 3, steeped, and
No. 4; in a short time, I began to have an appetite;
the first food that I took was a piece of smoked salmon,
and some ripe peach sauce. I soon recovered my
strength and was able to be about. This satisfied me
that I had formed a correct idea of this fatal disease;
that it was the consequence of losing the inward heat
of the body, and bringing it to a balance with the surrounding air; and the only method by which a cure can
be effected, is by giving such medicine as will increase
the fever or inward heat, to such a degree as to get the
determining power to the surface, by which means
perspiration will take place, and which is called the
turn of the fever; if this is not accomplished either by
medicine, or by nature being sufficient to overcome the
disease, mortification will be as certain a conseqence as
it would be if a person was strangled. The reason
why they lose their strength in so short a time, is because it depends wholly upon the power of inward heat;
and as much as they lose of that, so much they lose of
their strength and activity.

I had a good opportunity to prove these facts, and to
satisfy myself, by attending upon a Mr. M'Gowan, who
had the yellow fever. He was the teacher of the
Roman Catholic school, and an acquaintance of Mr.
Kavanagh, with whom I boarded, and who recommened
him to my care. He was attacked about noon, was
very cold, and had no pain; his eyes were half closed,
and appeared like a person half way between sleeping
and waking; he lost so much strength that in two hours
he was unable to walk across the room without stagger-
ing. I began with him by giving Nos. 2 and 3, to raise
the inward heat and clear the stomach, and in an hour
after getting him warm, he was in very extreme pain,
so much so that his friends were alarmed about him;
but I told them that it was a favourable symptom. After
being in this situation about an hour, perspiration began
and he grew easy; the next day he was out about his
business. The effect in these cases is exactly similar

to a person being recovered after having been drowned. The cold having overpowered the inward heat, all sensation or feeling ceases, and of course there is no pain; but as soon as the heat begins to increase so as to contend with the cold, sensation returns, and the pain will be very great till the victory is gained by heat having expelled the cold from the body, when a natural perspiration commences, and nature is restored to her empire.

I will here make a few remarks upon the food taken into the stomach, which is of the utmost importance to the preservation of health. While I was in New York, I took particular notice of their manner of living; and observed that they subsisted principally upon fresh provisions, more particularly the poorer class of people; who are in the habit in warm weather of going to market at a late hour of the day, and purchasing fresh meat that is almost in a putrid state, having frequently been killed the night previous, and being badly cooked, by taking it into the stomach, will produce certain disease; and I am convinced that this is one of the greatest causes that those fatal epidemics prevail in the hot season, in our large seaports. Mutton and lamb is often drove a great distance from the country, and having been heated and fatigued, then are cooled suddenly, which causes the fat to turn to water; and often when killed, are in almost a putrid state, and the meat is soft and flabby. Such meat as this, when brought into the market on a hot day, will turn green under the kidneys in two or three hours, and taken into the stomach will putrify before it digests, and will communicate the same to the stomach, and the whole body will be so affected by it, as to cause disorders of the worst kind. If people would get into the practice of eating salt provisions in hot weather and fresh in cold, it would be a very great preventive of disease. One ounce of putrid flesh in the stomach is worse than the effect produced by a whole carcass on the air by its effluvia. Much more might be said upon this important subject; but I shall defer it for the present, and shall treat more upon it in another part of the work. It is a subject that has been too much neglected by our health officers in this country.

While in the city of New York I attended an Irishman by the name of Doyle, who had the fever-and-ague. This disease gives a complete view of my theory of heat and cold; for it is about an equal balance between the two, heat keeping a little the upper hand. He had been afflicted with this distressing disorder about four months; he had the fits most of the time every day and was very bad. I began by giving him such medicine as I usually gave to increase the inward heat of the body, which subdued the cold, and gave heat the victory over it; and by strictly attending him in this way four days, he was completely cured. Being short of money I asked him for some compensation for my trouble; but he refused and never paid me a cent; observing that he must have been getting well before, for no one ever heard of such a disorder being cured in four days.

A gentleman whom I had formed an acquaintance with, by the name of James Quackenbush, who had the care of the state prison warehouse, finding how I had been treated, invited me to go to his house and live with him, which I thankfully accepted. I was treated with much kindness by him, for which he has my most sincere thanks.

On the 16th of September I started for home; and took passage on board a packet for Boston, where I arrived in five days; and on the 26th reached my home, after an absence of three months, and found my family well. I was often called on to practise in the neighbourhood; but declined most part of the applications in consequence of the treatment I had received from them, which has been before related. In November I went to Plum Island to collect medicine; on my way I called on Joseph Hale, Esq. of Pepperell, and engaged him to come down with his wagon in about three weeks, to bring back what medicine I should collect. I went by the way of Newburyport; and after being on the Island three or four days, collected such roots as I wanted and returned to that place. While there, being in a store in conversation with some persons, there came in a man from Salisbury mills, by the name of Osgood, who stated that he was very unwell, and that his wife lay at the point of death, with the lung fever; that she had been attended by Dr. French, who had given her over. One of the gentlemen standing by told him that I was a doctor, and used the medicine of our own country. He asked me if I would go home with him, and see his wife. As I was waiting for Mr. Hale, and had nothing to do, I told him I would, and we immediately started in the chaise for his home, which was about six miles. On our arrival he introduced me to his wife as a doctor who made use of the medicine of our country; and asked her if she was willing that I should undertake to cure her. She said if I thought that I could help her she had no objection. I gave my opinion that I could, and undertook, though with some reluctance, as I was in a strange place and no one that I knew. I proceeded with her in my usual method of practice, and in about fourteen hours her fever turned, and the next day she was comfortable, and soon got about.

This cure caused considerable talk among the people in the neigbourhood, who thought very favourably of me and my practice; but it soon came to the ears of Dr. French, who was very much enraged to think one of his patients, that he had given over, should be cured by one whom he called a quack; and attempted to counteract the public impression in my favour, by circulating a report that the woman was getting better and sat up the greatest part of the day before I saw her; but this was denied by the woman's husband, and known by many to be false.

While I remained in this place, waiting for Mr. Hale to come down with his wagon to carry home my medicine, I was called on to attend several cases, in all of which I was very successful; most of them were such as had been given over by the doctors. One of them was the case of a young man, who had cut three of his fingers very badly, so as to lay open the joints. Dr. French had attended him three weeks, and they had got so bad that he advised him to have them cut off as the only alternative. The young man applied to me for advice. I told him if I was in his situation, I should not be willing to have them cut off till I had made some further trial to cure them without. He requested me to undertake to cure him, to which I consented and began by clearing the wound of mercury, by washing it with weak lye; I then put on some drops, and did it up with a bandage which was kept wet with cold water. ' While I was dressing the wound, a young man, who was studying with Dr. French, came in and made a great fuss, telling the young man that I was going to spoil his hand. I told him that I was accountable for what I was doing, and that if he had any advice to offer I was ready to hear him; but he seemed to have nothing to offer except to find fault, and went off, after saying that Dr. French's bill must be paid very soon. I continued to dress his hand, and in ten days he was well enough to attend to his work, being employed in a nail factory. Soon after, I saw him there at work, and asked him how his fingers did; he said they were perfectly cured; he wished to know what my bill was for attending him. I asked him what Dr. French had charged, and he said he had sent his bill to his mother, amounting to seventeen dollars; I told him I thought that enough for us both, and I should charge him nothing. His mother was a poor widow depending on her labour and that of her son for a living. I remained in this place about two weeks, and the people were very urgent that I should stay longer; but Mr. Hale having arrived, I left them with a promise that I would visit them again in the spring. We arrived at Pepperell, where I remained several days with Mr. Hale, who was an ingenious blacksmith and a chemist, having been much engaged in the preparation of mineral medicine. He had an inquiring turn of mind and was very enthusiastic in his undertakings; although he prepared medicines from minerals, he acknowledged that he was afraid to use them on account of his knowing their poisonous qualities. I convinced him of the superiority of my system of practice, and instructed him in the use of my medicine, so that he engaged in it and soon had as much practice as he could attend to; being so well satisfied of its general application to the cure of all cases of disease, that he looked no more for it in his mineral preparations.

In the winter of 1807, I went with my wife to Jericho, Vermont, to visit my father and friends who lived

there.   While there I was called on to see a number
who were sick, among whom was a young man that had
been taken in what is called cramp convulsion fits.
He was first taken on Sunday morning, and continued in
fits most of the time till Tuesday; he was attended during this time by the best doctors that could be procured,
without doing him any good.   They could not get their
medicine to have any effect upon him; he continued in
convulsions most of the time; every part of him was as
stiff as a wooden image; after trying every thing they
could they gave him over.   His father came after me,
and just as we entered the room where the young man
was, he was taken in a fit.   His feet and hands were
drawn in towards his body, his jaws were set, his head
drawn back, and every part of him as completely fixed
as a statue.   The first difficulty was to get him to take
any thing; his jaws were set as tight together as a vise.
I took a solution of Nos. 1, 2 and 6, as strong as it
could be made, and putting my finger into the corner of
his mouth, making a space between his cheek and teeth,
poured some of it down; and as soon as it touched the
glands at the roots of his tongue, his jaws came open,
and he swallowed some of the medicine; which had
such an effect upon the stomach, that all the spasms
immediately ceased.   I left him some medicine with
directions, and he entirely recovered his health; I saw
him three years after, and he told me that he had not
had a fit since the one above described.   I was convinced from this circumstance, that the cause of all
cramps or spasms of this kind, is seated in the stomach,
and that all applications for relief in such cases should
be made there; as it will be of no service to work on
the effect as long as the cause remains.

  Before returning home, I was called on by Captain
Lyman, of Jericho, to advise with me concerning his
son, who had a fever sore on his thigh, with which he
had been afflicted for seven years.   He had been attended by all the doctors in that part of the country to
no advantage.   They had decided that the only thing
which could be done to help him, was to lay open his
thigh and scrape the bone.   I told him that I did not
see how they could do that without cutting the great

artery, which lay close to the bone, where they would
have to cut. He said he was satisfied that it would not
do, and was very urgent that I should undertake with
him. I told him that it was impossible for me to stay
at that time; but if his son would go home with me, I
would undertake to cure him; to which he consented,
and the young man returned with me; which was in the
month of March. I began with him by giving medicine
to correct and strengthen the system; bathed the wound
with my rheumatic drops, or No. 6, sometimes bathing
with cold water to strengthen it, and after proceeding in
this manner for about a month, he was well enough to
do some work; he remained with me till August, when
he was entirely cured, so that he was able to return to
his father's on foot, a distance of one hundred miles.

In the fall of this year, the dyssentary, or camp dis-
temper, as it was called, was very prevalent in the above
named town of Jericho; and was so mortal that all but
two who had the disease and were attended by the doctors died, having lost above twenty in a short time. The
inhabitants were much alarmed, and held a consultation,
to advise what to do; and being informed by the young
man above mentioned, that I was at home, they sent an
express for me, and I immediately made arrangements to
comply with their request. In twenty-four hours I started, and arrived there on the third day after, and found
them waiting with great anxiety for me, having refused
to take any thing from the doctors. I had an interview
with the Selectmen of the town, who had taken upon
themselves the care of the sick; they informed me that
there were about thirty then sick, and wished me to undertake the care of them. I agreed to take charge of
them on condition that I could have two men to assist me;
this was complied with, and I commenced my practice
upon thirty in the course of three days. The disorder
was the most distressing of any that I had ever witnessed.
One man had been speechless for six hours, and was supposed to be dying; but on my giving him some medicine
to warm him, he seemed to revive like an insect that was
warmed by the sun after having laid in a torpid state
through the winter. I had but little medicine with me,
and had to use such as I could procure at this place. I

found the cause of the disease to be coldness and canker ; the digestive powers being lost, the stomach became clogged so that it would not hold the heat.   I made use of red pepper steeped in a tea of sumac leaves, sweetened, and sometimes the bark and berries, to raise the heat and clear off the canker, which had the desired effect.   After taking this tea, those who were strong enough, I placed over a steam, as long as they could bear it, and then put them in bed.   Those who were too weak to stand, I contrived to have sit over a steam ; and this repeated as occasion required.   To restore the digestive powers, I made use of cherry stones, having procured a large quantity of them, that had been laid up and the worms had eaten off all the outside, leaving the stones clean.   I pounded them fine, then made a tea of black birch bark, and after cleaning them, by putting them into this hot tea, and separating the meats from the stone part, made a syrup by putting from two to three ounces of sugar to one quart of the liquor ; this was given freely and answered a good purpose.   I continued to attend upon my patients, aided by those appointed to assist me, and in eight days I had completely subdued the disease.   They all recovered except two, who were dying when I first saw them.   I gave the same medicine to the nurses and those exposed to the disease, as to them that were sick, which prevented their having the disorder.   The same thing will prevent disease that will cure it.

After finishing my practice at this place, I was sent for and went to the town of Georgia, about thirty miles distance, where I practised with general success for one week, and then returned to Jericho.   Those patients whom I had attended, were comfortable, and soon entirely recovered.   The doctors were not very well pleased with my success, because I informed the people how to cure themselves, and they have had no need of their assistance in that disorder since.   They circulated reports for twenty miles round, that I killed all that I attended ; but the people were all perfectly satisfied with my practice, and were willing to give me all credit for my skill, so their malice towards me was of no avail.

About this time being in the town of Bridgewater, Vt. I was called on to see a young man about eighteen years of age, who had lost the use of his arm by a strain; it had been in a perishing condition for six months. The flesh appeared to be dead, and he carried it in a sling; his health was bad. Being unable to stop to do any thing for him at this time, he was sent to my house. I began with him in my usual manner by giving him warm medicine, and bathed his arm with the oil of spearmint; in about ten days he was well enough to use his arm and do some work; in about two months he was entirely cured and returned home.

In the spring of the year 1807, I went to Salisbury, according to my promise when there the fall before. On my way there, I stopped at Pelham; the man at whose house I staid, insisted on my going to see his father-in-law, who had the rheumatism very bad, having been confined two months. I attended him three days, when he was able to walk some, by the assistance of a cane; he soon got about and was comfortable. While at this place I was sent for to a young woman, sick of a consumption; she had been a long time attended by a doctor, who seemed very willing for my advice; I carried her through a course of my medicine, and the doctor staid to see the operation of it; he seemed well pleased with my system of practice, and gave me much credit, saying that I was the first person he ever knew that could make his medicine do as he said it would. I was sent for to attend several cases of consumption and other complaints at this time, in all of which I met with success, and gave general satisfaction to the people.

After stopping at Pelham three weeks, in which time I had as much practice as I could attend to, I went to Salisbury Mills, where I was very cordially welcomed by all those who had been attended by me the season before. I was called on to practise in this place and Newburyport, and my success was so great that it caused much alarm among the doctors, and a class of the people who were their friends, who did all they could to injure me, and destroy my credit with the people. A considerable part of the patients, who were put under my care, were such as the doctors had given over, and those being cured by me, had a tendency to open the

6*

eyes of the people, and give them a correct understanding of the nature of their practice, and convince them that a simple and speedy cure was more for their interest and comfort, than long sickness, pain, and distress; besides having to pay exhorbitant doctors' bills, for useless visits and poisonous drugs, which have no other effect than to prolong disease, and destroy the natural constitution of the patient.

Among those doctors who seemed so much enraged against me, for no other reason that I could learn, than because I had cured people whom they had given over, and instructed them to assist themselves when sick, without having to apply to them; there was none that made themselves so conspicuous as Dr. French. I had considerable practice in his neighbourhood, and was very successful in every case; this seemed to excite his malice against me to the greatest pitch; he made use of every means in his power, and took every opportunity to insult and abuse me both to my face and behind my back. A few of the inhabitants who were his friends, joined with him, and became his instruments to injure me; but a large proportion of the people were friendly to me, and took great interest in my safety and success. The doctor and his adherents spread all kinds of ridiculous reports concerning me and my practice, giving me the name of the old wizzard; and that my cures were done under the power of witchcraft. This foolish whim was too ridiculous for me to undertake to contradict, and I therefore rather favoured it merely for sport; many remarkable circumstances took place tending to strengthen this belief, and some of the silly and weak-minded people really believed that I possessed supernatural powers. This will not appear so strange, when we take into view, that the people generally were ignorant of my system of practice, and when they found that I could cure those diseases that the doctors, in whom they had been in the habit of putting all their confidence, pronounced as incurable; and that I could turn a fever in two days, which would often take them as many months, they were led to believe that there was something supernatural in it.

A man who was one of the friends of Dr. French, and who had been very inimical to me, doing all in his power to injure and ridicule me, sent word one day by a child, that his calf was sick, and he wanted me to come and give it a green powder and a sweat. Knowing that his object was to insult, I returned for answer, that he must send for Dr. French, and if he could not cure it, I would come, for that was the way that I had to practise here. It so happened that the calf died soon after, and his youngest child was taken suddenly and very dangerously sick. Not long after he found another calf dead in the field, and about the same time his oldest son was taken sick. These things happening in such an extraordinary manner, caused him to reflect on his conduct towards me, and his conscience condemned him, for trying to injure me without cause. He had the folly to believe, or the wickedness to pretend to believe, that it was the effect of witchcraft; and wishing to make his peace with me, sent me word, that if I would let his family alone, he would never do or say any thing more to my injury. This I readily assented to; and his children soon after getting well, though there was nothing very extraordinary in it, as it might all be easily accounted for by natural causes; yet it afforded much conversation among the gossips, and idle busy-bodies in the neighbourhood; and was made use of by my enemies to prejudice the people against me. Being in company with a young woman who belonged to a family that were my enemies, she, to insult me, asked me to tell her fortune. I consented, and knowing her character not to be the most virtuous, and to amuse myself at her expense, told what had taken place between her and a certain young man the night before. She seemed struck with astonishment; and said that she was convinced that I was a wizzard, for it was impossible that I could have known it without the devil had told me. She did not wish me to tell her any more.

I practised in this place and vicinity a few months and returned home to attend to my farm for the rest of the season. While at home I was sent for, and attended in different parts of the country, and was very successful in my mode of practice, particularly in places where the

dysentery and fevers were most prevalent; never failing
in any instance of giving relief, and completely putting a
check to those alarming epidemics, which caused so much
terror in many places in the interior of the country.

In the year of 1808, I went again to Salisbury, and on
my way there, stopped at Pelham, and attended and gave
relief in several cases of disease.   On my arrival at
Salisbury Mills, where I made it my home, I was immediately called on to practise in that place and the adjacent towns.   Many came to me from different parts,
whose cases were desperate, having been given over by
the doctors, such as humours, dropsies, mortifications,
fellons, consumptions, &c.   Fevers were so quickly
cured, and with so little trouble, that many were unwilling to believe they had the disease.   My success was
so great that the people generally were satisfied of the
superiority of my mode of practice over all others.
This created considerable alarm with the doctors, and
those who sided with them.   Dr. French seemed to be
much enraged, and having failed to destroy my credit
with the people by false reports, and ridiculous statements of witchcraft, shifted his course of proceeding,
and attempted to frighten me by threats, which only
tended to show the malice he bore me; for no other
reason, that I could conceive of, as I had never spoken
to him, than because of my success in relieving those
he had given over to die.   He would frequently cause
me to be sent for in great haste to attend some one in
his neighbourhood, who was stated to be very sick; but
I saw through these tricks, and avoided all their snares.
It seemed to be his determination, if he failed in destroying my practice, to destroy me.   Being in company
one day at Salisbury village, with Mr. Jeremiah Eaton,
of Exeter, whose wife was under my care for a dropsical complaint, I was sent for four times to visit a young
man at the house of Dr. French; the last time a man
came on horseback in the greatest haste, and insisted
that I should go and see him.   I asked why Dr. French
did not attend him; he answered that he had rather
have me; being convinced from the appearance of
things, that it was an attempt to put some trick upon
me, I refused to go, and the man returned.   In a short

time after, Dr. French came into the village, and Mr. Eaton, who was present when they came after me, asked him what ailed the young man at his house; he said nothing, but that he was as well as any body. This revealed the whole secret. Mr. Eaton then asked him why he caused me to be sent for so many times, under a false pretence. He said to see if I dared to come into his neighbourhood; that he did not care how much I practised on that side of the river; but if I came on his, he would blow my brains out; that I was a murderer and he could prove it. Mr. Eaton observed that it was a heavy accusation to make against a man, and that he ought to be made to prove his words, or to suffer the consequence; that his wife was under my care, and if I was a murderer he ought to see it. Dr. French again repeated the words, with many threats against me, and showed the spite and malice of a savage.

Mr. Eaton and others of my friends considered my life in danger; and came immediately to me and related what had been said by the doctor; and advised me to be on my guard. I had to pass his house every day to visit my patients; but did not consider myself safe in going in the night, nor in the day time without some one with me. I continued in this manner for several days, and finding his malice towards me to be as great as ever, and still continuing his threats; with the advice of my friends, I was induced to have resort to the law for protection. I went to Newburyport and entered a complaint against him before a magistrate, who granted a warrant, and he was brought before him for a trial. My case was made out by fully proving his words; he asked for an adjournment for three hours to make his defence, which was granted. He then brought forward evidence in support of his character, and proved by them that he had always been a man of his word. The justice told him that he thought he proved too much, and to his disadvantage, for it had been fully proved that he had made the threats alleged against him, and to prove that he was a man of his word, went to satisfy the court that the complaint was well grounded. He was laid under two hundred dollar bonds to keep the peace and appear at the next court of common pleas.   He appeared at the next court, was ordered to pay all the costs, and was discharged from his bail.   This was an end of our controversy for that time ; but his malice continued against me long after ; seeking every means to destroy me and prevent my practising, that he could devise ; but proceeded with more caution, which caused me a great deal of trouble and much suffering, as will be hereafter related.

I continued to practise in this place, and had as many patients as I could possibly attend upon, notwithstanding the opposition I constantly met with from the doctors and their friends ; for with all their arts and falsehoods they were not able to prevent those labouring under complaints, which they had found could not be removed by the fashionable mode of treatment, from applying to me for relief; none of whom but what were either cured or received great relief by the practice.   Some of the most extraordinary cases I shall give a particular account of for the information of the reader.

Mr. Jabez True, the minister of Salisbury, was afflicted with what the doctors called nettle-rash, or what is commonly called St. Anthony's fire.   He stated to me that it was caused by fighting fire, about twenty-five years before, and that he had been subject to a breaking out ever since; which at certain times was very painful and troublesome, as it felt like the sting of bees, and would swell all over his body.   He had applied to all the doctors in those parts for their advice, but got no assistance from them.   I told him that he had heated himself to such a degree by violent exercise, and being exposed to the fire, that there was nearly a balance between the outward and inward heat, and then cooling too sudden, the inward heat had fallen as much below the natural state as it had been above it before, and the only way to effect a cure was to bring him into the same state as he was in when fighting the fire.   He wished me to undertake his case.   I carried him through a course of my medicine, and made use of every means in my power to raise the inward heat, pursuing my plan with all zeal for two days; when he became alarmed, and said he felt as though he should die, for he felt the same as he did when he was fighting the fire.   I then kept him in that situation as much as possible, and it went down gradually so as to hold a natural proportion of heat. My plan succeeded so completely, that he was perfectly cured and has enjoyed good health ever since. I attended upon his wife at the same time, who had been long in a consumption, and had been given over. She was perfectly cured; and they are now living in good health and are ready to testify to the truth of these statements.

Previously to my difficulty with Dr. French, as has been before mentioned, Mrs. Eaton and another woman by the name of Lifford, came to me at Salisbury Mills from Exeter. Their complaint was dropsy; and were both desperate cases, having been given over by the doctor who had attended them. Mrs. Eaton was swelled to such a degree, that she could not see her knees as she sat in a chair, and her limbs in proportion. I felt unwilling to undertake with them, as I considered there would be but little chance of a cure; and declined doing any thing for them, and sent them away, stating that there was no place that they could get boarded. They went away as I supposed to go home; but they soon returned, and said they had found a place where they could stay, and a young woman had agreed to nurse them. I undertook with them very reluctantly; but could not well avoid it. I gave them some medicine, and it operated favourably on both, especially on Mrs. Lifford; then gave strict orders to the nurse, to attend them attentively through the night, and keep up a perspiration; but she almost totally neglected her duty, spending her time with the young people. On visiting them in the morning, I was very much hurt to find my directions neglected. Mrs. Lifford was quite poorly; and stated to me that the nurse had neglected her, and that she had got her feet out of bed; her perspiration had ceased, and other symptoms appeared unfavourable.

I attended upon her through the day and did all I could to relieve her, but could not raise a perspiration again. She continued till the next night about midnight and died. My hopes of doing her any good were small; but think that if she had not been neglected by the nurse, there might have been some small chance for her, as the first operation of the medicine was so favourable. Her bowels were in a very bad state, and had been almost in a mortified condition for three weeks, and what passed her was by force, and very black.

This caused great triumph among my enemies, and Dr. French tried to have a jury on the body; but he could not prevail; for the circumstances were well known to many, and all that knew any thing about it, cleared me from all blame. The nurse said that I did all I could, and if there was any blame it ought to fall on her and not on me. So they failed in their attempt to make me out a murderer; but this case was laid up to be brought against me at another time. This shows what may be done by the folly of people, and the malice and wickedness of designing men, who care more for their own interested ends, than for the health and happiness of a whole community. The fashionable educated doctor may lose one half his patients without being blamed; but if I lose one out of several hundred of the most desperate cases, most of which were given over as incurable, it is called murder.

Mrs. Eaton remained under my care about three weeks, in which time she was reduced in size eight inches, she then returned home to Exeter. I had several cases of dropsy and consumption from the same town, about this time, who were all relieved; all of them were very solicitous for me to go to Exeter and practise. As soon as I could get the patients under my care in a situation to leave them, I left Salisbury Mills, and went to Exeter, and commenced practising in my usual way, and was applied to from all parts. I had not so many to attend as I had in some places; but they were all of the most desperate nature, such as had been given over by the doctors, in all of which I met with great success. Many of the cases had been attended by Dr. Shephard; he had attended with me upon his patients at Salisbury; was a very plain candid sort of a man, and treated me with much civility. I well remember his first speech to me, which was in the following words: "Well, what are you doing here, are you killing or curing the people?" I replied, you must judge about that for yourself. "Well," said he, "I will watch you, not for fear of your doing harm, but for my own information; I wish you well, and will do you all the good I can." I always found him candid and friendly, without any hypocrisy. He once called on me to visit with him one of his patients in the town where he lived, who had the rheumatism in his back and hips. The doctor had attended him about two months, and said he had killed the pain, but his back was stiff, so that he could not bring his hands below his knees. I attended him about forty-eight hours, and then went with him to see the doctor, which was half a mile; the doctor appeared to be much pleased to see him so well, and have the use of his limbs; for he could stoop and use them as well as he ever could. He said that he was as glad for the young man's sake as though he had cured him himself. He frequently came to see Mrs. Eaton, whom I was attending for the dropsy; and expressed much astonishment at the effect the medicine I gave had in relieving her of a disease which he had considered incurable. At one time when conversing with her upon her situation, and finding her so much better, having been reduced in size above fifteen inches, he expressed himself with some warmth on the occasion, saying that it was what he had never seen or heard of being done before, and what he had considered impossible to be done with medicine. Addressing himself to me with much earnestness, inquired how it was that I did it. I replied, you know doctor that the heat had gone out of the body, and the water had filled it up; and all I had to do was to build fire enough in the body to boil away the water. He burst into a laugh, and said that it was a system very short.

While practising in Exeter, I had many desperate cases from the different parts of the country, and from Portsmouth. One from the latter place I shall mention, being different from what I had before witnessed. A man applied to me who had the venereal, in consequence, as she stated, of having had a bad husband; which I believed to be true. She had been attended by the doctors in Portsmouth for nearly a year, who had filled her with mercury, for the purpose of curing

7

the disorder till the remedy had become much worse than the disease. Her case was alarming, and very difficult; she was brought on a bed, being unable to sit up; and seemed to be one mass of putrefaction. I proceeded with her in my usual way of treating all cases where the system is greatly disordered, by giving medicine to promote perspiration, steaming to throw out the mercury, and restore the digestive powers; and in three weeks she returned home entirely cured. Another woman came to me from the same place, who had been sick five years, which had been in consequence of having had the same disease, and the doctors had filled her with mercury to kill the disorder, as they called it, then left her to linger out a miserable existence. When she stated her case to me, I felt very unwilling to undertake with her, apprehending that it would be very uncertain whether a cure could be effected, having been of so long standing; but she insisted upon it so strongly, that I could not put her off. After attending upon her three weeks, however, her health was restored, and she returned home well; and in less than a year after, she had two children at one birth. She had not had a child for eight years before. This disease is very easily cured in the first stages of it, by a common course of medicine, being nothing more than a high stage of canker seated in the glands of certain parts of the body, and if not cured, communicates to the glands of the throat and other parts; by giving mercury the whole system is completely disordered, and although the disease may disappear, it is not cured; and there is more difficulty in getting the mercury out of the body of one in this situation, than to cure a dozen of the disease who have not taken this dangerous poison.

While in Exeter, I had a case of a young man, son of Col. Nathaniel Gilman, who was in a decline. He was about fourteen years old, and had been troubled with bleeding at the nose. They had made use of such powerful astringents, with corrosive sublimate snuffed up his nose, that the blood vessels in that part seemed to be shrunk up, and his flesh much wasted away; I carried him through a course of medicine, and gave an equal circulation of blood through the body, and stopped its course to the head; then raised a natural perspiration, restored the digestive powers, and regulated the system, so as to support the body with food instead of medicine. In a short time he recovered his health so that he commanded a company of militia at the alarm at Portsmouth, during the late war.

My success while at this place, and the many extraordinary cures I performed, gained me great credit among the people; but the medical faculty became much alarmed, and made use of every artifice to prejudice them against me. The foolish stories about witchcraft, which had been made a handle of at Salisbury, were repeated here, with a thousand other ridiculous statements for the purpose of injuring me; but I treated them with contempt as not worthy my notice, except in some instances, to amuse myself with the credulity of the ignorant, who were foolish enough to believe such nonsense. I will relate one circumstance for the purpose of showing upon what grounds they founded their belief of my possessing supernatural powers, and which caused much talk among the people at the time it happened. Mrs. Eaton, where I boarded, had a five dollar bill stolen out of her pocket book. She made inquiry of all the family, who denied having any knowledge of it. A girl that lived in the family denied it so strongly, that I thought she discovered guilt, and led me to believe that she had taken the money. I pretended that I could certainly discover who stole the money, which was believed by many; and told Mrs. Eaton in presence of all the family, that if I did not tell who took it by the next day at twelve o'clock, I would pay the amount lost myself. In the evening I had them all called into the room, and took the bible and read from the law of Moses the penalty for stealing; then took the purse and put it into the place and shut the book and gave it to Mrs. Eaton, with strict injunction to put it under her pillow and let no one touch it; and that the person who stole the money could have no peace nor rest till he or she confessed his or her guilt. They then all retired to bed. As soon as it was daylight in the morning the girl came down stairs crying, and went to the bed where Mrs. Eaton lay, and confessed that she took the money; saying that she had not slept any during the night, as I had said would be the case. It will be unnecessary to inform the reader, that this wonderful discovery was brought about by the effect of a guilty conscience on a credulous and weak mind.

While I was at Exeter, a woman brought her son to me, who had a fever sore, so called, on his hip; he had been in this situation so long, without any assistance, that his legs had perished, and he was so much wasted away by the continual discharge of the sore, and his nature had become so far spent, that I felt perfectly satisfied that a cure was impracticable, and declined undertaking with him. This honest declaration on my part very much affronted the boy's mother, and she turned against me and did me all the hurt she could, because I would not undertake to do what I knew was impossible for any one to accomplish. She went with her son to a fashionable doctor, who said he would cure him out of spite to me. They continued with the doctor several weeks, till the expense amounted to about fifty dollars; the lad continued to grow worse till he died. This woman seemed satisfied with having her son die, after spending fifty dollars, because it was done in a fashionable manner; but my refusing to undertake to cure him, was sufficient reason for her to circulate all kinds of false and ridiculous reports about me. However strange this may appear, it is no more strange than true, for this is but one out of many hundred similar cases, where I have received injury, when I was entitled to credit, by being honest and sincere in my endeavour to do what I conceived my duty towards my fellow creatures.

About this time, among the rest of my troubles, I met with a new difficulty with an apprentice that I had taken, by the name of William Little; whom I had taken from a state of poverty and sickness, cured him, and supported him for two years, until he had gained knowledge enough of my medicine and system of practice to be useful to me, he then proved dishonest. While I was absent from home, he collected all the money he could, and sold all my medicine, and then went off. On my return I found my debts collected and my medicine gone, so that I was obliged to go back immediately, to collect more before I could attend to my practice. This was the first time I had met with difficulty by employing agents; but since then I have had experience enough to satisfy me of the difficulty of trusting to other people; having found but very few of those I have been under the necessity of employing, who have proved trusty and honest. I have suffered much pecuniary loss in this way, besides in some instances, those I have assisted and given instruction to, so as to be useful in the practice, have become my enemies, and been made instrumental to destroy me.

A son of Mr. John Underwood, of Portsmouth, was brought to me while at Exeter, who had what is called a scalt head. He had been afflicted with it for nine years. The doctors had been applied to, to no purpose; and when he brought him to me, agreed to give a generous price if I would cure him. I took charge of him and after pursuing my usual plan of treatment three weeks, he returned home perfectly cured, and has not since had any appearance of the disease. This man had the meanness, in order to get clear of paying any thing for curing his son, to turn against me and my practice, although he had acknowledged that I had saved his life, and had recommended me to many others, whom I had relieved; yet to get clear of paying a trifling sum according to his agreement, he did all he could to injure me, and through his influence many were kept from being cured. He was taken sick, and notwithstanding he had said so much against my medicine, he applied to some who had the right of using it, and was relieved thereby.

Sometime towards the close of the summer, while I was at Exeter, I was sent for to go to Portsmouth to see a young man by the name of Lebell, who was in a very dangerous situation, supposed by his friends to be in a dying state, having been given over by Drs. Cutler and Pierpont at ten o'clock that morning. I arrived about two in the afternoon. He had been attended by the two doctors above named for upwards of a month to cure the venereal; they had filled him with mercury, so that he had swelled all over with the poison. The

7*

doctors pronounced it to be the dropsy. His legs had
been scarified to let off the water; the disorder and
the mercury had gained the power, and nature had submitted. I at once pronounced it to be a desperate case,
and told the French Consul, who had the care of him,
that I could give no encouragement that I could do him
any good; but he was very solicitous for me to do something for him. I told him the only chance was to raise
perspiration, and that twenty-four hours would determine his case; for he would either be better in that
time, or be dead. The idea of perspiration caused him
to urge me to try; and he said if I could effect it, he
would give me one hundred dollars; the doctors had
tried for a month and could not succeed. I gave him
some medicine, then put on the clothes by degrees,
until he was shielded from the air, and he sweat freely
in about an hour. The two doctors were present and
seemed astonished at my success; they walked the room,
talked low, then went out. I staid with him till six
o'clock, and the symptoms seemed to be favourable;
he sweat profusely, and spit much blood. I told the
nurse to keep him in the same situation till I returned,
went out and was gone about an hour, and come back
again with Mr. Underwood. When we came into the
room, found that the doctors had taken him out of bed
and sat him in a chair, and opened the window against
him. I told them that their conduct would cause his
death, and I would do no more for him; but should
give him up as their patient.

It appeared to me that they were afraid I should cure
him, and thus prove the superiority of my practice over
theirs, for they had tried a month to get a perspiration
without success, and I had done it in one hour. The
man fainted before I left the room. I went home with
Mr. Underwood and staid that night, and left them to
pursue their own course; the man died before morning. Instead of getting the hundred dollars as was
agreed, I never got a cent for all my trouble of coming
fifteen miles and returning back again on foot; and besides this loss, afterwards when I came to be persecuted by the faculty, the above two doctors gave their
depositions against me, in which I was informed they

swore that I killed this man, notwithstanding they had given him over to die the morning before I saw him, and they had taken him out of my hands, as above stated. On being informed that they were trying to support a complaint against me, I got the depositions of Mr. Underwood and others, who were knowing to the facts, to contradict these false statements; on finding that I was determined to oppose them, and prove what they had sworn to be all false, they thought proper to drop the matter; but I was informed they had sworn that my medicine was of a poisonous nature, and if it did not cause the patient to vomit soon after being taken, they would certainly die. It is unnecessary for me to contradict this, for its incorrectness and absurdity is too well known to all who have any knowledge of the medicine I use.

I was frequently in Portsmouth to visit those who had been sent to me to be attended upon at Exeter. Sometime in September in 1808, when there, I was called on to visit Mr. Richard Rice, who was sick with the yellow fever, as it was called. The reason for his sending for me, was in consequence of having heard the reports of the doctors, that I sweat my patients to death. He conceived an idea that if he could sweat, he should be better; but they would not allow him to be kept warm, taking the clothes off of him and keeping the windows and doors open; no fire was permitted in the room, while he was shivering with the cold. The plan was to kill the fever, and to effect this with more certainty, the doctor had bled him, and told his sister that he had given him as much ratsbane as he dared to give, and if that did not answer he did not know what would.

I began to give him medicine a little before night, and in one hour perspiration took place. He was so weak that he was unable to help himself. In the morning the doctor proposed to bleed him; but he was dismissed. I was with him till the symptoms were favourable, and then left him in the care of three persons whom I could confide in. After I was gone, Dr. Brackett came into the room where the patient was, in a great rage saying that they were killing him; for the mortification would soon take place in consequence of keeping

him so warm.   He was asked by one of those present, in
which case mortification was most likely to take place,
when the blood was cold and thick, or warm and thin.
He suspected some quibble and would not give an answer; and it was immaterial which way he answered;
for in either case he had no grounds to support an argument upon, but what might be easily refuted.   After he
had failed in the interference with those who had the
care of the patient, he went to his wife and other relations, and tried to frighten them; but he did not succeed,
for they were well satisfied with what was doing.

The patient was much out by spells, sometimes im-
agining himself to be a lump of ice; but my directions
were pursued by the person I left in charge of him during the night, keeping up a perspiration, in the morning
he was much relieved and had his right mind.   He had
no pain except in the lower part of the bowels; to relieve which he was very anxious that I should give him
some physic; I opposed this, being confident that it
would not do in such putrid cases.   He was so urgent,
however, I gave him some, which operated very soon,
and the consequence was, that it reinforced his disorder,
and threw him into the greatest distress.   He asked for
more physic, but I told him that I would not give him
any more, for I was satisfied of the impropriety of giving it in such cases, and I have never given any since.
It checked the perspiration, and drew the determining
-powers from the surface inward; so that I had to go
through the same process again of raising perspiration,
and vomiting, which was much more difficult than at
first, and it was with the greatest attention that I was
able to keep off the mortification for twelve hours that
he was kept back by taking this small dose of physic.
I kept up the perspiration through Friday and Saturday,
and on Sunday morning when I called to see him, he
was up and dressed; on asking how he did, he said as
strong as you are, and took me under his arm and carried me across the room.   On Monday he was down on
the wharf attending to his business.

This cure caused considerable talk in the town, and
because it was done so quick, the doctors said that there
was but little ailed him, and he would have got well

himself if he had taken the physic and been left alone; but those who saw it were convinced to the contrary; others doubted, and said among themselves, how can a man who has no learning and never studied physic, know how to cure disease. Mr. Rice, however, gave me credit for the cure, and was very grateful for it, and I made his house my home, when in Portsmouth, and was treated with much respect. He introduced me to his uncle, Alexander Rice, Esq. a man of respectability, and high standing in that place; who at first could not believe that so valuable a discovery could be made by a man without an education. I conversed with him upon the subject, and explained the principles upon which my system was founded; how every thing acted under the nature and operation of the four elements, and by one acting upon another caused all motion; how the element of fire by rarrifying water and air keeps the whole creation in motion; how the temperament of the body, by adding or diminishing heat and cold would promote either life or death. After hearing my explanation, he became satisfied of its correctness, and confessed that my natural gift was of more value than learning. He then made known to me his infirmities, and wished me to take the care of his family, and give him and his wife such information as would enable them to attend upon themselves and family in case of sickness. I readily agreed to this, and soon after carried some of the family through with the medicine, and gave them all the information in my power, of the principle, and the medicine with which it was done. Mrs. Rice undertook the management of the business; she was a kind and affectionate woman, possessing a sound judgment without fear. After she had gained the information, she wished me to attend to carrying her through a course of the medicine, for a bad humour, called the salt rheum, which she had been long afflicted with; she was attended a few times, which effected a complete cure.

Major Rice had been for many years subject to turns of the gout; and had been in some instances confined by it for six months at a time, and for six weeks not able to sit up, much of the time not able to lift his hand to his head. He had been constantly under the care of the most skilful doctors, who would bleed and blister, and physic him, till his strength was exhausted; after attending him in this way through the winter, they said he must wait till warm weather, before he could get about. When the warm weather come, he would crawl out in the sun side of the house, and in this way he gradually gained his strength; after this he was afflicted with a violent burning in the stomach, which was almost as troublesome as the gout.

After he had the right of my medicine, he had frequent turns of the gout; but no attack of this disease has continued more than twenty-four hours, before he was completely relieved; and he has been but little troubled with the burning of the stomach since. He has told me since, that if he could have been as sure of relief, when he was first subject to the disease, as he is now certain of it in twenty-four hours, he would have been willing to give all he was worth. This family has been so much benefitted by the use of the medicine, that no sum of money would be any temptation to them to be deprived of it. This man has never been lacking to prove his gratitude to me; in the time of my troubles his assistance was of the greatest importance to me, and I shall ever feel grateful to him and his family for their goodness.

Soon after I went to Portsmouth, I was sent for to go to Deerfield, where the dysentery prevailed, and had become very alarming. A young man by the name of Fulsom, came after me, and said that the doctor had lost every patient he had attended, that seven had died, and many were sick; that his father and two brothers were given over by the doctor that morning to die.

The young man seemed so anxious, and was so much frightened, that I concluded to go with him; the distance was twenty-eight miles. We started a little before night, and arrived there about ten o'clock. I found the father and the two sons, as bad as they could be and be alive; they were stupid and cold. I told the mother that it was very uncertain whether I could help them. She begged of me to save her husband's life if possible. I told her that I could not tell whether they were dying,

or whether it was the deadly effect of opium. I gave
them all medicine. The two children died in about
three hours; but Mr. Fulsom soon grew better by taking
my medicine. I had not only the sick to attend to, and
do every thing myself; but the opposition of all the
neighbourhood; there was eight of the family sick, and
if I went out of the house, some person would open the
doors and windows, which would cause a relapse; while
perspiration continued, they were easy, but as soon as
they grew cold, the pain would return and be very violent. In the morning I was preparing to come away;
but the father urged me so hard to stay, promising that
I should be treated in a better manner than I had been,
that I consented and remained with them about ten
days. I caught the disorder myself and was very bad;
on taking the medicine, the operation was so violent,
that the neighbours were much frightened, and left the
house, and were afraid to come nigh us, leaving us to
die altogether. I soon got better and was able to carry
Mr. Fulsom through for the first time; which relieved
him, and he soon got better. In the mean time a small
child was brought home sick, that had been carried
away to prevent it from taking the disorder. It was so
far gone, that the medicine would have no effect upon it,
and it soon died. All that were not in a dying situation before they took the medicine, were relieved and got well.
I attended some that had the disorder in other families, all
of whom got well; fifteen in the whole recovered and
three died. Two years after, the death of these three
children was brought against me on a charge of murder.

All that I ever received for my trouble in these cases,
was fifteen dollars; there was no credit given me for
curing the fifteen out of eighteen, when the doctor had
lost all that he attended; and although he had given
over three to die, I cured one of them twelve hours
after. When I left this place the doctor adopted my
mode of practice as far as he knew it, particularly in
sweating, and about one half lived. Notwithstanding
all this, the doctor, as I was informed, made oath that
the three children died in consequence of taking my
medicine; and the good minister of the parish, I was
also informed, testified to the same thing; though I am

confident that neither of them knew any thing about me
or my medicine. A judgment seemed to follow this
clergyman, for a short time after he had lent his aid in
promoting the prosecution against me, a circumstance
took place in his family, which if it had not been done by
a fashionable doctor, might have been called murder.
His wife was at times troubled with a pain in her face,
something like a cramp; a certain doctor said that he
could help her by cutting. He used the knife and other
instruments of torture for four hours, which stopped
her speech, and let loose the juices that filled the flesh
from her breast, so that the blood and water crowded
out of her ears in striving for breath. She remained in
this distressed situation about seven days and died.
This information I had from two respectable men, who
were present at the time of her sufferings and death.

I continued to practise in Portsmouth and vicinity
during this autumn, and while there, was sent for to go
to Salisbury to see a child that had been attended by a
woman for several days, who I had given information to,
but they said the perspiration would not hold; and they
wished for further information. On seeing the child, I
at once found that they had kept about an equal balance
between the outward and inward heat; when they gave
medicine to raise the inward heat and start the determining power to the surface, they at the same time kept
the outward heat so high as to counteract it. After ex-
plaining to them the difficulty, I raised the child up and
poured on to it a pint of cold vinegar, and it immediately revived. Applied no more outward heat, but only
to shield it from the air; and gave the warmest medicine inward, on the operation of which, the child grew
cold and very much distressed. As soon as the inward
heat had gained the full power, and drove the cold out,
the circulation became free, and the child was relieved
from pain and fell asleep; the next day the heat was as
much higher than what was natural, as it had been
lower the day before; and when heat had gained the
victory over cold, the child gained its strength and was
soon about, perfectly recovered.

I had not practised in Salisbury before, since I went
to Exeter, which was in June, and my returning there

seemed to give Dr. French great offence. He had been to see the child mentioned above, and tried to discourage the people from using my medicine; and threatened them that he would have them indicted by the grand jury, if they made use of any without his consent; his threats, however, had very little effect, for the people were well satisfied of the superiority of my practice over his. About this time the bonds for his good behaviour were out; I did not appear against him, and when the case was called the court discharged him and his bail, on his paying the cost. The action was brought on a complaint in behalf of the commonwealth; but I had caused another action of damage to be brought against him, which was carried to the Supreme Court, and tried at Ipswich the spring following. I employed two lawyers to manage my case, and brought forward two witnesses to prove my declaration, who swore that the defendant made the assertion, that I was guilty of murder and he could prove it. His lawyer admitted the fact, but pleaded justification on the part of his client, and brought witnesses on the stand to prove that what he had said was true. The young woman who nursed Mrs. Lifford, and by whose neglect she took cold, swore to some of the most ridiculous occurrences concerning the death of that woman, that could be uttered, which were perfectly contradictory to every thing she had before confessed to be the truth. Another young woman, the daughter of a doctor at Deerfield, made a statement to make it appear that I was the cause of the death of the three children, who died as has been before related. I had no knowledge of ever seeing this woman, and have since ascertained that she was not at the house but once during the sickness, and then did not go into the room where the sick were; and her exaggerated account must have been made up of what she had heard others say.

These things were a complete surprise to me, not thinking it possible that people could be induced to make such exaggerated statements under the solemnity of an oath. I could have brought forward abundance of testimony to have contradicted the whole evidence against me if there was time, but not expecting that the cause

8

would have taken the course it did, was unprepared.
There appeared to be a complete combination of the
professional craft against me, of both the doctors and
lawyers, and a determination that I should lose the
cause, let the evidence be what it might.   My lawyers gave up the case without making a plea; and
the judge gave a very partial charge to the jury, representing me in the worst point of view that he possibly
could, saying that the evidence was sufficient to prove
the facts against me, and that if I had been tried for
my life, he could not say whether it would hang me or
send me to the state prison for life.   The jury of course
gave their verdict against me, and I had to pay the
cost of the court.

The counsel for Dr. French asked the judge whether
a warrant ought not to be issued against me, and be
compelled to recognize to appear at the next court, to
which he answered in the affirmative.   This so frightened my friends, that they were much alarmed for my
safety, and advised me to go out of the way of my enemies, for they seemed to be determined to destroy me.
I went to Andover to the house of a friend, whose wife
I had cured of a cancer, where I was very cordially received, and staid that night.   The next day I went to
Salisbury Mills, and made arrangements to pay the cost
of my unfortunate law suit.

In the fall of the year 1806, I was sent for to go to
Beverly, to see the wife of a Mr. Appleton, who was
the daughter of Elder Williams, the Baptist Minister in
that town, and was very low in a consumption.   She
had formerly been afflicted with the salt rheum on her
hands, and had applied to a doctor for advice; he had
advised her to make use of a sugar of lead wash, which
drove the disease to her lungs, and she had been in that
situation for a long time, and very little hopes were entertained of her ever being any better.   I carried her
through a course of the medicine, with very good success.   I remained in Beverly about a week; and while
there, became acquainted with Mr. Williams, and also
Mr. William Raymond, to whom I afterwards gave information of my practice and he assisted me to attend
on my patients.   Then returned to Portsmouth, where

I was constantly called on to practise, and had all the most desperate cases put under my care, in all of which I met with very great success.

After staying here about two weeks, I returned to Beverly, to see Mrs. Appleton and other patients there, and found them all doing well; was called on to attend many desperate cases; in all of which I effected a cure, except one, who was dying before I was called on. While practising in Beverly, was called on by a Mr. Lovett, to attend his son, who was sick, as they supposed with a bad cold, some thought it a typhus fever. I was very much engaged in attending upon the sick at the time, and could not go with him; he came after me three times before I could go. On seeing him, found that he complained of a stiff neck, and appeared to be very stupid, and had no pain. His aunt who took care of him, said that he would certainly die, for he had the same symptoms as his mother who died a short time before. I gave some medicine which relieved him; the next day carried him through a course of the medicine, and he appeared to be doing well. Being called on to go to Salem, I left him in the care of Mr. Raymond, with particular directions to keep in the house and not expose himself. This was on Wednesday, and I heard nothing from him, and knew not but what he was doing well, till the Sunday afternoon following, when I was informed that he was worse. I immediately inquired of Mr. Raymond, and learned from him that he had got so much better, he had been down on the side of the water, and returned on Friday night; that the weather was very cold being in the month of December; that he had been chilled with the cold, and soon after his return had been taken very ill; he staid with him on Saturday night, and that he was raving distracted all night; that he had not given any medicine, thinking that he was too dangerously sick for him to undertake with.

I told the young man's father, that it was very doubtful whether I could do any thing that would help him; but that I would try and do all I could. I found that the patient was so far gone that the medicine would have no effect, and in two hours told him that I could not help his son, and advised him to call some other advice.; this was said in presence of Elder Williams, and Mr. Raymond. Mr. Lovett made answer that if I could not help his son, he knew of none who could; and was very desirous for me to stay with him all night, which I did, and stood by his bed the whole time. He was much deranged in his mind till morning, when he came to himself, and was quite sensible. I then again requested the father to send for some other doctor, as I was sensible that I could do nothing for him that would be any benefit. He immediately sent for two doctors, and as soon as they arrived, I left him in their care. The two doctors attended him till the next night about ten o'clock when he died. I have been more particular in giving the history of this case, because two years after it was brought as a charge against me for murdering this young man. The father and friends expressed no dissatisfaction at the time, in regard to my conduct, except they thought I ought not to have neglected the patient so long; but it was a well known fact, that I attended as soon as I knew of his being worse, and that the whole cause of his second attack was owing to his going out and exposing himself, and could not be imputed as any fault of mine.

In the latter part of December, 1808, I was sent for to attend Elder Bowles, the Baptist minister of Salem. I was introduced to him by Elder Williams, and found him in bed, and very weak and low, in the last stage of a consumption; all hopes of a recovery were at an end; his doctors had left him as incurable. He asked my opinion of his case; I told him that I could not tell whether there was a possibility of a cure or not till after using the medicine; being doubtful whether there was mortification or not. He was a man very much respected and beloved by his people, and the public anxiety was very great about him. He expressed a strong desire that I should undertake with him; but I declined doing any thing until he consulted his deacons and other members of his church, who were his particular friends, and their advice taken; which being done, they offered no objection, but wished him to act his own mind, and, whatever the result should be they would be

satisfied. He replied that he was convinced that he
could not live in his present situation more than a week,
and therefore his life could not be shortened more than
that time; and it was his wish that I should undertake
to cure him. His strength was so far exhausted that it
was with the greatest exertion and difficulty that they
could get him to sit up about three minutes in a day, to
have his bed made.

I gave his friends as correct an account of his disorder
and the operation of the medicine, as I could; and that
I did not wish to do any thing which might cause reflec-
tion hereafter; but they promised that let the result be
what it might they should be satisfied and would not
think hard of me. On these conditions I undertook,
and told them that twenty-four hours time would decide
whether he lived or died. I began to give the medicine
in the morning, which had a very calm and easy operation; the emetic herb operated very kindly, and threw
off his stomach a large quantity of cold jelly, like the
white of an egg; the perspiration moved gently on, and
was free; the internal heat produced by the medicine
fixed the determining power to the surface, and threw
out the putrefaction to such a degree that the smell was
very offensive. Mr. Bowles had a brother present who
was a doctor; he observed that he did not know whether
the medicine made the putrefaction, or whether it made
visible what was secreted in the body; but he was soon
convinced on that head, for when the medicine had
cleansed him, all this putrid smell ceased. While the
medicine was in the greatest operation, the perspiration
brought out the putrefaction to such a degree, that the
nurses in making his bed, were so affected with it, that she
fainted and fell on the floor. I attended on him for
about three weeks, in which time he was able to set up.
two or three hours in a day; his food nourished his
body, and his strength gained very fast, considering the
season of the year being unfavourable. I gave him my
best advice, and left directions how to proceed, and returned home to my family to spend the rest of the winter with them. I returned in the spring to see Mr.
Bowles, and found him so far recovered, as to be able to
ride out and in good spirits. He soon gained his health,

8*

and is now well and ready to give testimony of the facts as I have related them.

In the season of 1809, I suffered much. In the first part of the summer, I attended many patients of old complaints; in particular one case that I shall mention of a young woman in Kittery, in a consumption. She had been confined to her house four months; her flesh was exhausted and she had a violent stricture of the lungs, which she said seemed as though there was a string that drawed her lungs to her back; this caused a dry, hacking cough, which was very distressing. I could give her friends no encouragement of a cure; but the young woman and her friends were so urgent, that I undertook with her. Her courage was very great; and she took the medicine and followed all my directions with great perseverance. She said she wished that it might either kill or cure, for she did not desire to live in the situation she was then in. I left her medicine and directions, and occasionally visited her. My plan of treatment was followed with much attention and zeal for six months, before I could raise an inward heat that would hold more than six hours. She then had what was called a settled fever; and I gave her medicine to get as great an internal heat as I possibly could; this caused much alarm among her friends, as they thought she would certainly die. I told them that the heat holding, which was the cause of the fever, was the first favourable symptom that I had seen in her favour. She soon gained her health, to the astonishment of all her friends and acquaintances. She continued to enjoy good health till the next season, when she had another turn of the fever. I attended her in my usual way, and raised the heat till it completely overpowered the cold, when she was entirely cured, and has ever since enjoyed good health.

During this summer, a woman applied to me from a neighbouring town, who had the dropsy, and brought with her a little girl, who had the rickets very bad, so that she was grown much out of shape. I carried them both through a course of the medicine, attended them for three or four weeks, and then gave the woman information how to relieve herself, and the girl, by occasionally visiting them; they both recovered of their complaints;

and have enjoyed perfect health since. This woman paid me the most liberally of any that I had attended, and has on all occasions manifested her gratitude for the assistance I afforded her. Another woman from the same town applied to me, who had a cancer on her breast. She had been under the care of several doctors, who had by their course of practice made her worse. I undertook with her and by giving medicine to check the canker and promote perspiration, effectually relieved her from the disease. Many other desperate cases, such as consumptions, dropsies, cancers, &c. most of which had been given over by the doctors, were attended by me about this time, which it will be unnecessary for me to particularize; all of them were either completely cured or essentially relieved and made comfortable by the system of practice. One case I shall, however, state, being rather of an extraordinary nature, to show the absurdity of the fashionable manner of treating disease by the doctors of the present day.

A young lady applied to me who had been much troubled with bleeding at the stomach. She stated to me that she had been bled by the doctors forty-two times in two years; and that they had bled her seven times in six weeks. So much blood had been taken from her, that the blood vessels had contracted in such manner that they would hold very little blood; and the heat being thereby so much diminished, the water filled the flesh, and what little blood there was rushed to her face, while all the extremities were cold; this produced a deceptive appearance of health, and caused those who judged by outward appearances, to doubt whether there was any disease; so that she had not only to bear her own infirmities, but the reproaches of her acquaintances. I kindled heat enough in the body to throw off the useless water, which gave the blood room to circulate through the whole system, instead of circulating as it had done before, only in the large blood vessels, and they being much extended by not having heat enough to give it motion, leads the doctors into the erroneous idea, that there is two much blood, and resort to the practice of bleeding, which reduces the strength of the patient, and increases the disease. There is no such

thing as a person having too much blood, no more than
there is of having too much bone, or too much muscle,
or sinews; nature contrives all things right.   The blood
may be too thick, so as not to circulate, and is liable to
be diseased like all other parts of the body; but how
taking part of it away can benefit the rest, or tend in
any way to remove the disease, is what I could never
reconcile with common sense.   After I had carried this
woman through a full operation of the medicine, and
got the heat to hold, so as to produce a natural perspiration, she at once exhibited a true picture of her situation; instead of appearing to be so fleshy and well as
she had done, she fell away and became quite emacia-
ted; but as soon as the digestive powers were restored
so that food could nourish her body, she gained her
strength and flesh, and in a short time was completely
restored to health.

I was about this time called to attend a woman who
was very severely attacked with the spotted fever.   The
first appearance of it was a pain in her heel, which soon
moved up to her hips and back, from thence to her
stomach and head; so that in fifteen minutes her sight
was gone, and in less than half an hour she was senseless and cold; about this time I saw her and examined
well the cause of the disease; I was well satisfied that
it was the effect of cold having overpowered the inward
heat.   By confining her from the air, giving her Nos.
1 and 2, and keeping her in a moderate steam, she in a
short time came to her senses; and the symptoms were
exactly similar to a drowned person coming to, after
having life suspended by being under water.   As soon
as the perspiration became free, all pain ceased, and
she was quite comfortable; in twenty-four hours the
disease was completely removed, and she was able to attend to her work.

The same day I had another case of a child which
the doctor had given over.   When I came to this child
it was senseless, and I expected in a mortified state; I
gave it the hottest medicine I could get, with the emetic;
it lay about six hours silent, before the medicine had
kindled heat enough to cause motion in the stomach and
bowels, when it began to revive, and what came from it

was black and putrid ; the bowels just escaped mortification.   The child was soon well.   These two cases
were both cured in twenty-four hours time.

When the spotted fever first appeared in Portsmouth,
the doctors had five cases and all of them died.   I had
five cases similar, all of which lived.   Because my patients did not die, the doctors said they did not have the
fever.   In this they had much the advantage of me, for
there could be no doubt of theirs all having it, as death
was, in most of the cases under their care, on their side
and decided the question.   I have had a great number
of cases of the spotted fever under my care, and in all
of them used the remains of heat as a friend, by kindling
it so as to produce heat enough in the body to overpower
and drive out the cold ; and have never failed of success,
where there was any chance of a cure.

Sometime this season I was sent for to attend Captain
Trickey, who was very sick ; I examined him and was
confident that I could not help him, and took my hat
in order to leave the house.   His family insisted on my
stopping and doing something for him ; but I told them
that I thought he was in a dying state, and medicine
would do no good.   I told his son that in all probability, he would not be alive over twenty-four hours, and
that he had better go for some other help, for I could
do him no good.   I told the wife that I should give no
medicine myself, but as they had some in the house
that they knew the nature of, she might give some of it
to her husband, which she did.   Two doctors were sent
for ; the first one that arrived bled him, and he soon
breathed very short, and grew worse ; the other doctor
came, and said that his breathing short was in consequence of the medicine I had given him ; but by this
he did not gain credit, for all the family knew to the
contrary ; and the woman soon after told me of his
speech.   The patient continued till the next day about
ten o'clock and died.   Soon as he was dead the doctors
and their friends spared no pains to spread the report in
every direction, that I had killed this man with my screw
auger, a cant name given to my emetic herb, in consequence of one of my patients when under the operation
of it, saying that it twisted in him like a screw auger.

This was readily seized upon by the doctors, and made use of for the purpose of trying to destroy the reputation of this medicine by ridicule; they likewise gave similar names to several other articles of my medicine for the same purpose, and represented them as the names by which I called them. They had likewise given me several names and titles, by way of reproach; such as the sweating and steaming doctor; the Indian doctor; the old wizzard; and sometimes the quack. Such kind of management, had a great effect on the minds of many weak minded people; they were so afraid of ridicule, that those whom I had cured were unwilling to own it, for fear of being laughed at for employing me.

The circumstance of the death of the above mentioned Capt. Trickey, was seized upon by the doctors and their friends, and the most false and absurd representations made by them through the country, with the intention of stopping my practice, by getting me indicted for murder, or to drive me off; but my friends made out a correct statement of the facts, and had them published, which put a stop to their career for that time. I continued my practice, and had a great number of the most desperate cases, in most of which I was successful. The extraordinary cures I had performed, had the tendency to make many people believe, that I could cure every one who had life in them, let their disease be ever so bad; and where I had attended on those who were given over as incurable, and they died, whether I gave them any medicine or not, the report was immediately circulated that they were killed by me, at the same time the regular doctors would lose their patients every day, without there being any notice taken of it. When their patients died, if appearances were ever so much against their practice, it was said to be the will of the Lord, and submitted to without a murmur; but if one happened to die that I had any thing to do with, it was readily reported by those interested in destroying my credit with the people, that I killed them.

I could mention a great number of cases of the cures that I performed, if I thought it necessary; but my intention is to give the particulars of such only as will have the greatest tendency to convey to the reader the most correct information of my mode of practice, without repeating any that were treated in a similar manner, to those already given. I shall now proceed to give the particulars of one of the most important circumstances of my life, in as correct and impartial a manner as I am capable of doing from memory ; in order to show what I have suffered from the persecutions of some of the medical faculty, for no other reason, as I conceive, than that they feared my practice would open the eyes of the people, and lessen their importance with them ; by giving such information as would enable them to cure themselves of disease without the aid of a doctor ; and from many others, who were governed altogether by the prejudices they had formed against me by the false reports that had been circulated about my practice, without having any other knowledge of me. Many of the latter, however, have since been convinced of their error, have a very favourable opinion of my system, and are among my best friends.

After practising in those parts through the season of 1809, I went home to Surry, where I remained a few weeks, and returned back to Salisbury ; on my way there, I made several stops in different places where I had before practised, to see my friends and to give information to those who made use of my medicine and practice. On my arrival at Salisbury, my friends informed me that Dr. French had been very busily employed in my absence, and that he and a Deacon Pecker, who was one of the grand jury, had been to Salem, to the court, and on their return had said that there had been a bill of indictment found against me for wilful murder. They advised me to go off and keep out of the way ; but I told them I should never do that ; for if they had found a bill against me, the government must prove the charges, or I must be honourably acquitted. About ten o'clock at night Dr. French came to the place where I stopped, with a constable, and made me a prisoner in behalf of the commonwealth. I asked the constable to read the warrant, which he did ; by this I found that Dr. French was the only complainant, and the justice who granted the warrant ordered me before him to be examined, the next morning. I was then taken by the constable to Dr. French's house, and keepers were placed over me to prevent me from escaping. While at his house and a prisoner, Dr. French took the opportunity to abuse and insult me in the most shameful manner that can be conceived of, without any provocation on my part; he continued his abuse to me till between two and three o'clock, when he took his horse and set out for Salem to get the indictment. After he was gone, I found on inquiry of the constable, that after he had been before the grand jury and caused me to be indicted, he came home before the bill was made out, and finding that I was at Salisbury, fearing I might be gone, and he should miss the chance of gratifying his malicious revenge against me, he went to a brother doctor, who was a justice of the peace, before whom he made oath, that he had probable ground to suspect, and did suspect, that I had with malice aforethought, murdered sundry persons in the course of the year past, whose names were unknown to the complainant; upon which a warrant was issued against me, and I was arrested, as before stated, in order to detain and keep me in custody, till the indictment could be obtained.

In the morning I was brought before the said justice, and he not being ready to proceed in my examination, the court was adjourned till one o'clock; when I was again brought before him, and he said he could not try me until the complainant was present, and adjourned the court again till near night. The constable took me to his house in the mean time, and put me in a back room and left me alone, all of them leaving the house. When they came back, some of them asked me why I did not make my escape, which I might very easily have done out of a back window; but I told them that I stood in no fear of the consequence, having done nothing whereby I ought to be punished; that I was taken up as a malefactor, and was determined to be convicted as such, or honourably acquitted. Just before night, Dr. French arrived with a Sheriff, and ordered me to be delivered up by the constable to the Sheriff; and after Dr. French had again vented his spleen upon me by the most savage abuse that language could express, saying that I was a murderer, and that I had murdered fifty, and he could prove it; that I should be either hung or sent to the State prison for life, and he would do all in his power to have me convicted. I was then put in irons by the sheriff, and conveyed to the jail in Newburyport, and confined in a dungeon, with a man who had been convicted of an assault on a girl six years of age, and sentenced to solitary confinement for one year. He seemed to be glad of company; and reminded me of the old saying, that misery loves company. I was not allowed a chair or a table, and nothing but a miserable straw bunk on the floor, with one poor blanket which had never been washed. I was put into this prison on the 10th day of November, 1809; the weather was very cold, and no fire, and not even the light of the sun, or a candle; and to complete the whole, the filth ran from the upper rooms into our cell, and was so offensive that I was almost stifled with the smell. I tried to rest myself as well as I could, but got no sleep that night, for I felt something crawling over me, which caused an itching, and not knowing what the cause was, inquired of my fellow sufferer; he said that it was the lice, and that there was enough of them to shingle a meeting-house.

In the morning there was just light enough shone through the iron grates, to show the horror of my situation. My spirits and the justness of my cause prevented me from making any lamentation, and I bore my sufferings without complaint. At breakfast time I was called on through the grates to take our miserable breakfast; it consisted of an old tin pot of musty coffee, without sweetening or milk, and was so bad as to be unwholesome; with a tin pan containing a hard piece of Indian bread, and the nape of a fish, which was so hard I could not eat it. This had to serve us till three o'clock in the afternoon, when we had about an equal fare, which was all we had till the next morning. The next day Mr. Osgood came from Salisbury to see me, and on witnessing my miserable situation, he was so much affected, that he could scarcely speak. He brought me some provisions, which I was very glad to receive; and when I described to him my miserable lodgings, and

9

the horrid place I was in, he wept like a child.　He asked liberty of the jailor to furnish me with a bed, which was granted, and brought me one, and other things to make me more comfortable.　The next day I wrote letters to my family, to Dr. Fuller, and to Judge Rice, stating to them my situation.

The bed which was brought me, I put on the old one, and allowed my fellow sufferer a part of it, for which he was very thankful.　I had provisions enough brought me by my friends for us both, and I gave him what I did not want; the crusts and scraps that were left, his poor wife would come and beg, to carry to her starving children, who were dependent on her.　Her situation and that of her husband were so much worse than mine, that it made me feel more reconciled to my fate; and I gave her all I could spare, besides making his condition much more comfortable, for which they expressed a great deal of gratitude.

In a few days after my confinement, Judge Rice came to see me, and brought with him a lawyer.　On consulting upon the case, they advised me to petition to the Judges of the Supreme Court to hold a special court to try my cause, as there would be no court held by law, at which it could be tried, till the next fall, and as there could be no bail for an indictment for murder, I should have to lay in prison nearly a year, whether there was any thing against me or not.　This was the policy of my enemies, thinking that they could keep me in prison a year, and in all probability I should not live that time, and their ends would be fully answered.

I sent on a petition agreeably to the advice of my friends, and Judge Rice undertook to attend to the business and do every thing to get the prayer of the petition granted.　He followed the business up with great zeal, and did every thing that could be done to effect the object.　I think he told me that he or the lawyer, Mr. Bartlett, had rode from Newburyport to Boston fifteen times in the course of three weeks, on the business.　At length Judge Parsons agreed to hold a special court at Salem, on the 10th day of December, to try the cause, which was one month from the day I was committed. My friends were very attentive and zealous in my cause, and every preparation was made for the trial.

During this time the weather was very cold, and I suffered greatly from that cause, and likewise from the badness of the air in our miserable cell, so that I had not much life or ambition. Many of my friends came to see me, and some of them were permitted to come into the cell; but the air was so bad and the smell so offensive, that they could not stay long. My friend, Dr. Shephard, came to see me, and was admitted into our dungeon. He staid a short time, but said it was so offensive he must leave me; that he would not stay in the place a week for all Newburyport. On Thanksgiving day we were taken out of our cell and put in a room in the upper story, with the other prisoners, and took supper together; they consisted of murderers, robbers, thieves, and poor debtors. All of us tried to enjoy our supper and be in as good spirits as our condition would permit. The most of their complaints were of the filthiness and bad condition of the prison, in which we all agreed. Before it was dark I and my companion were waited upon to our filthy den again. There was nothing in the room to sit upon higher than the thickness of our bed; and when I wrote any thing, I had to lay on my belly, in which situation I wrote the Medical Circular, and several other pieces, which were afterwards printed.

After I had been in prison about two weeks, my son-in-law came to see me. I had before my imprisonment sent for him to come to Portsmouth on some business, and on hearing of my being in prison, he immediately came to Newburyport to see me. He seemed much more troubled about my situation than I was myself. I felt perfectly conscious of my innocence and was satisfied that I had done nothing to merit such cruel treatment; therefore my mind was free from reproach; for I had pursued the course of duty, which I conceived was allotted me by my Maker, and done every thing in my power to benefit my fellow-creatures. These reflections supported me in my troubles and persecutions, and I was perfectly resigned to my fate.

About this time, a lawyer came into the prison and
read to me the indictment, which was in the common-
form, that I, with malice aforethought, not having the
fear of God before my eyes, but moved by the instiga-
tion of the devil, did kill and murder the said Lovett,
with lobelia, a deadly poison, &c.; but feeling so perfectly innocent of the charges, which the bill alleged
against me, it had very little effect upon my feelings;
knowing them to be false, and that they had been
brought against me by my enemies, without any provocation on my part.

In the morning of the day that was appointed for me
to be removed to Salem for trial, I was taken out of my
loathsome cell by the jailor, who gave me water to
wash myself with, and I was permitted to take my breakfast by a fire, which was the first time I had seen any
for thirty days, and could not bear to sit near it in consequence of its causing me to feel faint.   As soon as I
had eaten my breakfast, the iron shackles were brought
and put on my hands, which I was obliged to wear till I
got to Salem.   The weather was very cold, and the
going bad; we stopped but once on the way, the distance being about twenty-six miles.   On our arrival, I
was delivered over to the care of the keeper of the prison
in Salem, and was confined in a room in the second
story, which was more comfortable than the one I had
left.   I was soon informed that Judge Parsons was sick,
and had put off my trial for ten days; so I had to reconcile myself to the idea of being confined ten days
more without fire.   However I was not without friends;
Elder Bowles and Capt. Russell came to see me the first
night, and Mrs. Russell sent her servant twice every day
with warm coffee, and other things for my comfort, for
which I have always been grateful; and Mrs. Perkins,
whom I had cured of a dropsy, sent for my clothes to
wash against the day of my trial.

Many of my friends came to Salem to attend my trial;
some as witnesses, and others to afford me any assistance
in their power.   A few days before my trial, Judge
Rice and Mr. Bartlett, whom I had employed as my
lawyer, held a consultation with me, as to the arrangements necessary to be made; when it was decided that

it would be best to have other counsel; and Mr. Story was agreed upon, who engaged in my cause. I had also engaged Mr. Bannister, of Newburyport, to assist in the trial; but he was of no benefit to me, and afterwards sued me for fifty dollars, at fifty miles distance, to put me to great expense. In order to be prepared for the trial, my counsel held a consultation together, and examined the principal witnesses in the defence. Mr. Bowles, Judge Rice, and several others gave great satisfaction as to the value and usefulness of the medicine, and the variety of cures that had been performed with it within their knowledge. Dr. Fuller, of Milford, N. H. was present and made many statements in my favour, as to the value of the medicine, and advised to have Dr. Cutler, of Hamilton, summoned, which was done. Every thing was done by my friends that was in their power, to assist me and give me a chance for a fair trial, for which I shall always feel very grateful.

On the 20th day of December, 1809, the Supreme Court convened to hear my trial, at which Judge Parsons presided, with Judges Sewall and Parker, assistant Judges. The case was called about ten o'clock in the morning, and the chief justice ordered me to be brought from the prison and arraigned at the bar for trial. I was waited on by two constables, one on my right and the other on my left, in which situation I was brought from the jail to the court-house and placed in the bar. The court-house was so crowded with the people, that it was with much difficulty we could get in. After I was placed in the criminal seat, a chair was handed me and I sat down to wait for further orders. Here I was the object for this great concourse of people to look at; some with pity, others with scorn. In a few minutes I was directed to rise and hold up my right hand, to hear the indictment read, which the grand jury had upon their oaths presented against me. It was in common form, stating that I had with malice aforethought, murdered Ezra Lovett, with lobelia, a deadly poison. I was then directed by the court to plead to the indictment, guilty or not guilty; I plead not guilty, and

9*

the usual forms in such cases, were passed through, the
jury called and sworn, and the trial commenced.

The Solicitor General arose, and opened the case on
the part of the Commonwealth, and made many hard
statements against me, which he said he was about to
prove ; he stated that I had at sundry times killed my
patients with the same poison.   The first witness called
to the stand on the part of the government, was Mr.
Lovett, the father of the young man that I was accused of killing.   He made a tolerable fair statement of
the affair in general, particularly of coming after me
several times before I could attend ; though I think he
exaggerated many things against me, and told over
several fictitious and ridiculous names, which people
had given my medicine, by way of ridicule, such as
bull-dog, ram-cat, screw-auger, and belly-my-grizzle ;
all of which had a tendency to prejudice the court and
jury against me ; and I also thought that he omitted to
tell many things in my favour, that must have been
within his knowledge ; but there was nothing in his
evidence that in the least criminated me, or supported
the charges in the indictment.

The next witness called was Dr. Howe, to prove that
I had administered the poison alleged in the indictment.   He stated that I gave the poison to the said
Lovett, and produced a sample of it, which he said was
the root of lobelia.   The Judge asked him if he was
positive that it was lobelia ; he said he was, and that
I called it coffee.   The sample was handed round for
the court to examine, and they all appeared to be afraid
of it, and after they had all satisfied their curiosity,
Judge Rice took it in his hand and ate it, which very
much surprised them.   The Solicitor General asked
him if he meant to poison himself in presence of the
court.   He said it would not hurt him to eat a peck
of it, which seemed to strike the court with astonishment.   Dr. Howe was then called at my request for
cross-examination, and Mr. Story asked him to describe lobelia, how it looked when growing, as he had
sworn to it by the taste and smell.   This seemed to put
him to a stand, and after being speechless for several
minutes, he said he had not seen any so long, he should

not know it if he should see it at this time. This so completely contradicted and did away all that he had before stated, that he went off the stand quite cast down.

Dr. Cutler was called on to inform the court what the medicine was that Dr. Howe had declared so positively to be lobelia, and after examining it, he said that it appeared to him to be marsh-rosemary, which was the fact. So far, all they had proved against me was, that I had given the young man some marsh-rosemary, which Dr. Cutler had declared to be a good medicine.

Some young women were brought forward as witnesses, whom I had no knowledge of ever seeing before. They made some of the most absurd and ridiculous statements about the medicine, that they said I gave the young man, that were probably ever made in a court of justice before; some of which were too indecent to be here repeated. One of them said that I crowded my puke down his throat, and he cried murder till he died. This was well known to be a falsehood, and that the story was wholly made up by my enemies, as well as what had been before stated by those women, for the purpose of trying to make out something against me. I had two unimpeachable witnesses in court ready to swear that I never saw the young man for more than fourteen hours before he died, during all which time he was in the care of Dr. Howe; but by not having an opportunity to make my defence, in consequence of the government not making out their case against me, could not bring them forward.

John Lemon was the next witness brought forward on the part of the Commonwealth, and was directed to state what he knew about the prisoner at the bar. He stated that he had been out of health for two years, being much troubled with a pain in his breast, and was so bad that he was unable to work; that he could get no help from the doctors; that he applied to me and I had cured him in one week; and that was all he knew about the prisoner at the bar. By this time Judge Parsons appeared to be out of patience, and said he wondered what they had for a grand jury, to find a bill on such evidence. The Solicitor General said he had more evidence which he wished to bring forward.

Dr. French was called, and as he had been the most busy actor in the whole business of getting me indicted, and had been the principal cause, by his own evidence, as I was informed, of the grand jury finding a bill against me, it was expected that his evidence now would be sufficient to condemn me at once; but it turned out like the rest, to amount to nothing. He was asked if he knew the prisoner at the bar; he said he did. He was then directed to state what he knew about him. He said the prisoner had practised in the part of the country where he lived, with good success; and his medicine was harmless, being gathered by the children for the use of the families. The judge was about to charge the jury, when the Solicitor General arose and said, that if it was not proved to be murder, it might be found for manslaughter. The Judge said, you have nothing against the man, and again repeated that he wondered what they had for a grand jury.

In his charge to the jury, the Judge stated that the prisoner had broken no law, common or statute, and quoted Hale, who says, any person may administer medicine with an intention to do good; and if it has the contrary effect from his expectation, and kills the patient, it is not murder, nor even manslaughter. If doctors must risk the lives of their patients, who would practise? He quoted another clause of law from Blackstone, who says, where no malice is, no action lies.*

* As the learned Judge could find no law, common or statute, to punish the accused, he directed or advised those present to stop this quackery, as he called it, and for this purpose, to petition the Legislature to make a law that should make it penal for all who should practise without license from some medical college; to debar them of law to collect their debts; and if this should not answer, to make it penal by fine and imprisonment. This hint, thus given by the Judge, was seized upon first in Massachusetts; from thence it has spread to nearly all the States in the Union. From this source may be traced all those unconstitutional laws which have been enacted in relation to this subject, and all those vexatious suits which I have had to attend in many of the States, from Massachusetts to South Carolina, more or less almost every year since. But I have been able to break them down by my patent being from higher authority, which Judge Parsons could not prevent, or perhaps he never thought of. He however made his own report, and handed it to the reporter,

The charge being given to the jury, they retired for about five minutes and returned into court and gave in their verdict of Not Guilty.

I was then honourably acquitted, without having had an opportunity to have my witnesses examined, by whom I expected to have proved the usefulness and importance of my discovery before a large assembly of people, by the testimony of about twenty-five creditable men, who were present at the trial; besides contradicting all the evidence produced against me. After the trial was over, I was invited to the Sun Tavern to supper, where we enjoyed ourselves for the evening. When we sat down to the table, several doctors were present, who were so offended at my being acquitted, that they left the table, which made me think of what the Scripture says, that "the wicked flee when no man pursueth, but the righteous are bold as a lion."

During the evening I consulted with my friends upon the subject of prosecuting Dr. French and making him pay damages for his abuse to me when a prisoner at his house, in saying that I had murdered fifty, and he could prove it; and after having had a fair chance, and having failed to prove one, it was thought to be a favourable opportunity to make him pay something for his conduct towards me, in causing me so much suffering, and for the trouble he had made me and my friends. A prosecution was agreed upon, and to bring the action in the county of York. Judge Rice agreed to be my bail, and likewise he undertook to pay my lawyers and witnesses for the above trial, and paid Mr. Bartlett forty dollars that night. Mr. Story was paid twenty dollars by a contribution of my friends in Salem. I staid at Mrs. Russel's that night; I had but little sleep, for my mind was so much agitated, when I came to consider what I had gone through, and the risk I had run in escaping the snares of my enemies, with the anxiety of my family till they got the news of my acquittal, that sleep fled from my eyelids, and I was more confused than when in prison.

which is published in the 6th volume of Massachusetts' Reports, and is resorted to by all the enemies of the practice, for a defence against the system.

The next day I went to `Sailsbury, and stopped with
Mr. Osgood, where I was first arrested.   Mrs..Osgood
and a young woman who had been employed by me as
a nurse, assisted to clean my clothes, and clear me of
some troublesome companions I had brought with me
from the prison ; and when I had paid a visit to all my
old friends, who were very glad to see me, I went to
Portsmouth, to recover my health, which was very much
impaired, by being confined forty days in those filthy
and cold prisons, in the coldest part of a remarkably
cold winter.   My friends attended upon me, and carried
me through a regular course of medicine; but the first
operation of it had little effect, in consequence of my
blood being so much chilled, and it was a long time before I could raise a perspiration that would hold.   I am
confident that I should not have lived through the winter
in prison, and believe that this was their plan; for which
reason they managed to have me indicted for murder ;
knowing in that case there could be no bail taken, and
there would be no court at which I could be tried, for
nearly a year, I should have to lay in prison during that
time, and that I should probably die there ; or in any
case, they would get rid of me for one year at least,
whether there was any thing proved against me or not ;
and in that time the doctors and their dupes would be
enabled to run down the credit of my medicine and put
my practice into disrepute among the people ; but I
have been able, by good fortune and the kind assistance
of my friends, to defeat all their plans.   Most of those
that have been instrumental in trying to destroy me and
my practice, have had some judgment befall them as a
reward for their unjust persecutions and malicious conduct towards me.   I was credibly informed that Deacon Pecker, one of the grand jury that found a bill
against me, went with Dr. French, to hunt up evidence
to come before himself, in order to have me indicted.
A short time after I was put in prison, he had a stroke
of the palsy, and has remained ever since, one half
of his body and limbs useless.   Dr. French, one
year after I was acquitted, was brought to the same
bar in which I was placed, and convicted for robbing a grave yard of a dead body, which it was re-

ported he sold for sixty dollars. He lost all his credit, and was obliged to quit his country.*

In the month of January of 1810, I returned home to my family, and staid till I had in some measure recovered my loss of health by imprisonment. In March I returned to Portsmouth, and after taking the advice of my friends made arrangments for prosecuting Dr. French. The prosecution was commenced and he was summoned before the court of common pleas, in the County of York. Judge Rice undertook the principal management of the business, and became my bail. The action was called and carried to the Supreme Court by demurer, which was to set at Alfred, in October. I attended with my witnesses, and expected to have gone to trial; and after waiting several days to know what the defence was going to be, the counsel for the defendant made their plea of justification. I found that their plan was to prove that I had murdered sundry persons whom I had attended, and by that means to make it out that any one had a right to call me a murderer; and that for this purpose, Dr. French had been to every place where I had practised, collecting every case of the death of any that I had attended in this part of the country, and had made out eight cases, all of which have been before mentioned in this narrative, most of whom had been given over by the doctors as past cure, and the others known to be desperate cases. He had obtained the depositions of all that were prejudiced against me, and had collected a mass of evidence to support his defence. After finding what their plan was, it was thought necessary for me to go to all the places where they had been, and get evidence to contradict these highly coloured and exagerated statements, and was under the necessity of requesting a delay of the trial for one week, which was granted. I proceeded immediately and took the depositions of those who were knowing to the facts; but found that these were not sufficient and went again to Deerfield and summoned two

* I do not pretend that these things followed on account of their treatment to me; but I only state them as matters of fact; for so it happened.

men to appear at court and give their verbal testimony. When I had got ready to come to trial, the defendant was not ready, and got, it put off to the next term, which would be holden at York the next year.   In the spring before the setting of the court, I went to the clerk's office to find what the depositions were that were filed against me ; and the whole appeared to be a series of exaggerated statements, made by those who were governed by their prejudices, without having but very little, if any, knowledge of the facts, more than what they obtained by hearsay.   This caused me to redouble my diligence to get witnesses to appear on the stand to contradict their testimony, on each case they had alleged against me.

On the day appointed for the trial, every thing was prepared on my part to have a fair hearing.   Judge Parsons was on the bench, and seemed, as I thought, to be determined to have the case go against me ; for he appeared to know every thing that was to be in the defence beforehand.   I made out my case by proving the words uttered by the defendant, which were in my declaration.   They then proceeded in the defence, to make out the eight cases of murder, which were alleged against me.   The first was the case of a man by the name of Hubbard, of Eliot, who had been dead above two years, the particulars of which I have before stated. The witness brought to support this case, told a very lamentable and highly coloured story ; and I brought on the stand a very respectable witness, who completely contradicted the whole statement.

The next cases brought up were the three children of Mr. Fulsom, of Deerfield, the particulars of which have been before related.   A number of depositions were read, which the defendant had obtained of those that had been my enemies, and who knew nothing of the matter more than hearsay reports among themselves.   They gave a very highly coloured account of my treatment of the children ; so much so, that it would appear by their stories, that I had taken them in health, and had roasted them to death ; never saying a word about the fifteen that I cured, some of which had been given over by the doctors.   To rebut the evidence

that was produced to prove that I had killed those
children, I brought on to the stand, two respectable witnesses, who were knowing to all the circumstances, being present at the time of my attending the family.
They gave a correct and particular account of all the
circumstances as they took place; of the situation of
the family when I first saw them, and the violence of
the disorder; how the doctors had lost all their patients
that had been attacked with the disorder before I came;
with the number that I cured by my mode of practice;
and that the doctors afterwards adopted my plan, and
saved the lives of a number by it. The Judge interrupted them and read some of the depositions over again;
but these witnesses stated, that they were not true, and
went on to give some of the particulars of the opposition I met with in my practice from those very persons,
whose depositions had been read, when the Judge seemed put out, and attempted to stop them, saying they had
said enough. They said that having sworn to tell the
whole truth, they felt it their duty to do it.

They next brought on the case of a woman who had
died at Beverly, that I had attended, and with it the
case of Ezra Lovett, whom I had been tried for murdering. I was very glad to have this case brought up
again, as I wished to have an opportunity to prove all
the facts relating to it, which I had been prevented from
doing on my trial, in consequence of being acquitted
without making any defence. The evidence brought
forward to support this case, were the depositions of
those who had testified against me on my trial at Salem;
they were pretty near the same as then given. After
those depositions were read, I had called on to the stand
Elder Williams and Mr. Raymond, who gave all the particulars of my attending upon the young man, as has
been before related, which completely contradicted all
the depositions they had read in the case. The Judge
interrupted these witnesses and read the deposition of
the girl, who stated that I crowded my pukes down the
patient's throat and he cried murder till he died. They
both positively testified, that there was not a word of it
true; for when he died, and for twelve hours before,
he was under the care of Dr. Howe, during which

10

time I did not see him. As to the woman in Beverly, whom they tried to make out that I murdered, it was proved by these witnesses, that she was in a dying condition when I first saw her, and that I so stated it as my opinion at the time, and that my medicine would not help her.

The next case was that of Mrs. Lifford, who died at Salisbury, the particulars of which have been before given. The evidence brought to prove this case of murder, was the deposition of the woman who nursed her, and by whose neglect the patient took cold, after the medicine had a very favourable operation, and appearances were much in her favour; in consequence of which she had a relapse, and I could not produce any effect upon her by the medicine afterwards. This woman confessed at the time, that she was the only one to blame, and that no fault ought to be attached to me; but she afterwards was influenced by Dr. French to turn against me, and made threats that she would swear to any thing to injure me. After her deposition was read, I brought witnesses on the stand, who completely contradicted every thing contained it it; but the Judge read her deposition to the jury, and directed them to pay attention to that in preference to the witnesses on the stand.

The eighth and last case was that of the son of Thomas Neal, of Portsmouth, who was very violently attacked, and was attended by Dr. Cutter. I was called on at night to attend him, and thought there was a possibility of helping him; but the man with whom he lived, would not consent that I should do any thing for him, and I went away, after telling them that he would be either worse or better before morning, and if he was worse he would die. I was called to visit him in the morning, and was informed that he was worse, and that his master had consented to have me attend upon him. I told his father it was undoubtedly too late; but he insisted upon it so much, I attended, and told them the chance was very small for doing him any good, as I considered it a desperate case. After being very hardly urged by his friends, I gave him some medicine, but it had no effect, and about sun-down he died. The doctor who attended him was brought forward to prove that I murdered the patient. If I recollect rightly, he swore that the patient had the dropsy in the brain, and that the disorder had turned and he was in a fair way to recover ; but I came and gave him my poison pukes and killed him. I brought forward evidence who swore to the facts as I have above related them; and that the doctor would give no encouragement of helping the patient. The father of the young man gave his evidence, and stated that his son was in a dying situation when I gave him medicine ; but the Judge interrupted him, and asked if he was a doctor, to which he answered no. He then said the doctor has stated that his disorder had turned, and he was getting better; are you going to contradict the doctor? and thus managed to do away his testimony.

I have thus given a brief sketch of the evidence in the eight cases, which were attempted to be proved as murder, in order to make out justification on the part of the defendant, with my defence to the same, in as correct a manner as I am able from memory ; and am confident that every circumstance as I have related it, can be substantially proved by living witnesses. After the evidence was gone through, the lawyers on both sides made their pleas, making the case on my part as good and as bad as they could. The Judge then gave his charge to the jury, which was considered by those who heard it, to be the most prejudiced and partial one that had been ever heard before. He made use of every means to raise the passions of the jury and turn them against me.; stating that the defendant was completely justified in calling me a murderer, for if I was not guilty of wilful murder, it was barbarous ignorant murder; and he even abused my lawyers for taking up for me, saying that they ought to be paid in screw-augers and bull-dogs. The people that were present were very much disgusted at his conduct, and they expressed themselves very freely upon the subject; it was said by some, that our courts, instead of being courts of justice, had become courts of prejudice. One man said that he hoped Judge Parsons would never have another opportunity to act on a cause; which prediction turned out true, for he

soon after had a stroke of the palsy, and as I am informed, died before the next court met. The jury brought
in their verdict of justification on the part of the defendant, and throwed the whole costs on me, which
amounted to about two thousand dollars.

When I found how the case was going to turn, I
went to Portsmouth, and soon after made arrangements
to pay the costs. Judge Rice was my bail and undertook to pay all the bills that I had not paid at the time.
On my settlement with him I owed him six hundred
dollars for money that he had advanced on my account;
for which I had no way to secure him, but by giving
him a mortgage of my farm; which I did, and it was
put on record, and never known to any of my friends
till I had paid it up. He charged nothing for all his
time and trouble, through the whole of my persecution s
and trials, for which and for his kindness and friendship on all occasions, I shall ever consider myself under
the greatest obligations.

Sometime in the spring of the year previous to this
trial at York, a young man came to me at Portsmouth,
by the name of Alfred Carpenter, from the town where
my family lived; he was recommended to me by his
neighbours, as being lame and poor, and wanted my assistance. I took him out of pity and instructed him in
my mode of practice, under the expectation that it would
be a benefit to him and thereby he would be able to
assist me in attending the sick.

About the first of June, 1811, I received a letter from
Eastport, where I had been the fall before and shown
some of my mode of practice. Some of the people in
that place were so well satisfied with it, that seven men
had subscribed their names to the letter, requesting me
to come there and practise in the fevers, which prevailed in those parts. I left the care of my business at
Portsmouth, with Mr. Carpenter, my apprentice, and
immediately took passage for Eastport, where I arrived
about the middle of June. I was very gladly received
by those who had wrote to me, and by those with whom
I had become acquainted when there before. I agreed
to practise under the protection of those who had sent
for me, until I had convinced them of its utility, to

which they consented, and promised me all the assistance in their power. I was soon called on to practise, and had all the most desperate cases that could be found, in all of which I met with very great success. The first cases I attended in presence of the committee, were five desperate cases of consumption. These patients were all relieved in three weeks, and were all living this present year, 1831. While attending these people, I was called upon to attend a young man on board a vessel; who had his foot bruised to pieces by a block falling from mast-head, weighing thirteen pounds. It being done five days before I saw him, it was mortified, and the whole body in convulsions. I took off three toes and set the fourth, and cured him in five weeks with the usual practice. While attending him, I had to pass a doctor's shop. A scythe was thrown at me, point first, about the distance of two rods. It passed between my feet without doing any injury. In consequence of this assault, I sent word to all the doctors who had opposed me, that for the politeness with which they had treated me, I would compensate them by taking off the burden of being called up at night, and thus breaking their rest, and would give them the chance of laying in bed until noon, without being disturbed by their patients.

I was called on the night following to attend a woman in child-bed. I attended according to my promise, and let them rest; and if I had remained there, they might have rested until the present time, as I attended to all branches in practice.

There was, I think at that time, five practising doctors on the Island, among whom my success in curing the sick caused great alarm; and I soon experienced the same determined opposition from them, with all the arts and plans to destroy me and my practice, that I had experienced from the same class of men in other places. In order to show some of their conduct towards me, I shall relate the particulars of some of the cases I attended; but most of the numerous cases which I had under my care, were so nearly similar to those that have been already given, and my mode of treating them being about the same, that it will be unnecessary to repeat them.

10*

I was sent for to visit a Mrs. Lovett, who was the daughter of Mr. Delisdernier, at whose house I attended her. She had the dropsy, and had been under the care of one of the doctors, till he had given her over as incurable. I went to see her in company with the doctor; but we could not agree as to the cause and remedy. I asked him several questions concerning the power of the elements, and the effect of heat on the human system. He answered that the elements had nothing to do with the case. After giving him my ideas on the subject, which all appeared to be new to him, I told him that the contending powers in this case was between the fire and water; and if I could get heat enough in the body to make the water volatile, it could not stay in the body. He said that any thing warm would not answer for her. I then asked him how he thought the hottest medicine would do. He said it would produce immediate death. I then told him that if I did any thing for her, I should administer the hottest medicine I could give. Finding there would be a disadvantage on my part in doing any thing for her, as the doctor and I could not agree, I left the house. I was followed by the father and mother and the doctor, who all insisted on my returning; but I told them that notwithstanding the doctor had given her over, if I was to attend her and she should die, they would say that I killed her. They promised that let the consequences be what they might no blame should be alleged against me. Upon which I agreed that I would stop on condition that two of my friends should be present as witnesses to what was said, and see the first process of the medicine, which was agreed to and they were sent for, and heard the statements of the doctor and family. A Capt. Mitchell, from New York, was also present, and heard the conversation between me and the doctor; and being pleased with the principles that I laid down, which excited his curiosity so much that he expressed a wish to be present and see the operation of the medicine, and staid accordingly.

The doctor pretended to be going away till after I had given the first medicine, and appeared to be very busy going out and coming in, and had much conversation with Mrs. Lovett, the husband's mother, who was

the nurse. After the first medicine had done, which
operated very favourably, I gave directions what to do,
and particularly to keep the patient in perspiration
during the night and left medicine for that purpose; we
then went home. In the morning I called to see her
and to my surprise found her sitting with the window
up, and exposed to the air as much as possible; on
examination I found that no medicine had been used.
On inquiry I found that the doctor had been in frequently to see her; and on asking why they had not
followed my directions, the nurse appeared very cross,
and said she would not take any of my medicine. I
told them that they had not killed her, but I did not
thank them for their good will any more than if they
had done it. I was about leaving the house, as I found
my directions would not be attended to by the nurse,
but Capt. Mitchell was very urgent for me to continue.
I told him that if he would attend upon her and see the
medicine given and every thing done according to my
directions, I would continue, to which he agreed. I
left the patient in his care and he attended her faithfully through the day; at night I visited her and found the
swelling began to abate. He continued his care of her,
and in three days she was able to go up and down stairs,
and in one week she was well. By the influence of
the doctor, the woman and the husband, all turned against
me, and I never received any thing for my trouble but
their abuse and slander. The woman's father and Capt.
Mitchell, however, gave me all credit for the cure, and
they both purchased a right.

About a year after, at a private assembly of women,
this Mrs. Lovett, the mother-in-law of the sick woman,
gave an account of the whole transaction, and stated
that there was a private interview between her and the
doctor, and it was agreed to go contrary to my directions, and the doctor said she would die in the course
of the night; and that he should take me up for murder,
and that she must be an evidence. This appeared to
be almost incredible, that they should be so void of all human feelings, as to be willing to have the woman die, in
order to have the opportunity to take me up for murder; but two women who were present when she told

the story, gave their depositions proving the facts as above stated.

I continued my practice on this Island, at Lubec, and on the main, paying my most particular attention to those who sent for me, and wanted information. I practised under their inspection about five weeks, and then told them that I had done enough for a trial, to prove the use of the medicine, and should do no more till I knew whether a society could be formed. They expressed their entire satisfaction, and wished to have a society formed; a meeting was called for that purpose, and sixteen signed the articles at the first meeting. After this, a meeting was held every week, at which a lecture was given for the purpose of giving information, and for the admission of members; and eight each week was added during the summer. In the fall I went back to Portsmouth to attend to my business there, and see to the the society which had been formed in that place.

After staying in Portsmouth a few weeks to give information to the people, and procuring a stock of medicine I made arrangements to return to Eastport; and sometime in the month of October, I set sail for that place, taking with me my apprentice and Stephen Sewell. On my arrival I introduced Mr. Carpenter as my apprentice and got Mr. Sewell into a school as an assistant; in which he had fifteen dollars a month, and all his leisure time he attended to gain information of the practice. I took a small shop and put into it a good assortment of medicine, and attended to practice till I had got Mr. Carpenter introduced among the people.

While practising here, I frequently heard of the abuse and scandal towards me and my practice, from Mrs. Lovett, the old woman before mentioned, as the nurse of her son's wife, whom I cured of the dropsy. This old woman was a singular character, and was called a witch by the people; I have no faith in these kind of things, yet her conduct, and certain circumstances, that took place, were very extraordinary, and puzzled and astonished me more than any thing I had ever met with, and which I have never been able to account for to this day. Mr. Carpenter was attending a man, where this woman often visited, who had the consumption, and his child, which was sick and had fits. He came to me and said that the medicine he gave would not have its usual effect; that the emetic instead of causing them to vomit, would make them choak and almost strangle. I attended them myself, and on giving the medicine it would operate on the man, and not on the child at one time, and the next time on the child and not on him. Sometimes the child would lay in fits, for a whole night, and nothing would have any effect upon it; in the morning it would come out of them and appear to be quite bright and lively. I had never known the medicine to fail of producing some effect before, where the patient was not so far gone as not to have life enough left to build upon. I can give no reason for this strange circumstance, satisfactory to myself, or which would be thought reasonable by the readers. The old woman, before mentioned, was frequently in and out of the house where the man and child were, and seemed to be very much interested about them; when she was gone the child would frequently go into violent fits, and when I steamed it, it was said the old woman would be in great distress. It caused much conversation among the neighbours; they believed it to be the power of witchcraft; and that the old woman had a control over the destinies of the man and child, and was determined to destroy them in order to get her revenge on me. I have no belief in these things; but must confess that her strange conduct, and the extraordinary circumstances attending the whole affair, baffled me more than any thing I had ever met with before. I was unable to do any thing for these two patients, except sometimes by a temporary relief; they continued to grow worse, and finding it not in my power to do them any good, I left them, and they both soon after died.

Whether the extraordinary circumstances attending the two cases above stated, were caused by a stratagem of the doctors, in which the old woman was made their agent, to injure me by causing in some way or other poisonous medicines to be administered to them in order to prevent my medicine from having any salutary effect, is what I do not feel disposed to assert as a fact; but the many cases in which I have been certain that such things have been done by the faculty, and their enmity and uniform opposition to my practice, both at this place and elsewhere, as well as the confession made by the old woman, would tend strongly to confirm such a belief. I could mention a great number of facts in addition to what I have said in regard to this affair, if necessary, which appeared very extraordinary to me and all who witnessed them; but I think that enough has been said on the subject, and shall leave it to the public to decide between us.   There were five doctors at Eastport when I went there, who had a plenty of business; but my success was so great, and the people became so well satisfied of the superiority of my system of practice over theirs, that they were soon relieved from most of their labours; and in a short time after, three of them had to leave the place for want of employment.

I made arrangements to go back to Portsmouth to spend the winter, and to leave Mr. Carpenter with the care of my business and practice at Eastport, under the protection of John Burgin, Esq. a man who has been particularly friendly to me on all occasions. I told him if he would be faithful in my business and in selling medicine, that he should have half the profits after the money was collected; and in December I took passage for Portsmouth. We had a long and tedious passage of eighteen days; the vessel took fire and our lives were exposed; but we were fortunate enough to extinguish it without much damage. I stopped in Portsmouth and practised some time, then went to see my family, where I remained the rest of the winter, in which time I was employed in collecting and preparing medicine. I returned to Portsmouth in the spring of 1812, and after making the necessary arrangements, I set sail for Eastport, where I arrived about the first of May. I made a settlement with Mr. Burgin, and paid him sixty-three dollars for the board of Mr. Carpenter, and for shop rent. Then furnished the shop with a complete stock of medicine, to which I added cordials and spirits, the whole of which amounted to about twelve hundred dollars. There was a great call for medicine this spring, and also for practice.

After arranging my business, I concluded to return to Portsmouth; a short time before I came away, a Mr. Whitney came to me for assistance, and purchased a right. About the same time, a Mr. McFadden applied also for assistance, who had the consumption. I left them both under the care of Mr. Carpenter, and immediately sailed for Portsmouth, where I arrived in safety. Soon after my arrival there, I found there was going to be a war with Great Britain; in consequence of which, I returned immediately back to Eastport to settle my affairs in that place. In a short time after my arrival there, the declaration of war came on, and I made the best arrangements of my business I could, leaving Mr, Carpenter with directions, if there should any thing happen in consequence of the war, so as to be necessary for him to leave the Island, to come to Portsmouth. Before leaving the place, I called on him for some money, and all he could pay me was sixty-four dollars, which was but one dollar more than I had paid for his board and shop rent. The people were in such confusion it was impossible to get a settlement with any one. I left Mr. Whitney and Mr. McFadden in his care, and left the Island about the middle of June, and arrived in Portsmouth in forty-eight hours, where I remained the greater part of the summer; during which time I had constant practice, and formed some regulations for the society, which was established there, for the purpose of greater facility in communicating information of my system of practice to the people who wished my assistance. In the fall of this year I published my pamphlet of directions, as many were urgent that I should not leave the place destitute of the knowledge of my practice and medicine. Many persons who had been the most urgent for me to give them information, now became the most backward, and complained that the restrictions were too hard with regard to their giving the information to others; some of whom had never done the least thing to support the practice or me. When any of them were sick they were ready enough to call on me for assistance; and if I relieved them quick, they thought it worth nothing, and they run out against my practice, saying I deserved no pay.

This sort of treatment I have met with from a certain class of people in all places where I have practised. I was treated with much attention when they were in danger from sickness; but when I had cured them I was thought no more of. This kind of ingratitude I have experienced a pretty large share of during my practice.

In the month of October, having got my business arranged, and a stock of medicine prepared, I returned to Eastport. On my arrival there I went to my shop, and found that Mr. Carpenter had gone home, and Mr. McFadden and a Mr. Harvey, left very sick, and only a boy to take care of them and the shop. Mr. McFadden was very low with a consumption, and unable to lay down. I found there was no regulations of the business in the shop, and the property I had, chiefly gone. I was obliged to pay every attention to the sick men that had been left in this manner without assistance; I attended Mr. Harvey, and got him well enough to go home in a few days; and Mr. McFadden was so put to it for breath and was so distressed, that I had to be with him night and day for six weeks and three days, when Mr. Carpenter returned. Previous to this, I found that Mr. McFadden had put his farm into the hands of Mr. Carpenter as security for his attending him in his sickness; and as he had no relations the remainder to go to him and me. On inquiry into the business I found that he had taken a deed in his own name and that all the bills and accounts for his practice and medicine in my absence were in his own name. I asked him for a settlement and he refused; I then asked him what he meant by his conduct; he said he owed me nothing, and bid me defiance, saying if I chose I might take the steps of the law. I could not conceive what he meant by treating me in this manner, till after making further inquiry, I found that he had formed a connection in a family; that he had been advised to take the course he did, and as I had no receipt for the property, or any written agreement to support my claim, he could do with me as he pleased, and keep every thing for his own benefit. The night after he returned, and before I had any knowledge of his intentions, he had robbed the shop of all the ac-

counts, notes, bills, and all other demands, so that I
knew no more about the business than a stranger.

I frequently tried to get a settlement with Carpenter;
but he said he had none to make with me. Mr. Mc-
Fadden died shortly after, and Carpenter came forward
and claimed all his property, saying that it was all willed to him. I asked him why it should be willed to him,
when I had borne the expense and done the principal
part of the labour in taking care of him in his sickness.
He said I must look to him for my pay. I told him that
it was very singular that my apprentice had become my
master in one year; he denied that he was my apprentice, and said that he was a partner; but I had said in
order to encourage him to be faithful and do well by me,
he should have half the profits of the practice, and that
I had no idea of his having the whole of my property,
because I made him this promise. All I could say I
found would have no effect, for the more I tried to reason with him, the more obstinate and impudent he was.
He even went so far as to say that the shop and all that
was in it was his, and that I had nothing to do with it;
he called a witness and forbid my having any concern in
the shop. I found there was no other way for me, but
to turn him out and get rid of him in the best manner I
could; to effect which I applied to the owner of the shop
and got a writing to prove my claim to the possession,
and immediately took measures to get rid of him. He
made all the opposition, and gave me all the trouble he
could; he went into the shop while I was absent, and
began to throw the property out into the street; but I
soon put a stop to his career, and secured the property
from his reach. He still held all my books and accounts,
which put my business into such confusion that I was unable to collect any of the demands that were due; and
the only remedy I had was to advertise him as my apprentice, and forbid all persons having any dealings with
him on my account, or settling with him. My loss by
the dishonest conduct of this man was very considerable,
besides the injury to my feelings from his base ingratitude to me; for I had taken him from a state of poverty
and distress; supported him for a long time when he was
of very little benefit to me; and had instructed him in my

system of practice, and given him all the information in my power; had introduced him into practice, and given him every encouragement to enable him not only to assist me in supporting my system of practice, but to benefit himself; and after all this, for him to turn against me and treat me in the manner he did, was a deeper wound to my feelings than the loss of my property.

After having got clear of Carpenter, I hired a young man whom I had cured and given information to, and put him into the shop, and agreed to pay his board for one year, and then returned to Portsmouth. As Carpenter had bid me defiance, and threatened to sell my rights, and give information to any one who would buy of him; and likewise I found that there was another plot got up to destroy me; a petition had been sent on to the Legislature, to have a law passed against quackery, in which I was named; and there can be no doubt but that the whole object of it was to stop my practice; I was at a stand, and put to much perplexity to know what course it was best to steer. I found I had enemies on every hand, and was in danger of falling by some one of them. Every thing seemed to conspire against me; but I had some friends who have never forsaken me; my courage remained good, and my spirits were never depressed; and it appeared to me that the more troubles I had to encounter, the more firmly I was fixed in my determination to persevere unto the last.

When I had maturely considered the subject in all its bearings, and exercised my best abilities in devising some plan by which I could extricate myself from the dangers which threatened me on every hand; and to prevent those rights, which twenty years labour, with much suffering and great expense had given me a just claim to, from being wrested from me; I finally came to the conclusion that there was only one plan for me to pursue with any chance of success; and that was to go on to Washington, and obtain a patent for my discoveries; and put myself and medicine under the protection of the laws of my country, which would not only secure to me the exclusive right to my system and medicine, but would put me above the reach of the laws of any state.

After coming to the conclusion to go on to the seat of government and apply for a patent, made all necessary preparation for the journey, and started from Portsmouth on the 7th of February, and arrived at Washington on the 23d. The next day after my arrival, I waited on Capt. Nicholas Gilman, of Exeter, showed him my credentials, and asked his advice, what I must do to obtain my object. He said that he thought it could not be made explicit enough to combine the system and practice, without being too long; he however advised me to carry my petition to the patent office; which was then under the control of Mr. Monroe, Secretary of State. I went to the patent office, and found that Dr. Thornton was the Clerk, and presented him my petition. He asked me many questions, and then said I must call again; I called again the next day, and he said the petition was not right; that I must specify the medicine, and what disorder it must be used in; he said that those medicines in general terms to cure every thing, was quackery; that I must particularly designate the medicine, and state how it must be used, and in what disease I then waited on Martin Chittenden, late governor of Vermont, who was at Washington, and asked his assistance; he was from the same town where my father lived, and readily consented. We made out the specifications in as correct a manner as we could, and the next day I carried them to the patent office, and gave them to Dr. Thornton; he complained much about its being too short a system, and put me off once more. I applied again and asked him for my patent; but he said I had not got the botanic names for the articles, and referred me to Dr. Mitchell, of New York, who was in the House of Representatives. I applied to him, and requested him to give the botanic names to the articles mentioned in my petition. He wrote them, and I carried them to Dr. Thornton; but he was unable to read some of the names, one in particular, he said, I must go again to Dr. Mitchell, and get him to give it in some other words, and not tell him that he could not read it. I went, and the doctor wrote the same word again, and then wrote, or "Snap-dragon;" which I carried to Dr. Thornton, and requested him to put in the patent my names, and record it for himself, snap-dragon, or any other name he chose.   He then talked about sending me to Philadelphia, to Dr. Barton, to get his names.

I found he was determined to give me all the trouble he could, and if possible to defeat my getting a patent, and I intimated that I should go with my complaint to Mr. Monroe, upon which he seemed a little more disposed to grant my request, and said he would do without Dr. Barton's names.   He then went to work to make out the patent, and when he came to the article of myrrh, he found much fault about that, and said it was good for nothing.   I told him that I paid for the patent, and if it was good for nothing it was my loss.   After much trouble, I got it made out according to my request, and the medicine to be used in fevers, colics, dysenteries and rheumatisms ; he then asked me if I wanted any additions, and I told him to add, "the three first numbers may be used in any other case to promote perspiration, or as an emetic," which he did.   I then had to go to the treasury office and pay my money and bring him duplicate receipts.   After all this trouble, I at length succeeded in obtaining my patent according to my request, which was completed and delivered to me on the third day of March, 1813.

The next day after I had completed my business, was the day of inauguration of the President of the United States ; and I had the curiosity to stay and see the ceremonies on that occasion.   After the ceremonies were over I went to the stage office and found that the seats were all engaged for a fortnight ; and was obliged to stay till the 13th before I could get a passage. I then took passage in the stage and came on to Philadelphia, where I remained several days for the purpose of seeing Drs. Rush and Barton, to confer with them upon the subject of introducing my system of practice to the world.   I spent considerable time with Dr. Barton ; but Dr. Rush was so much engaged, that I was unable to have but little conversation more than stating my business.   He treated me with much politeness ; and said that whatever Dr. Barton agreed to, he would give his consent, so that my business was chiefly with the lat-

ter gentleman. I asked him many questions concerning
my system and patent, and requested his advice of the
best mode of introducing it. He advised me to make
friends of some celebrated doctors, and let them try the
medicine and give the public such recommendation of it
as they should deem correct. I told him that I feared
that if I should do so, they would take the discovery to
themselves and deprive me of all credit or benefit from
my labours; and asked him if he thought that would
not be the case. He said it might with some, but he
thought there were some of the profession honourable
enough not to do it. I asked him if he would make a
trial of it himself, and give it such credit as he should
find it to deserve. He said that if I would trust it in
his hands, he should be pleased, and would do justice
to me and the cause. I accordingly left some of the
medicine with him, with directions how to use it; but
before I received any return from him he died; and Dr.
Rush also died sometime previous; by which means I
was deprived of the influence of these two men, which
I was confident would otherwise have been exerted in
my favour.

During my interviews with Dr. Barton, we had much
conversation upon the subject of the medical skill, and
he being quite sociable and pleasant, I expressed myself
very freely upon the fashionable mode of practice, used
by the physicians of the present day. He acknowledged
there was no art or science so uncultivated as that of
medicine. I stated to him pretty fully my opinion of
the absurdity of bleeding to cure disease; and pointed
out its inconsistency, inasmuch as the same method was
made use of to cure a sick man as to kill a well beast.
He laughed and said it was strange logic enough.

While in the city of Philadelphia, I examined into
their mode of treating the yellow fever; and found to
my astonishment that the treatment prescribed by Dr.
Rush was to bleed twice a day for ten days. It appeared to me very extraordinary to bleed twenty times to
cure the most fatal disease ever known; and am confident that the same manner of treatment would kill one
half of those in health. This absurd practice being
followed by the more ignorant class of the faculty, mere-

11*

ly because it has been recommended in some particular
cases by a great man, has, I have not the least doubt, destroyed more lives than has ever been killed by powder
and ball in this country in the same time. Those I
met in the streets who had escaped the fatal effect of
bleeding, mercury, and other poisons, carried death in
their countenance ; and on conversing with them, they
said they had never been well since they had the fever ;
that they took so much mercury and opium, they were
afraid that they were in a decline.

After remaining in Philadelphia about two weeks, I
went in the stage to New York, where I obtained a passage in a coaster, and arrived in Portsmouth on the 5th
day of April. Immediately after my arrival at Portsmouth, I gave public notice in the newspapers, of my
having obtained a patent, and forbid all persons trespassing upon it under the penalty of the law in such
cases provided ; and prepared and published a handbill,
in which I gave a description of the nature of disease
on the constitution of man ; and also the conditions of
disposing of the right of using my system of practice ;
and taking a number of the handbills with me, sat out
for Eastport, where I arrived about the first of May.
On my arrival the handbills were circulated among the
people, which caused considerable stir among them,
particularly with the doctors, who seemed surprised that
I had obtained a patent. I again called on Mr. Carpenter for a settlement, but could obtain none, for his
friends advised against it, telling him that he could still
pursue the practice in spite of my patent, by calling the
medicine by different names. I furnished my shop with
a stock of medicine, and made an agreement with Mr.
Mowe, the young man that I had employed since Carpenter was dismissed, to continue the practice for me,
and take charge of my business at this place. My ex-
penses for his wages, board, and shop rent, was about
one dollar per day ; and the amount of the practice
and sale of medicine, was about one hundred dollars
per month.

While at Eastport, I met with a loss, which I will
mention, to show the hard fortune I had to contend with.
Wishing to send one hundred dollars to my friend Judge

Rice, in part payment for what I owed him, took two fifty dollar bills and went to the post-office and gave them to the post master, with a letter directed to Alexander Rice, Esq. Portsmouth, requesting him to secure them in the letter in a proper manner and send it on. The letter was never received in Portsmouth, and no traces of it could be found. I had strong suspicions that the post master at Eastport destroyed the letter and kept the money. I made arrangements to inquire further into his conduct, but shortly after he fell from a precipice and was killed, which put a stop to pursuing the subject any further; so it turned out a total loss to me.

After settling my business in Eastport, I returned to Portsmouth, where I stopped but a short time; and taking Mr. Sewell with me, went to Portland to introduce my practice in that place. On our arrival I advertised my patent in the newspapers, and had handbills printed and circulated among the people, giving the conditions on which I should practise, and the manner of selling family rights, to those who wished the use of my practice and medicine; and that I should attend to no case except such as wished to purchase the rights, to give them information, and prove the utility of the medicine. I gave the information to Mr. Fickett, where we boarded, and a right of using the medicine for himself and family; and gave information to several of his workmen. Soon after making myself known, I had a great number of desperate cases put under my charge, all of which were cured or essentially relieved. My success in the cases I attended, most of which were such as had been given over by the doctors, caused great alarm among those professional gentlemen who are styled regular physicians; and I experienced the same opposition from them that I had met with in other places. I was followed by them, or their spies, and all kinds of false and ridiculous reports were circulated among the people to frighten and prejudice them against me and my medicine.

Soon after coming to this place, I was called on by Capt. John Alden, to attend his wife, who was in a very alarming situation. She was in a state of pregnancy, and had the dropsy, and was then as she supposed, several weeks over her time. She had been in the same situation once before, and was delivered by force, and came very near losing her life; the doctors gave it as their opinion that if she should ever be so again, she would certainly die. I told him that I did not attend on any except those who wished to purchase the right, in which cases I would give them the information. I explained to him the principles upon which my system was founded, and he purchased a right; after which I attended upon his wife, and found her very low; she had not laid in bed for three weeks, being so put to it for breath when she lay down, was obliged to get immediately up again. I carried her through a course of the medicine every day for five days, during which she was reduced in size about eight inches; her travail then came on natural, and in about two hours she was delivered of a daughter, and they both did well. She was able to come down stairs in one week, and in two weeks was well enough to be about the house. This cure so alarmed the doctors, that they circulated a story at a distance, where the facts were not known, that I was so ignorant of this woman's situation, that I killed her immediately; but the woman and her husband gave me all credit for the cure, and appeared very grateful to me for it.

During the summer a son of Capt. Alden was violently seized with the spotted fever; he was taken very suddenly, when at the pump after water, fell and was brought into the house senseless. I attended him, and his jaws being set, administered a strong solution of Nos. 1, 2, and 6, by putting my finger between his cheek and teeth, and pouring in the medicine; squeezing it round to the back of his teeth, and as soon as it reached the roots of his tongue, his jaws came open; I then poured down more of the medicine, and soon after swallowing it, his senses came to him, and he spoke; he appeared like a person waking out of a sleep. As soon as the warm effect of the medicine was over, he relapsed, and life seemed to go down with the heat. I found that I could not restore him till I could rarify or lighten the air; I laid him across the laps of three persons, shielding him from external air with a blanket, and put under him a pan with a hot stone in it about half immersed in hot water; while over this steam, again gave the medicine, which raised a perspiration; and as the heat raised inside, life gained in proportion; and when the perspiration had gained so as to be equal to a state of health, the natural vigour of life and action was restored.

I was called on to attend a woman who had a relax, and in a few visits restored her to health. One night about midnight I was sent for to visit this woman in consequence of their being alarmed about her, the cause of which I could never learn; for on my arrival she was as well as usual. I returned immediately home and was soon after taken in a violent manner with the same disease; and was so bad as not to be able to do any thing for myself. Mr. Sewell attended upon me and did all he could, which had no effect. I was persuaded that I should not live three days unless I could get some relief. I had no pain and every thing I took passed through me in two minutes; nothing seemed to warm me. I sent and obtained some butternut bark, boiled it, and took some as strong as it could be made; as soon as it began to operate I followed it with brandy and loaf sugar burnt together, till it became a syrup; this soon put me in pain; I then followed my general rule of treatment, and was soon relieved.

While at Portland I was sent for to see a Mr. Mason, who was very sick, and it was expected that he would not live through the night. He had been attended by the doctors of the town, for a sore on his nose, which was much inflamed; they had given him so much saltpetre to kill the heat that they almost killed him. I had the hardest trial to save his life of any one I ever attended.; and was obliged to carry him through a course of medicine two or three times a week for three months, besides visiting him every day. The doctors said he would certainly die, and if he did, they meant to take me up for murder; and every means were resorted to, by discouraging him and other ways, to prevent his getting well; and when he got so as to be about, and it was decided that he was going to recover under the operation of the medicine, one who pretended to be his friend gave him a bottle of pepper vinegar; I had made a free use of this article in his case, and he took some of what was given him by this friend, and he soon grew worse.   The man who gave him the pepper vinegar often inquired how he did, and when told that he was worse, he would say that I should kill him.   I could not ascertain the reason of this patient being affected in the manner he was, till Mr. Sewell took some of the same, and was immediately taken in the same manner as the sick man.   He took medicine and got over it, and, a short time after, took some more, and was attacked in a similar manner.   I then began to mistrust that there was something in the pepper vinegar, and on examining it, was satisfied that it had been poisoned to destroy the patient in order to take advantage of me.   I was obliged to carry them both through a course of the medicine, and they afterwards had no such turns.

This patient, after about three month's close attention, gained so as to enjoy a comfortable state of health.   The undertaking was very tedious on my part; I should be hardly willing to go through the same process again, for any sum whatever.   The destructive effects of salt-petre is the worst of any poison I ever undertook to clear the system of.   The only method I have found successful, is to give No. 1 and No. 2, and throw all of it out of the stomach that can possibly be done; and by steaming keep the heat of the body above it; all other poisons can be eradicated by the common course of medicine.   I was called on to attend the sick from all quarters; but few of them were able to purchase the information, and many who had it have never paid any thing.   The people generally were well satisfied with its utility; my friends were very zealous in introducing it among the people; but my opponents were not slack in doing every thing in their power to prejudice the public against me and the medicine.   The doctors seemed much troubled at the success of the practice, many having been cured who were given over by them.   One woman, who had been unable to walk for about nine months, after having been confined, and the doctors could not help her, was attended by Mr. Sewell, and in a short time restored to a comfortable state of health, which gave them great offence; and some of them published in the newspapers,

part of my trial for murder, in order to prejudice the
public against me. I prepared an answer, but they had
so much influence with the printers, that I was unable
to get it inserted ; they had the meanness to circulate the
report that I acknowledged the fact, because I did not
answer their statement. Thus have the faculty, by such
unprincipled conduct, managed to keep the people blind
to the benefit they might receive from the use of the
medicine, for the purpose of keeping up their own credit
and making them tributary to themselves, without regard to the public good.

This season I went to Eastport and collected some
money to pay my friend Rice ; and thinking to make
some profit, laid it out in fish, and sent it to Portland,
consigned to my friend Fickett. When I went there
myself, sold the fish to him. I afterwards made a settlement with him, and took his note for one hundred and
sixty-three dollars, which he agreed to pay Judge Rice ;
as he was going to Boston in a short time, and he would
call on him at Portsmouth for that purpose. I then went
home to see my family, and in about six months after,
returned to Portsmouth, and on calling on Judge Rice,
found to my surprise that Mr. Fickett had not paid the
money, that he had failed, and there was no chance for
me to get any thing of him. So I was again disappointed in my expectations of paying this demand, and it appeared to me that all my hard earnings would be sacrificed to pay the expense of persecutions ; but my friend
Rice was very indulgent; and instead of complaining,
did all he could to encourage me and keep up my spirits.

In the fall of the year 1813, I started from Portland
to go to Eastport ; and took Mr. Sewell with me, in order
to try to get a settlement with Mr. Carpenter ; as he
knew all the particulars of the agreement between us.
After suffering many hardships, and being at great expense, in consequence of having to go part of the way
by water, and part by land, owing to the war that then
existed, we arrived there on the 12th day of November.
On my arrival I made inquiry concerning my affair with
Carpenter, and ascertained what proof I could obtain to
support an action against him for the property he had
wronged me out of; and after making an unsuccessful

attempt to get my account books out of his hands, brought an action against him for the property left in his possession; this being the only way in which I could bring him to an account. After much time and expense, I at last obtained a judgment against him, got out an execution, which was levied on the land he had unjustly got a deed of, and it was finally appraised to me; and after having to get a writ of ejectment to get Mr. Tuttle out of possession of it, who claimed it under a pretended deed from Carpenter, to prevent it from being attached, I at last got the farm which had cost in getting it more than it was worth; so I had to put up with the loss of all my earnings at Eastport for two years, with the loss of medicine sold by Carpenter, all of which amounted to not less than fifteen hundred dollars.

I returned to Portland, where I remained to attend to my practice and the society that had been formed there, for considerable time; and after settling and arranging my business as well as I could, left Mr. Sewell in charge of all my affairs there, and in January, 1814, returned to Portsmouth, which place I made the principal depot of my medicines; having previous to my returning from the Eastward, made arrangements with my agents to supply them, and all others who had purchased the rights, with such medicine as they might want, by their applying to me for them. I had laid in a large stock, the value of which I estimated to be about one thousand dollars. I went to Boston and Salem to procure some articles that could not be obtained elsewhere, in order to complete my stock; when absent the great fire took place at Portsmouth, and all my stock of medicine was consumed. This was a very serious loss to me, not only in a pecuniary point of view, but it disarranged all my plans, and put it out of my power to supply those who I knew depended upon me for all such articles as were most important in the practice. The season was so far advanced that it was impossible to obtain a new recruit of most of the articles; and I was obliged to collect a part of what had been sent to different places, in order to be able to supply in the best manner I could, such demands for medicine, as I should be called on for. In doing this I was put to great trouble and expense, and in order to make myself whole, was under the necessity of raising the price of the medicine fifty per cent; this caused much grumbling and complaint from the members of the societies in different places, and was taken advantage of by my enemies to injure me all they could.

I sent in the estimate of my loss, by the committee, who had the charge of the money contributed to the people in different parts, for the relief of the sufferers by the fire, and afterwards called on them, with an expectation of receiving my share; but they said my loss was of such a nature that they could not give me any thing, as I should be able to collect another supply the next season, and I never received a cent from them. In addition to my loss by the fire, and other difficulties I had to encounter, and while I was at Portsmouth using all my exertions to replenish my stock of medicine, and assist those who were suffering from disease and needed the benefit of my practice, I received information from Portland, that the doctors had obtained one of my books of direction, which was published expressly for the information of those who purchased the right of using my system of practice, and had some knowledge of it by verbal and other instruction, had printed an edition of it, and advertised them for sale at $37\frac{1}{2}$ cents a copy. They stated in their advertisements, that "this invaluable work which had heretofore been selling for twenty dollars, may now be had for thirty-seven and a half cents;" and sent them to all places where my societies had been formed, and my practice had been introduced, for the purpose of putting me down and preventing the use of my medicine; but after all this pitiful attempt to do me the great injury which they so fondly anticipated, they gained nothing by it, except it was the contempt of all the honest part of society, who were knowing to the circumstances. To put a stop to these practices, and prevent the public from being imposed upon, I caused a notice to be published in the Portsmouth and Portland papers, cautioning the people against buying these books, or making use of the medicine, and trespassing on my patent, under the penalty of the law in such cases provided; and also offered a reward of fifty dollars to any one who would give information of any doctor, who

12

should trespass on my patent, and ten dollars for any one who should be found guilty of selling the books. This put a stop to the sale of the books, and prevented them from doing me any injury by this trick; for those concerned in this disgraceful manœuvre, were compelled to acknowledge that my agents could sell more books at twenty dollars, than they could at thirty-seven and a half cents.

I continued in Portsmouth, after the loss I met with from the fire, informing the people in that place and vicinity, until I collected another assortment of medicine, during which time fifty members were added to the society there. I appointed Mr. John Locke as my agent in Portsmouth, and the society accepted of him as such, to take the management of the practice and supply them with medicine; I agreed to allow him twenty-five per cent on the sale of rights, and in eighteen months he added about forty members to the society. He conducted himself with the greatest propriety in performance of all the duties assigned him, and in this, as well as in all other concerns, which I had with him, has given me the highest satisfaction. I mention this tribute of praise to his fidelity, the more readily, as he is one of the very few whom I have put confidence in, that I have found honest enough to do justice to me and the people. It has generally been the case, with those I have appointed as agents, that as soon as they have been sufficiently instructed to attend to the practice with success, and give satisfaction to the people, that they have made it a matter of speculation; and have, by all the means that they could devise, attempted to get the lead of the practice into their own hands, and deprive me of the credit and profits of my own discovery; and when I have found out their designs, and put a stop to their career, by depriving them of their agency, they have uniformly turned against me and done every thing in their power to injure me and destroy the credit of the medicine.* This kind of conduct has been a very serious evil, and has caused me much trouble and expense, besides destroying the confidence of the people in the

* A further notice will be taken of this agent in another place.

beneficial effects of the medicine and practice, and keeping back the information necessary for its being properly understood by them. This, however, has not been the case with all that I have entrusted with the care of my business as agents, for some of them have been uniformly honest and faithful, both to me and to those to whom they have given the information.

While Mr. Locke, was acting as my agent at Portsmouth, he gave offence, by his faithful and upright conduct, to some members of the society, who wanted to reap all the advantages and profits without any labour or expense. They made complaint to me of his conduct, and wished him turned out; but on asking them for their charges against him, they said he speculated on the medicine, and sold it one third higher than I did. I told them that I had been obliged to raise the price in consequence of my loss by the fire, and that he was not to blame for it. They, however, persisted in their complaints, and after finding that they could not make me turn against him, they turned against me. After making further inquiries into the subject, I satisfied myself of their reasons for wishing Mr. Locke turned out of the agency. A man by the name of Holman, whom I had four years previous cured of a consumption, as has been before related, and to whom I had given the information, and authorized to form a society at Hopkinton, where he had practised three years without making me any returns, had returned to Portsmouth, and practised with Mr. Locke, as an assistant. This man formed a plan to have Mr. Locke turned out, in order to get his place himself, and had managed so as to gain over to his side a number of the society, who joined with him in effecting this object. They made use of all kinds of intrigue to get the control of the practice out of my hands, by offering to buy the right for the county, and many other ways; but I understood their designs, and refused all their offers.

At the next annual meeting of the society, Holman was chosen their agent without my consent, and I refused to authorize him to give information; for he had deceived me before, by saying on his return to Portsmouth, that he could not form a society at Hopkinton,

which I had found out to be false; and many other
things in his conduct had caused me to be much dissatisfied with all he did, that I declined having any thing
further to do with him. ' He persisted in practising, and
in eighteen months, by his treacherous conduct, run
down the credit of the medicine and practice, and broke
up the society, after it had, the eighteen months previous, got under good way by Mr. Locke's agency, and
was in a very prosperous condition.   I had good reason
to believe that Holman was employed by my enemies to
break me up in this place, and destroy the credit of the
medicine ; for when I was absent, I ascertained that he
gave salt-petre and other poisons, under the pretence
that by giving it the night before it would prepare the
stomach for my medicine to be taken in the morning.
This was like preparing over night to build a fire in
the morning, by filling the fire-place with snow and
ice.   After preparing the stomach in this way, the medicine would have no beneficial effects ; and he would
then place the patient over a steam, which caused them
to faint.   In this way he proved to the members of the
society that my mode of practice was bad, and thus used
his influence to destroy the credit of my medicine in
their minds, and make them believe that I had deceived
them.   His practice turned out very unsuccessful, and
he lost many of his patients.   He had lost more in six
months, than I had lost in six years, which I imputed
entirely to his bad conduct.

After my return, finding how things were situated in
regard to the practice, that all the credit I had gained
by seven years labour, had been destroyed in eighteen
months, led me to make a particular inquiry into the
cause.   On visiting his patients I found some of the pills
made of salt-petre, and also some opium pills, which he
had been in the habit of administering secretly to his
patients under the name of my medicine ; and after collecting an assortment of his poison, I called a meeting
of the society, and proved to them that he had made
use of these poisons under the pretence of giving my
medicine ; and also that he had confessed to have given
tobacco when called on to administer my medicine ; all
of which satisfied the society so well of the baseness of

the conduct of their agent, that they immediately passed a vote dismissing him from his agency. A committee was appointed to investigate the whole of his conduct, and publish a statement of the same, in order to do away the false impression that had been made on the public mind, and convince them that the bad success of this man's practice, had been owing to his own wicked conduct, and not to any fault in the medicine. I was never able, however, to get this committee to meet and attend to the duty assigned them by the society, although they confessed themselves satisfied of the truth of my charges against Holman, and of the injury I had sustained by his conduct; and after waiting six months, and finding that they were more willing that I should suffer, than that the blame should fall where it justly belonged, I left them to their more fashionable practice, and withdrew all my medicine from the place.

In the spring of the year of 1814, I wrote to Mr. Mowe, my agent at Eastport, to leave that place, in consequence of the war becoming troublesome, and come to Portsmouth. He came up in May. I took him with me and went to Surry, where we continued through the summer, and he assisted me in carrying on my farm and collecting an assortment of medicine. In August we went to Onion River, where my father resided, to make a visit, and collect some articles of medicine, that could not be obtained in Surry. After my return, Mr. Mowe went to Portsmouth, and I remained at home till after the harvesting was over, then went to Portsmouth, to collect medicine and attended to some practice. Some time in December, I returned home and found an express had been there for me to go to Guildford, sent by Mr. Davis, whom I had attended the year before at Portsmouth. I went with all speed and found his wife sick with a consumption. I attended her a few days to give them information, and sold him the right of using the medicine; and also sold some rights to others; I then returned to Portsmouth, and sent Mr. Mowe to Guildford to practise and give information to those who had purchased the rights, where he remained till spring.

During the time Mr. Mowe was at Guildford, he was very successful in the practice, and made some remark-

12*

able cures.   Great opposition was made to his practice, by the doctors, and all the false representations made about it that they could invent, to prejudice the minds of the people against the medicine and stop its being introduced among them.   After this another plan was got up to injure me ; societies were formed in the manner I had formed mine, and members were admitted for two dollars ; the only information given them was to furnish each member with one of the pamphlets, containing my directions, which had been stolen from a woman and published at Portland, without my knowledge.   In this manner my system of practice, in the hands and under the superintendence of those who were endeavouring to destroy me, became popular in Guildford and the towns adjacent ; and had become so important, that a general invitation was given throughout the neighbouring towns for the people to come and join them in the great improvement of restoring the health of mankind.   Thus did these professional gentlemen tamper with my rights and the credulity of the people, for the pitiful purpose of injuring me, by pretending to sell all my information for two dollars, for which I asked twenty ; and in their hands called it honourable scientific knowledge.   After these trespasses had become open and general, and the people had been invited to join in it, my agent at Guildford, wrote me a letter giving information of the transaction, and I went there to see to it; on my arrival, I conversed with those who had purchased their rights of me or my agent ; they informed me of the facts as above related, and said that they had been solicited to join the society, that had been formed ; and they wished my advice, whether they should attend a general meeting which was to be held in about a fortnight.   I told them that they had better attend ; they then asked me if they should be asked for information, what they should do about giving it ; I told them that I thought people joined societies to get information, and not to give it.   I employed an attorney to proceed against those who trespassed, and have them punished according to law, in such cases provided, and returned to Portsmouth.   And here the matter rested, as I heard of no further trespass in that quarter.

In the month of February, 1815, I had an application
to go to Philadelphia and introduce my societies and system of practice in that city. Thinking it not proper to
go alone, I made an agreement with Mr. John Locke, to
go with me; and after we got every thing prepared, he
started on the seventh in the morning to go in the stage,
and I chose to go by water, and sailed the same day in
a vessel for New York. We had a long and tedious
passage, suffering very much from the cold. We had a
gale of wind which blew us off into the Gulf Stream,
and we were two hundred miles south of our port; on
getting into a warmer latitude the weather became
warmer, when we were enabled to get clear of the ice,
with which the vessel was much burdened, and could
set some sail; and we arrived at New York after a very
rough passage of seventeen days.

During the passage, one of the crew had frozen his
hands and feet very badly, and when we had got where
the weather became warmer, he was in the most extreme
pain. He said that it seemed as though the bones of
his hands and feet were coming in pieces; his suffering
was so great that the tears would run from his eyes, and
the sweat down his cheeks with the pain. I was requested by the captain and crew to do something to relieve him. I agreed to do the best I could for him, in
the cold and comfortless situation we were in. There
was no place to keep a fire under decks, and the weather
was so rough that we could seldom keep any in the
caboose on deck. I was obliged to administer the medicine according to my judgment in the best manner I
could. In the first place I procured handkerchiefs and
cloths enough to wrap his hands and feet up in several
thicknesses, then wet them well with cold water, and
wrapped his hands and feet as well as I could, wetting
them with cold water, and put him in his birth, covered
well with blankets, and gave him the warmest medicine
to take I had with me, and repeated it to keep the inward heat sufficient to cause a free circulation in the
limbs; and if his hands and feet grew painful, poured
cold water on the cloths; and continued this course of
treatment, of keeping the inward heat above the outward, by raising the one and letting down the other, till

I got the fountain above the stream; and in about two hours, freed him from all pain, to the surprise and astonishment of all the hands on board.   When I come to take off the cloths, the blood had settled under the nails and under the skin, which came off without any blister being raised, and before we arrived at New York, he was able to attend his watch.

It was said by the captain and crew that this was the most remarkable cure they had ever known; and that if he had been attended in the common form, he would have lost his toes if not his feet, besides suffering much pain and a long confinement.   It will be necessary to remark, that the greatness of this cure consisted in its simplicity; any person could have performed the same, who had come to years of discretion, by adopting the same plan, and many times be the means of saving the amputation of limbs.   There is no mystery in it, the whole plan consists in keeping the determining power to the surface, from the fountain of the body, which is the stomach; from which all the limbs receive their support and warmth, and when you cannot raise the fountain sufficient to give nature its proper course, you must lower the stream, or outward heat, by keeping the heat down on the limbs, and raising the inward heat, when there can no mortification ever return from the limbs to the body, any more than a log can float against a stream.

In the case above stated, before I began to do any thing for the man, I duly considered his situation; he had been almost chilled to death by the extreme cold weather, so that his limbs had very little warmth from the body, not enough to bring them to their feeling; until the warm weather raised a fever on the limbs faster than in the body, and in proportion as the heat in the extremities is raised above that in the body, by applying hot poultices or other similar applications, so much will the whole system be disordered, and the parts that have been injured will be extremely painful, and by a continued application of such means, the fever or outward heat will increase by the current being turned inward, till mortification takes place, when the limbs have to be taken off to save life; and in most cases the body has become so much disordered, that they die after all.   This may, I am confident, be avoided by understanding my plan of treatment and pursuing it with zeal, particularly in all cases of burns or freezing.

On my arrival at New York, I found Mr. Locke, who had come in the stage, and had been waiting for me ten days. The next morning we started in the stage for Philadelphia, where we arrived that evening, and went to a boarding house and put up for the night. In the morning we went in search of Elder Plummer, with whom I had engaged the fall before, to go to Philadelphia; we found him in the course of the forenoon, and he expressed much joy at our arrival. He preached a lecture that evening, and appointed a meeting at the same place the next evening for me; at which I attended and gave a lecture; there was a large collection of people attended this meeting, and I gave a full and explicit explanation of the principles upon which my system is founded. There were two medical students present, and while I was endeavouring to give a view of the formation of the animal creation out of the four elements; that heat was life, and cold death; and that the blood was necessary to life, as being the nourishment of the flesh, and inasmuch as it was taken away, so much was life and health diminished, one of them interrupted me and said, that cold was a promotion of life, and that bleeding was beneficial to preserve life also. I answered him by stating, that admitting his doctrine to be true, an animal that had the blood taken from it and was frozen, would be the liveliest creature in the world. This unexpected retort caused a laugh, and the two medical gentlemen left the room. I then went on and concluded the explanations I wished to make, which gave general satisfaction to the people present; and sixteen signed the articles of agreement that night, to obtain the knowledge of the medicine and practice, to whom I engaged to give information by lectures. We remained there about a week, in which time about twenty bought the right.

When we had completed our business at Philadelphia, we went on to Washington, where we remained several days, and had a view of the ruins of the public buildings, which had been destroyed by the British, when they took possession of that city, about six months previous to our being there.   While at the capitol, I had an interview with General Varnum, and some conversation passed between us concerning the pipsisway, which had been found useful in a case of cancer for which I attended his wife when practising at Pelham, in the year 1807.   He said that it having been found so useful in all cancerous cases, he thought it ought to be published in the newspapers or almanac, for the benefit of those who were afflicted with this dangerous disease, and expressed a wish that I would do it.   I told him that I thought it would be better for him to publish it than for me, and he consented ; and the next year he published it in the almanac, which was the cause of much speculation in this article, and of which I shall give some account in another part of this work.

After staying in Washington a few days, we went to Alexandria, where we remained about a week, in which time I collected some cyprus bark, which is known there by the name of poplar, and what we call poplar, is by them called quaking-asp, on account of the constant shaking of its leaves.   While at this place I fell in company with Capt. Davis, of Portsmouth, and agreed to take passage with him and return to that place.   Arrangements were made for Mr. Locke to return by land ; and I directed him to stop at Washington and get a copy of my patent, then to go on to Philadelphia and remain there as long as it should be necessary to give information to those who purchased the rights, or any that should wish to purchase them in that city, and after paying proper attention to them, to return to Portsmouth.   I then went on board the vessel and we set sail ; and, after a long passage, arrived safe at Portsmouth about the same time that Mr. Locke got there.

During this summer, I visited Eastport, Portland, Charlestown, South Reading and other places where societies had been formed, or rights sold to individuals, to give information to the people ; and in all places where I went, found the book of directions, which had been clandestinely obtained and published by the doctors and others, to injure me by stopping the sale of rights, selling at 37½ cents.   I was under the necessity of putting an advertisement in the papers, cautioning the people against this imposition, which put a stop to their sale; but great pains were taken by my enemies to circulate them among the people; and this is the way that some of my articles of medicine came to be made use of through the country in colds, such as cayenne, ginger, &c. In 1815 I published another edition of my book of directions, and secured the copy right; but this was reprinted at Taunton, and I advertised it as before, and stopped its progress.

In the fall of the year 1815, I went to Cape Cod to procure some marshrosemary, and collected a quantity, carried it to Portsmouth and prepared it for use. This is the last time I have collected any of this article, and as it becomes scarce, think I shall make no more use of it. It is too cold and binding, without using a large share of bayberry bark and cayenne with it, to keep the saliva free. I have found other articles as substitutes, which answer a better purpose, such as hemlock bark, which I have of late made use of and found very good, white lily roots, witch-hazle and raspberry leaves; and sumach berries; the last article is very good alone, steeped and sweetened, and is as pleasant as wine; it is good for children in cases of canker, especially in long cases of sickness when other articles become disagreeable to them.

In the spring of the year 1816, I went again to Cape Cod for medicine, and found that the spotted fever, or what was called the cold plague, prevailed there, and the people were much alarmed, as they could get no help from the doctors. I told them I had come after medicine where they were dying for want of the knowledge how to use it. They were desirous for me to try my practice and satisfy them of its utility. A young man in the next house to where I was, being attacked with the fever the day before, I went to see him, and the family expressed a wish to have me try my medicine. I put a blanket round him and put him by the fire; took a tea spoonful of composition, and added more No. 2 and as much sugar, put it in a tea cup, and poured to it a wine glass of hot water, when cool enough to take, added a tea spoonful of the rheumatic drops; he took it and in fifteen minutes was in a free perspiration; he was then put in bed and a hot stone wrapped in wet cloths put to his feet to raise a steam. I then left him in the care of his friends, with some medicine to be given during the night; they kept the perspiration free all night, and in the morning heat had gained the victory, the canker was destroyed, and he was comfortable and soon got well.

I attended three other persons in one house, who had been sick a longer time, and had taken other medicine, so that it was more difficult to cure them. I steeped No. 3, and poured off half a-tea cupful and sweetened it, and added half a tea spoonful of No. 2, when cool enough to take, put in one tea spoonful of No. 1, and gave it to each of the patients, repeating it once in fifteen minutes, till they had taken it three times, whether they puked or not in that time, kept a hot stone wrapped in wet cloths at their feet to keep up a steam; while they were under the operation of the puking and sweating, gave them as much cider or water to drink as they required; when they had done vomiting, gave milk porridge freely. As soon as they had done sweating, and their strength had returned, got them up and steamed them as long as they could bear it; then rubbed them over with spirits, water or vinegar, changed their clothes, and they went to bed, or sat up as their strength would permit. I will here remark for the information of the reader, that when the patient is so bad as not to be able to get up, they must be steamed in bed as hot as they can bear it, then set them up on end, rub them as before mentioned, and change their clothes and bed clothes. This last direction is important to be attended to, for if their own clothes are changed without changing the bed clothes, they will absorb a part of the filth that has been discharged through the pores, and add to what remains of the disorder. This precaution is all important in every case of disease, and should be paid particular attention to, in order to guard against taking back any part of what has been thrown off by the operation of the medicine. The nurse or those who attend upon the sick, are also in danger from the same cause, and should be particularly careful to guard against taking the disorder by breathing in the foul vapour from

the bed clothes, and standing over the patient when under the operation of the medicine, the principal effect of
which is to throw off by perspiration and other evacuations, the putrefaction that disease has engendered in
the body. To guard against this, take some hot bitters,
and keep a piece of ginger root in the mouth, occasionally swallowing some of it, when most exposed ; also
take a tea spoonful of Nos. 2 and 3, steeped in hot
water, when going to bed ; one ounce of prevention, in
this way is worth a pound of cure when sick.

After relieving these four cases, I was sent for to attend a woman, who had been sick for a long time ; I
declined attending any more unless they would buy tha
right.   This displeased her so much, because I was not
willing to practise and cure all of them for nothing, that
she abused me for my declining to attend her.   Two
men bought the rights, and they asked me how much I
would take for the right of the whole town.   I offered
it to them for the price of twenty rights , but they said
that the sickness had so much abated that the alarm was
nearly over, and declined my offer.   This disease first
appeared in Eastham the fore part of February, in which
month twenty-seven died, in March, fourteen, and five
in April, making in the whole, forty-six in three months
in this small place.   I left some medicine with those who
had purchased the rights, and returned to Boston.

Within a week after my return from Cape Cod, I received a letter from Eastham, to come there as soon as
possible ; I took a stock of medicine and went on there
as quick as I could ; and on my arrival found that the
fever had again made its appearance among the people,
with double fatality.   I soon found enough ready to
purchase the twenty rights, for which I had offered to sell
the right of the whole town.   I attended on many of
those who had the disease, in company with the two men
who had purchased the right of me when here before,
and instructed them how to carry the patients through a
course of the medicine ; and they attended and gave information to others ; when they could meet together, I
gave information by lectures ; those who got the information attended wherever they were wanted.   I pursued
my usual mode of treatment, by administering the medi-

13

cine to promote a free perspiration, and when necessary,
steamed and gave injections, cleansed the stomach, and
cleared off the canker; the success in curing this alarming disease was very great.   I staid about two weeks,
during which time there were attended with my medicine, thirty-four cases, of whom only one died, the rest
got well.   At the same time, of those who were attended by the regular doctors, eleven out of twelve died, making in the whole upwards of fifty deaths in a short time in
this place, which was about one twelfth part of the inhabitants that were at home.   The truth of the above
statements is authenticated by the certificates of the
Selectmen of the town, and other respectable inhabitants,
which will be inserted in another part of the work.

During my stay this time, I attended the husband of
the woman who had abused me when here before, at the
house of his sister; she came there while I was attending upon her husband, and treated me and him in a
most abusive manner, saying that she would die sooner
than take any of my medicine, or have any thing to do
with me.   After she had vented her spite to her own
satisfaction, she went home, was taken sick on the way,
and was one of the last who died with the fever at
this time.   The people generally, treated me with kindness and respect, and took great interest in my cause;
and the success of my system of practice, in relieving them from this alarming disease, gave universal
satisfaction.

I formed those who purchased the rights, into a society; and they chose a committee, whom I authorized as
agents to sell rights and medicine; but this caused a
jealousy among the rest of the members, who said I gave
privileges to some more than to others.

I have formed four societies, and given them certain
privileges, by allowing them part of the profits on the
sale of rights and medicine; but as soon as there was
any funds, it has always created uneasiness among the
members.   Some of the ignorant and selfish, would call
for their dividends, as though it was bank stock, instead
of feeling grateful for the advantages they enjoy by having their diseases cured, and their minds relieved from
the alarming consequences of a disease, with a trifling

expense. I have since altered my plan, and now have
but one society. Every one who purchases a right for
himself and family, becomes a member of the Friendly
Botanic Society, and is entitled to all the privileges of a
free intercourse with each other, and to converse with
any one who has bought a right, for instruction and assistance in sickness, as each one is bound to give his
assistance, by advice or otherwise, when called on by a
member. In this way much more good can be done,
and there will be much more good-will towards each
other, than where there is any money depending.

I had now been in practice, constantly attending upon
those labouring under disease, whenever called on, for
about thirty years; had suffered much both in body and
mind, from the persecutions I had met with, and my un-
wearied exertions to relieve the sick; and to establish
my system of practice upon a permanent basis, that the
people might become satisfied of its superiority over that
which is practised by those styled regular physicians;
putting it in their power to become their own physicians,
by enabling every one to relieve themselves and friends,
from all disease incident to our country, by making use
of those vegetable medicines, the produce of our own
country, which are perfectly safe and easily obtained;
and which, if properly understood, are fully sufficient in
all cases of disease, where there can be any chance of
cure, without any danger of the pernicious, and often
fatal consequences attending the administering those
poisons that the fashionable doctors are in the habit of
giving to their patients.

After having discovered a system, and by much labour
and constant perseverance reduced it to practice, in a
manner that had given general satisfaction to all who
had become acquainted with it, and having secured the
same by patent, in order that I might reap some benefit
from my discovery, to support me in my old age, having
by a long series of attendance on the sick, both as physician and nurse, become almost worn out, I came to the
determination to appoint some suitable person, who would
do justice to me and the cause, as a general agent, to
take the lead in practice, and give the necessary information to those who should purchase the rights, which

would enable me to retire from practice and receive a
share of the profits as a reward for my long sufferings.
After considerable inquiry, I became acquainted with
Elias Smith, who was recommended as a man in whom
I could confide, and who was every way qualified as
a suitable person to engage in the undertaking.   I
found him in Boston, and in very poor circumstances;
having been for many years a public preacher, but in
consequence of his often changing his religious principles and engaging in different projects in which he had
been unsuccessful, he was now without a society or any
visible means of supporting himself and family.   He
readily engaged with me, and promised to do every thing
in his power, to promote my interest and extend the usefulness of my system of practice.

I sold him a family right in December, 1816, and was
in his family during the winter, for the purpose of instructing him in the practice, to qualify him to attend
upon the sick, and give information to others.   I put the
utmost confidence in his honour, and spared no pains in
communicating to him, without any reserve whatever, all
the knowledge I had gained by my experience, both by
practice and verbal instruction; under the expectation,
that when he became sufficiently acquainted with the
system and practice, I should be rewarded for my trouble, by his faithfully performing his duty towards me,
according to his promise.   I shall make no remark upon
my being disappointed in all my expectations in regard
to Mr. Smith's conduct, and the treatment I received
from him after he had gained a knowledge of the practice from me, to enable him to set up for himself; but
shall proceed to give a short account of what took place
during my connexion with him.

The first case I attended with him was in his own
family.   His son had the itch very badly, so that he was
nearly one half of him one raw sore.   They had tried
the usual remedies without any benefit.   I showed him
the use of No. 3, to wash with, to stop the smart of the
sores; then took some rheumatic drops and added about
one fourth part of spirits of turpentine and washed him
with it; this is very painful when applied where the skin
is off; to prevent which mix with it some of the wash

made of No. 3; at the same time of applying the above, give some of the composition, especially when going to bed; and occasionally give about fifteen of the drops, shaken together, on loaf sugar. By pursuing this treatment one week this boy was entirely cured.

The next case, which was the first we attended together out of his house, was a young woman, who had the ague in her face. I showed him the whole process of curing this complaint; which was done by putting a small quantity of No. 2 in a cloth, and placing it between her cheek and teeth; at the same time giving her some of Nos. 2 and 3 to take, and in two hours she was cured.

I was constantly with him in practice from February till June; during which time we attended many bad cases with great success. A Mrs. Grover came to his house to be attended, who had the dropsy. She had been given over by her doctor as incurable, and was so much swelled as to be blind, and her body and limbs in proportion. Mr. Smith undertook her case under my direction, and carried her through a course of the medicine every day for nine days, and then occasionally once or twice a week till she was cured. She was thus attended under my inspection for three weeks, and in four was entirely cured; for which she gave Mr. Smith about forty dollars. In this case I did a great part of the labour and he got the pay. About the third time of carrying her through a course of the medicine, I was absent; her symptoms appeared unfavourable, and he got frightened; a nurse woman, to whom I had given information, and who had more experience than he had, came to his assistance, and by using injections relieved her, and prevented mortification. The circumstance of this woman proving that she was forward of him in information, seemed to fix in Mr. Smith's mind a dislike to her ever after, as his subsequent treatment of her will show, the particulars of which will be hereafter related.

Another case was of a man that came to his house, who was in a declining way, and had taken a great quantity of physic before he came, which would not operate. On taking my medicine, as soon as he began to be warm,

13*

so as to cause motion in his bowels, the physic he had
before taken operated and run him down with a relax;
then the dysentery set in, and he suffered much with
pain, and had discharges of blood.   I gave Mr. Smith
directions to use injections, to clear his bowels of canker
and prevent mortification; but he neglected it until I
had told him three days in succession.   He then got
alarmed and sent for me; but before I arrived he had
given an injection, which had relieved the patient.   He
remained and was attended about three weeks, and went
home in a comfortable state of health.   This man paid
Mr. Smith about thirty dollars.

About the same time a man by the name of Jennings
applied to Mr. Smith, who had lost the use of one of his
arms by the rheumatism.   He had been attended by the
doctor for nine months, and had been given over by him
as incurable.   His arm was perished, and he was in poor
circumstances, having paid all he had to the doctor; he
wanted relief, but said he could pay nothing for it unless
he was cured, so that he could earn something by his
labour.   Mr. Smith asked me if I was willing to assist to
cure him on these terms, to which I agreed.   We carried him through a course of the medicine and steaming
twice or three times a week for four weeks, when a cure
was effected.   The last time he was carried through
was on election day, and he expressed a wish to go on
the common in the afternoon, to which I gave encouragement.   The medicine was done about ten o'clock;
he was then steamed and washed all over with pepper-
sauce.   He complained bitterly of the heat and threw
himself on the bed; I took a spoonful of good cayenne,
and put in two spoonfuls of pepper-sauce and gave it to
him to take.   This raised the inward heat so much
above the outward, that in two minutes he was quite
comfortable; and in the afternoon he went on the common.   His arm was restored and he was well from that
time; he afterwards, as I have been informed, paid Mr.
Smith forty dollars for the cure.

A Mrs. Burleigh came to his house about this time,
who had the rheumatism very badly, so that her joints
were grown out of place; and I assisted in attending
her.   She had never taken much medicine, which made

it the easier to cure her, as we had nothing to do but
remove the disease, without having to clear the system
of poisonous drugs, as is the case in most of those who
apply for relief in complaints of long standing. She
was carried through the medicine several times and
steamed ; the last time I attended her, and gave the
medicine three times as usual, which raised a lively perspiration and a fresh colour, showing an equal and natural circulation; but did not sicken or cause her to vomit,
as is the case most generally. I mention this to show
that the emetic qualities of the medicine will not oppe-
rate where there is no disease. She was then steamed
and washed, and went out of doors, being entirely cured
of her complaint.

Sometime the last of April or first of May, a woman
that was a relation of the nurse, who assisted Mr. Smith,
and of whom I have before spoken, hired a room of him
and moved into his house, and the nurse lived with her.
She had more experience than he had ; I had put the
utmost confidence in her, and she had in many instances
proved her superiority in a knowledge of the practice
over him. A singular circumstance took place, the particulars of which I shall relate, and leave the reader to
make his own inferences. Sometime in May, while I
boarded with Mr. Smith, I lost my pocketbook, which
contained upwards of thirty dollars in bank bills, and
notes to the amount of about five hundred dollars. I
made strict search for it and advertised it in the papers,
but have never gained any information of it or the contents to this day. It was in my coat pocket, and I could
think of no way in which I had been exposed, or could
lose it, except in his house. I lost it between Friday
night and Monday morning, during which time I attended a woman in his chamber, and several times had my
coat off, which appeared to me to be the only time that
it could be taken or that I could lose it. The only
persons present in the room were Mr. Smith and his
wife, and the nurse ; I had no suspicions of any person
at the time. About ten days after, being alone with Mr.
Smith, he asked me if I ever mistrusted the nurse being
dishonest. I told him no, for if I had I should not have
introduced her as a nurse. He then said that there had

been a number of thefts committed since she had been in
the house, both from him and other people, and named
the articles and circumstances. He further said, that
the girl who lived with him had said that she thought
the nurse was as likely to take my pocketbook as to
take the things she had undoubtedly stolen.   The circumstances which he related and the interest he seemed
to take in my loss, convinced me beyond a doubt that
this woman had taken my property.   During this conversation with him, he said, that if she did not move out
of the house he would.   The consequence was that the
family moved out of his house, and I dismissed the nurse
from having any more to do with my practice.   Since
Mr. Smith has taken to himself the lead in my system
of practice, he has acknowledged that he has become
convinced beyond a doubt, that this woman was not
guilty of taking the things which she had been accused
of; without assigning any reason, as I have been able to
learn, for his having altered his opinion.

During the time the above circumstances happened, his
son Ira came home, after being absent about four years;
but was not treated with that affection a child expects
to receive in a father's house, he was sent off to seek
lodgings where he could.   About twelve o'clock he returned, not being able to obtain lodgings, and called up a
young man who boarded with Mr. Smith, made a bitter
complaint, on account of the treatment he received from
his father, which he attributed to be owing to the influence of his mother-in-law; he took a phial and drank
from it, and soon after fell on the floor.   The young
man being alarmed, awaked his father and informed him
of the circumstance; before he got to his son he was
senseless, and stiff in every joint.   I was in bed in the
house, and Mr. Smith came immediately to me, and requested my assistance, said that he expected Ira had
killed himself. He showed me the phial and asked what
had been in it; I told him it had contained laudanum.
I got up as soon as possible, and on going down, met
Mr. Smith and the young man bringing Ira up stairs.   I
directed them to lay him on the hearth, and took a bottle
from my pocket, which contained a strong preparation
of Nos. 1, 2, and 6; took his head between my knees,

his jaws being set, and put my finger between his cheek
and teeth, and poured in some of the medicine from the
bottle ; as soon as it reached the glands .of his throat,
his jaws became loosened, and he swallowed some of it ;
in five minutes he vomited ; in ten he spoke ; in one
hour he was clear of the effects of the opium, and the
next day was well. After this the affection of the father
seemed in some measure to return ; he clothed him,
took him to Taunton, and introduced him into practice
as an assistant. He did very well till his mother-in-law
arrived there, when a difficulty took place between them,
and he went off. His father advertised him, forbidding
all persons from trusting him on his account. He was
absent four years, when he returned again to his father's
house, and was received in the same cold and unfeeling
manner as before, was not allowed to stay in the house,
but was obliged to seek an asylum among strangers. He
staid in town several days, became dejected, in consequence, as he said, of the treatment he had met with at
his father's house, went over to Charlestown, took a
quantity of laudanum, and was found near the monu-
ment senseless ; was carried to the alms-house, where
he died.

The morning after he died, his father came to see
the corpse, and, as I was informed by a person who
heard it, said that if he had been present one hour before he died he could have saved his life ; for, said he,
" I once administered medicine to him and saved his
life when he had taken a similar dose," and, putting his
hand on his pocket, said, " I always carry medicine in
my pocket for that purpose." He neither took him
home, nor put in the paper the cause of his death. The
notice in the paper was, " Died suddenly, in Charlestown, Ira Smith, son of Elias Smith, Boston."

After Ira went away the last time, I frequently heard
Mrs. Smith say that if she could only hear that Ira was
dead, she should be satisfied. The season before he returned, an account of his death appeared in the Palla-
dium of Boston, stating that Ira Smith died in Upper
Canada. How this account originated is yet unknown,
as Ira said he had never been there. However, his
father seemed to make great lamentation at this unfor-

tunate news, and mentioned it in one of his sermons in
Clark Street.   In the spring following I saw Ira in New
York, and informed Mr. Smith's family that I had seen
him ; but he did not proclaim it in the meeting as he did
the news of his death.   Neither did he exclaim, in the
words of an ancient father of a prodigal, " My son who
was dead, is alive, and who was lost, is found."
   In June following Ira came to me, instead of going to
his father's house.   I found him lodging two nights,
and then got him into business in Col. House's printing
office, where he worked some days before he went to his
father's house.   When calling there to see his brothers
and sisters, he said something took place between him
and his step-mother, which so disgusted him that he
threatened before the workmen in the office to destroy
his own life.   They laughed at his pretensions, but he
insisted on doing the deed, which he did in a few days
after, and thus ended this disgraceful tragedy.
   I continued with Mr. Smith, as has been before mentioned, giving him instruction, till the first of June, when
I appointed him agent, with authority to sell family
rights and medicine.   An agreement was drawn up and
signed by both parties, in which it was stipulated, that
I was to furnish him with medicine, and allow him twenty-five per cent. for selling ; and he was to have fifty per
cent. for all the rights he sold ; which was ten dollars for
each right, for giving the necessary information to those
who purchased, and collecting the pay.   His principal
dependance at this time was upon me and the practice,
for his support.   He paid me one half of what he received for family rights as he sold them.   The first of
July, I contemplated going home to get my hay ; but
Mrs. Smith expecting to be confined soon, was very
urgent that I should stay till after she was sick, which
detained me three weeks.   I staid accordingly, and attended her through her sickness, for which they gave
me great credit and praise at the time.   I then went
home to attend to my farm and get my hay ; after which
I returned to Boston, and in the fall went to Cape Cod,
to attend to some business there, and on my return to
Boston, I found Mr. Smith's youngest child sick with
the quinsy, or rattles ; he had done all he could, and

given it over to die. The women had taken charge of the child, after he had given it up, and had given it some physic. When I saw the child I gave some encouragement of a cure, and they were very desirous for me to do something for it. I told them they had done very wrong in giving physic, for it was strictly - against my orders to ever give any physic, in cases where there was canker. They observed that there was no appearance of canker. I told them it would never appear when they gave physic, for it would remain inside, till mortification decided the contest.

I began with the child by giving No. 2, which caused violent struggles and aroused it from the stupid state in which it had laid, until the moisture appeared in the mouth; then gave some No. 3, steeped, and Nos. 1 and 2, to start the canker, and cause it to vomit. This soon gave relief. The women who were present, accused me of the greatest cruelty, because 1 brought the child out of its stupid state, and restored its sense of feeling, by which means the life of the child was saved. The next morning its mouth was as white as paper with canker; they were then all satisfied that I knew the child's situation best, and that I had saved its life. I considered the child so much relieved, that the father and mother would be able to restore it to perfect health, left it in their care and went out of town. I returned the next day about noon, and found that they had again given it up to die; its throat was so filled with canker that it had not swallowed any thing for four hours. I was in suspense whether to do any thing for the child or not; but told the father and mother I thought if it was mine, I would not give it up yet; they wished me to try. I took some small quills from a wing, and stripped them, except about three quarters of an inch at the point, tied several of them together, which made a swab, dipped it in canker tea, and began by washing the mouth; then rinsing it with cold water; then washed with the tea again, putting the swab down lower in the throat which caused it to gag, and while the throat was open, put it down below the swallow, and took off scales of canker, then rinsed again with cold water. Soon as it could swallow, gave some tea of No. 2, a tea spoonful at a time, and it soon began to struggle for breath, and appeared to be in great distress, similar to a drowned person coming to life. In its struggling for breath discharged considerable phlegm from its nose and mouth; I then gave some more of the emetic with canker tea, which operated favourably; in two hours it was able to nurse, and it soon got well, to the great joy of the father and mother, who said that the life of the child was saved by my perseverance.

Soon after this child got well, which was in the fall of the year 1817, Mr. Smith moved to Taunton. Previous to his removal, a man from that place by the name of Eddy, applied to him to be cured of a bad humour, caused by taking mercury. I assisted in attending upon him part of the time. Mr. Smith began with him, and on the turn of the disorder, the man and he got frightened and sent for me. He had been kept as hot as he could bear, with the medicine, for six hours, which increased the heat of the body sufficient to overpower the cold, the heat turned inward and drove the cold on the outside; this produces such a sudden change in the whole system, that a person unacquainted with the practice would suppose they were dying; but there is no danger to be apprehended, if proper measures are taken and persevered in by keeping up the inward heat. In such cases steaming is almost indispensable; for which reason I have been obliged to steam the patient in most cases where the complaint has been of long standing, especially when much mercury has been taken, as nothing will make it active but heat. This man soon got well and returned home.

I furnished Mr. Smith with a stock of medicine, and in the winter paid him a visit, found him in full practice, and Mr. Eddy assisting him. I carried with me a quantity of medicine, renewed his stock, and stored the remainder with him. He had sold several rights, and was very successful in his practice, which caused great alarm among the doctors; they circulated all kinds of false and ridiculous reports about his practice, to break him up; but not succeeding, they raised a mob and twice broke open Mr. Smith's house, in his absence, and frightened his family.

In the spring of this year, Mr. Smith moved to Scituate, to preach there and attend to practice; and the medicine left with him, I consigned to Mr. Eddy, by his recommendation. The amount of the medicine was about one hundred dollars, and I sent him a note for twenty dollars, which he collected, and afterwards went off, and I lost the whole amount. During this season I went to Plymouth to visit some there who had bought family rights, and returned by the way of Scituate, in order to visit Mr. Smith, look over his books, and have some settlement with him. I had let him have medicine as he wanted it, trusting him to give me credit for what he sold or used. I think he had given me credit, so that the balance due me at this time, for what he had, was four hundred dollars. He was unable to pay me any thing, and I returned to Boston.

Mr. Smith afterwards removed his family to Boston, and in the fall of the year 1818, he said that he was not able to pay me any money, but he would let me have such things as he could spare. I was disposed to be as favourable towards him as I could, and took what he chose to offer at his own price. He let me have two old watches at one hundred dollars, and an old mare at eighty, which was for medicine at cash prices. I gave him all the chance of selling rights and medicine, in hopes that he would be able to do better by me. I often had requested him to deliver lectures on my system of practice, as this had been a favourite object with me in appointing him agent; but never could prevail with him to do any thing in that way. Another important arrangement I had made with him was, that he was to assist me in preparing for the press, a work to contain a narrative of my life, and a complete description of my whole system. I had written it in the best manner I could, and depended on him to copy it off and prepare it in a correct manner to be printed; but he put me off from time to time, and was never ready to attend to it. All this time I never had any suspicion of his having a design to wrong me, by usurping the whole lead of the business, and turning every thing to his own advantage.

I continued to keep medicine at his house, which he had free access to, and took it when he pleased, giving

14

me credit for it according to his honesty. There was two or three thousand dollars worth at a time, in the house. He charged me three dollars·per week for board, for all the time I was at his house, after he returned from the country ; and he had given me credit for only eighty dollars for medicine the year past. On a settlemeńt with him at this time, 1819, he owed me about four hundred dollars; I asked him for a due bill for the balance, but he refused to give one ; and said that Mr. Eddy had received two hundred dollars worth of the medicine, for which he had received nothing, and he ought not to pay for it. I agreed to lose one half of it, and allowed one hundred dollars, the same as if I had received cash of him. I took a memorandum from his book of what was due me, which was all I had for security. In the fall of the year 1820, I had another settlement with Mr. Smith, and he owed me about four hundred dollars, having received no money of him the year past. He told me that all the property he had was a horse and chaise, and that if I did not have it, somebody else would. I took the horse and chaise at three hundred dollars, and the hundred dollars I agreed to allow on Mr. Eddy's account, made us, according to his accounts, about square, as to the medicine he had given me credit for. He made out a statement of fifty-seven family rights that he had sold at twenty dollars each, twenty-three of which he had never paid me any thing for ; his plea for not paying me for them was, that he had not received his pay of those who had bought them. His agreement with me was, that he should account to me for ten dollars, for each right sold, and he was to have ten dollars each for collecting the money and giving the necessary information to the purchasers.

In the winter of 1819, I went to Philadelphia, and previous to my going made arrangements with Mr. Smith to publish a new edition of my book of directions; we revised the former edition, and made such additions as we thought would be necessary to give a complete and full description of my system, and the manner of preparing and using the medicine ; and I directed him to secure the copy-right according to law. I left the whole care with him, to arrange the matter, and have it printed. On my return to Boston in March, he had got it done; but in a manner very unsatisfactory to me, for he had left out twelve pages of the most useful part of the remarks and directions, and it was otherwise very incorrectly and badly printed. I asked him the reason of this, and he said a part of the copy had got mislaid, and the printer had not done his work well. I had no idea at the time, that he had any design in having this pamphlet printed in the manner it was; but his subsequent conduct would justify the belief, that he had previous to this, formed a plan to usurp the whole of my system of practice, and turn every thing to his own advantage; for he has since attempted to satisfy the public, that my system was no system; and has brought forward this very book, which was printed under his own inspection, and arranged by him, as a part of his proof, that I was incapable of managing my own discoveries, and of communicating the necessary information in an intelligible manner to make my system of practice useful to those who purchase the rights. It is a well known fact, that some of the most essential parts of the directions was to be verbal; and I had allowed him ten dollars each, to give the proper instructions to all those to whom he sold the rights.

Another circumstance that I have recently found out, goes to show a dishonesty in design, to say the least of it. He deposited the title page of the above mentioned pamphlet, and obtained a certificate from the clerk, in the name of Elias Smith, as proprietor, and caused it to be printed in the name of Samuel Thomson, as author and proprietor. What his intentions were in thus publishing a false certificate, I shall not attempt to explain; but leave the reader to judge for himself. If I had been taken away, he possibly might have come forward and claimed under it a right to all my discoveries, and eventually to substitute himself in my place as sole proprietor. From that time he neglected the sale of rights, and turned his attention mostly to practice and preparing his own medicine. During the summer of 1820, he employed Mr. Darling to assist him in practice, and prepare medicine, and while with him he prepared thirty-eight bottles of the rheumatic drops, which by agreement he was to

have of me ; he also directed him to take the materials
from my stock, which was in his house, and prepare
twenty-five pounds of composition, and this was kept a
secret from me.   The reason he gave Mr. Darling for
not having medicine of me according to his agreement,
was, that he owed me so much now that he was afraid
he should never be able to pay me.   I thought his taking the preparing and selling my medicine to himself,
was a very singular way to pay an old debt.

In May 1820, Mr. Smith collected together those in
Boston who had bought rights of me or my agents, and
formed them into a society, under a new name ; he wrote
a constitution, which they signed ; and the members
paid one dollar entrance, and were to pay twelve and a
half cents per month assessment, for which he promised
them important instructions and cheap medicine.   He
was appointed president and treasurer, and after he had
obtained their money, the meetings were discontinued,
and the society was broken up in the course of nine
months.   In this he appears to have taken the lead of
all those who had purchased the right of me, and make
them tributary to himself.

In November I returned from the country and found
that he had advertised, without my knowledge or consent, in the Herald, a periodical work published by him
at that time, " proposals for publishing by subscription,
a book to contain the whole of the system and practice
discovered by Samuel Thomson, and secured to him by
patent.   The price to subscribers to be five dollars.   By
Elias Smith."   This mostly stopped the sale of rights,
for no one would purchase a right of me or my agents at
twenty dollars, when they had the promise of them at
five.   I went to him to know what he meant by his conduct, in issuing these proposals ; he plead innocence,
and said he had no improper design in doing it.

I was now under the necessity of doing something in
order to counteract what had been done by Mr. Smith,
in publishing the above proposals; and came to the determination to issue new proposals for publishing a narrative of my life as far as related to my practice, with a
complete description of my system of practice in curing
disease, and the manner of preparing and using the med-

icine secured to me by patent; the price to subscribers to be ten dollars, including the right to each of using the same for himself and family. Mr. Smith undertook to write the proposals and get them printed; after they were struck off, I found he had said in them, by Samuel Thomson and Elias Smith; all subscribers to be returned to him. I asked him what he meant by putting his name with mine; he said in order to get more subscribers. I said no more about it at that time, and let them be distributed.

When I settled with him the last time, I asked him what he would charge me to prepare my manuscript for the press; he said he thought we were to write it together; I asked him what made him think so; he said because his name was on the proposals with mine; I admitted this; but told him the reasons he had assigned for putting his name to it without my consent or knowledge. He then intimated that he thought he was to be a partner with me; I asked him what I ever had of him to entitle him to an equal right to all my discoveries. To this he made no reply; but said he would write it, and we would agree upon a price afterwards. I told him no; I must know his price first. He said he could not tell within fifty dollars. I then told him we would say no more about it. This conversation, together with his conduct in regard to the proposals, convinced me beyond all doubt, that his design was to destroy me, and take the whole business to himself. I felt unwilling to trust him any longer, and took all my books and manuscripts from his house. His subsequent conduct towards me has fully justified all my suspicions, and left no room for a doubt, that his intentions were to take every advantage of me in his power, and usurp my whole system of practice.

My system of practice and the credit of my medicine, was never in a more prosperous condition, than when I began with Mr. Smith, to instruct him in a knowledge of all my discoveries and experience in curing disease; and appointed him agent. The people wherever it became known, were every day becoming convinced of its utility, and the medicine was in great demand; family rights sold readily, and every thing seemed to promise complete success in diffusing a general knowledge of the practice among all classes of the people ; but under his management, the whole of my plans have been counteracted, and my anticipations in a great measure have been frustrated. By his conduct towards me, in his attempt to take the lead of the practice out of my hands, and destroy my credit with the public, has not only been a serious loss to me in a pecuniary point of view, but the people at large are deprived of the blessings that might be derived by a correct knowledge of my discoveries ; and have it in their power to relieve themselves from sickness and pain with a trifling expense, and generations yet unborn be greatly benefitted thereby.

I tried to get a settlement with Mr. Smith, for the medicine he had prepared and sold, and also for the rights he had not accounted to me for, with the affairs that remained unadjusted between us; but could not get him to do any thing about it ; and finding there was no chance of obtaining an honourable settlement with him, about the first of February, 1821, I took all my medicine from his house and discontinued all connexion or concern with him. I was then, after waiting about four years for him to assist me in writing, which was one of my greatest objects in appointing him agent, obliged to publish a pamphlet, in which I gave some of the principles upon which my system was founded, with explanations and directions for my practice, and also to notify the public that I had appointed other agents, and caution all persons against trespassing on my patent.

He continued to practise and prepare medicine, bidding me defiance. I made several attempts to get an honourable settlement with him, without success. I employed three persons to go to him and offer to settle all our difficulty by leaving it to a reference; but he refused to do any thing ; continued to trespass, and made use of every means to destroy my character by abusive and false reports concerning my conduct, both in regard to my practice and private character. Finding that I could get no redress from him, I put an advertisement in the papers, giving notice that I had deprived him of all authority as my agent ; and cautioning the public against receiving any medicine or information from him

under any authority of mine. He redoubled his diligence in trespassing, and prepared the medicine and advertised it for sale under different names from what I
had called it. I found there was no other way for me to
do, but to appeal to the laws of my country for justice,
and brought an action against him for a trespass on my
patent, to be tried at the Circuit Court, at the October
term, 1821.   The action was continued to May term,
when it was called up and the Judge decided that the
specifications in my patent were improperly made out,
not being sufficiently explicit to found my action upon.
In consequence of which I had to become non-suited,
and stop all further proceedings against him, till I could
make out new specifications and obtain a new patent
from the government.

Mr. Smith has lately published a book in which he
has given my system of practice with directions for preparing and using the vegetable medicine secured to me
by patent, and my plan of treatment in curing disease as
far as he knew it.   In the whole of this work there is
not one principle laid down or one idea suggested, except what is taken from other authors, but what he has
obtained from my written or verbal instructions; and still
he has the effrontery to publish it to the world as his own
discovery, without giving me any credit whatever, except
he has condescended to say that "Samuel Thomson has
made some imperfect discoveries of disease and medicine, but has not reduced any thing to a regular system."   This assertion will appear so perfectly ridiculous
to all those who have any knowledge of my practice,
that I shall forbear making any comment upon it.   It is
true that he has made alterations in the names of some
of the preparations of medicine ; but the articles used
and the manner of using them, are the same as mine.   It
is also a well known fact, that he had no knowledge of
medicine, or of curing disease, until I instructed him ;
and if what he says be true, the effect has been very remarkable, in as much as his magnetical attraction has
drawn all the skill from me to himself, by which he has
taken upon himself the title of Physician, and left me
nothing but the appellation of Mr. Thomson, the imperfect projector.

I have been more particular in describing Mr. Smith's conduct, because it has been an important crisis in the grand plan for which I have spent a great part of my life, and suffered much, to bring about; that of establishing a system of medical practice, whereby the people of this highly favoured country may have a knowledge of the means by which they can at all times relieve themselves from the diseases incident to our country, by a perfectly safe and simple treatment, and thereby relieve themselves from a heavy expense, as well as the often dangerous consequences arising from the employing those who make use of poisonous drugs and other means, by which they cause more disease than they cure; and in which I consider the public as well as myself have a deep interest. I have endeavoured to make a correct and faithful statement of his conduct, and the treatment I have received from him; every particular of which can be substantiated by indisputable testimony if necessary. I now appeal to the public, and more particularly to all who have been benefitted by my discoveries, for their aid and countenance, in supporting my just rights against all encroachments, and securing to me my claims to whatever of merit or distinction I am honourably and justly entitled. While I assure them that I am not to be discouraged or diverted from my grand object by opposition, or the dishonesty of those who deal deceitfully with me; but shall persevere in all honourable and fair measures to accomplish what my life has principally been spent in fulfilling.

ADDITIONS

To the Second Edition....Nov. 1825.

SINCE the first edition of my narrative was published, some circumstances have occured which I think worth relating; and shall, therefore, continue to give the reader an account of all those things relating to my system of practice, and the success it has met with, up to the present time.

After having failed in my attempt to obtain justice, by prosecuting Elias Smith for trespass, as has been before related, I found it necessary to adopt some new plan of procedure in order to meet the universal opposition I have in all cases met with from not only the medical faculty, but from all those who belong to what are called the learned professions. Judge Story decided that the action could not be sustained, because the specifications in my patent were not so explicit as to determine what my claim was. He said it contained a number of recipes, which no doubt were very valuable; but I did not say what part of it I claimed as my own invention. How far this opinion was governed by a preconcerted plan to prevent me from maintaining my claim as the original inventor of a system of practice, and proving its utility in a court of justice, it would not be proper for me to say; but I have an undoubted right to my own opinion on the subject; besides I had it from very high authority at the time, that this was the fact, and that I should always find all my efforts to support my claim, frustrated in the same manner. When I obtained my patent, I had good legal advice in making out the specifications, besides, it was examined and approved by the Attorney General of the United States; and it was said at the time of the trial, by several gentlemen learned in the law, to be good; and that the very nature and meaning of the patent was, that the compounding and using the articles specified in manner therein set forth, was what I claimed as my invention.

There was, however, no other way for me to do, but to obtain another patent ; and immediately after the above decision, I set about getting one that would meet the objections that had been made to the first.   In making new specifications, I had the assistance of several gentlemen of the law, and others, and every precaution was taken to have them according to law ; but whether my second patent will be more successful than the first, time must determine.   It embraces the six numbers, composition or vegetable powders, nerve powder, and the application of steam to raise perspiration; and to put my claim beyond doubt, I added at the end as follows, viz. "The preparing and compounding the foregoing vegetable medicine, in manner as herein described, and the administering them to cure disease, as herein mentioned, together with the use of steam to produce perspiration, I claim as my own invention."   My second patent is dated January 28, 1823.

In obtaining a patent, it was my principal object to get the protection of the government against the machinations of my enemies, more than to take advantage of a monopoly ; for in selling family rights, I convey to the purchaser the information gained by thirty years practice, and for which I am paid a sum of money as an equivalent.   This I should have a right to do, if there were no patent in the case.   Those who purchase the right have all the advantages of my experience, and also the right to the use of the medicine, secured to me by patent, and to the obtaining and preparing it for themselves, without any emolument to me whatever.   And in all the numerous cases where I have sold rights, there have been very few instances where any objections have been made to paying for them, where notes, had been given, and these were by those who had been persuaded by men opposed to me and my practice, and who had interested views in doing me all the injury they could ; but where suits have been commenced to recover on notes given for rights, it has been decided that the demand is good in law, and the plea set up of no value received, is not valid; because the information given, and the advantages received, is a valuable consideration, without any reference to the patent right. In all cases where a person possesses valuable information from his own experience or ingenuity, there can be no reason why he should not have a right to sell it to another as well as any other property, and that all contracts made in such cases should not be binding, provided there is no fraud or deception used.

When a suitable opportunity offers, I shall avail myself of my patent rights, for the purpose of stopping the people being imposed upon by those who pretend to practise by my system, having no authority from me, and have not a correct knowledge of the subject; but are tampering with all kinds of medicine to the injury of their patients and the great detriment of the credit of my system of practice; for when they happen to be successful, they arrogate to themselves great credit for the cure; but when the patients die, it is all laid to the door of my system. The doctors are ready enough to avail themselves of these cases, and to publish exaggerated accounts of them, to prejudice the minds of the people against me. Whenever I again make an attempt to vindicate my rights, by appealing to the laws of my country, I am determined, if possible, to take such measures as shall give me a fair chance to obtain justice. All I ask is, to have a fair opportunity to prove my medicine to be new and useful, which is all the law requires to make the patent valid. In doing this, I shall spare no expense to have the most able counsel in the country engaged, and shall not stop at any decision against me, till carried to the highest judicial tribunal in the country.

It is a matter of much gratulation to me, and a balm for all my sufferings, that my system-of practice is fast gaining ground in all parts of the country. The people wherever it is introduced, take a lively interest in the cause, and family rights sell rapidly; and all who purchase give much credit to the superior and beneficial effects of the medicine above all others. The prejudices of those who have been opposed to it seem to be fast wearing away before the light of reason and common sense. A number of gentlemen eminent for their scientific researches and usefulness in society, have become advocates for the cause; and although they may not be perfectly converted so as to give up all their former opinions, yet they allow that the system is ingenious and philosophical, and that the practice is new and safe.

In introducing my new mode of practice to the people of this country, I have never sought the patronage or assistance of the great; and the success it has met with has been altogether owing to its own merit. There has been no management or arts used to deceive or to flatter the vanity of any one; but in all cases have endeavoured to convince by demonstrating the truth, by the most plain and simple method of practice, to effect the object aimed at, and to cure disease by such means as I thought would cause the least trouble and expense. This, probably, has been one of the greatest causes of the opposition I have met with from the people; for they have been so long in the habit of being gulled by designing men, and the ostentatious show of pompous declarations and high sounding words, backed by the recomendations of those they have flattered and deceived, that nothing brought forward in a plain and simple dress seems worthy of notice. If I had adopted a more deceptive plan, to suit the follies of the times, I might have been more successful; but I am satisfied I should have been less useful.

There is one thing which I think cannot be matter of doubt, that I have been the cause of awakening a spirit of inquiry among the people of this country, into the medical practice and the fashionable manner of treatment in curing disease, from which great benefits will be derived to the community. Many new contrivances and plans have been introduced by different men, to produce perspiration by steam and other methods, by the use of vegetables, which unquestionably have taken their origin from my practice. When I began to make use of steam, a great deal of noise was made about it throughout the country, and I was called the *steaming* and *sweating* doctor, by way of ridicule. It was even stated by the doctors, that I steamed and sweat my patients to death. This no doubt led some ingenious men to investigate the subject by experiments, and on discovering that it was useful in restoring health to the afflicted, particularly in scrofulous complaints, different contrivances have been introduced to apply steam to the sick. Jennings' vapor bath was highly recommended and considerably used a few years ago; but it has been found not to be safe in cases where there is a high state of inflammation, without the use of my medicine to first produce an equilibrium in the system. A man by the name of Whitlaw, has lately introduced what he calls his medicated vapor bath, which has made considerable stir among the medical faculty.

It seems that this Mr. Whitlaw, from what I can learn of him from his publications, about six years ago went from this country to England, and there introduced a new system of practice, and became celebrated in curing all kinds of scrofulous complaints and diseases of the glands, by means of his method of applying steam and the use of decoctions from American vegetables. How he got his knowledge, or what first induced him to fix upon this plan, I know not; but it seems, as far as I can understand him, that he has adopted my system of practice as far as he has been able to get a knowledge of it. He says something about gaining his knowledge from an Indian in this country; but this is too stale to require any notice. One of the great principles upon which my system is founded, is, that all disease originates in obstructions in the glands, and if not removed becomes scrofulous; and the only remedy is to remove the obstructions by raising perspiration by steam and hot medicine. In all my practice, for nearly forty years, there has been nothing that I have succeeded more completely in, than the cure of scrofulous complaints, such as salt-rheum, St. Anthony's fire, scalt head, cancers, king's evil, rheumatism and consumption.

It appears that the above gentleman has met with great success in England, and that he has had the support and patronage of many of the first men in the kingdom, who have liberally contributed to the support of an asylum for the cure of the poor, and that his success has given universal satisfaction. And it also appears that he has met with abuse from the medical fac-

ulty, both there and in this country. This was to be expected, and is the best evidence of its utility. I feel no
enmity towards those who are benefiting by my discoveries, and it gives me much pleasure to think that I have
been instrumental in introducing a new system of medical practice, by which I feel confident so much benefit
will be derived by relieving in a great measure, the sum
of human misery.   But I think those gentlemen who
have gained any knowledge from my practice, for which
I have suffered so much for introducing, ought, in justice,
to allow me some credit for the discovery.

It has been my misfortune to meet with not only opposition in my practice, but to suffer many wrongs from
some with whom I have had dealings, and this in many
cases where those who have attempted to injure me were
among those that I considered under obligations to me.
I have related a number of cases in the course of my
narrative ; but the disposition in many, still seems to
continue.   In selling family rights, I have always been
as liberal to purchasers as they could wish, particularly
where I was convinced their circumstances made it in-
convenient for them to pay the money down ; and have
been in the habit of taking notes payable at a convenient
time.   This has occasioned me considerable loss ; but
in most cases the purchasers have shown a disposition to
pay if in their power, have treated me with a proper respect, and have been grateful for the favour ; with these
I have been satisfied, and no one has had reason to com-
plain of my want of generosity towards them.   There
have been some, however, who have taken a different
course, and have not only refused to comply with their
contract, but have, notwithstanding they have continued,
to use the medicine, turned against me and have tried to
do me all the harm in their power.   Such conduct has
caused me some considerable vexation and trouble.

At the time I failed in my attempt against Elias Smith,
in consequence of the decision against the correctness
of the specifications of my patent, as has been before
related, I had a number of notes for rights sold, among
them were two against a person, who had previously
expressed great zeal in my cause, for a right for himself, and one for his friend. During the pending of the

trial, he took sides with Smith; and after the decision, came to the conclusion, or, as I suppose, was told by Smith, that the notes could not be collected by law, and refused to pay them. I did not wish to put him to cost, and therefore let the business rest, in hopes he would think better of it and pay me according to contract; but after waiting until the notes were nearly outlawed, and he still refusing to pay, I put one of them in suit, and the action was tried before the Boston Police Court. The defence set up was, that the contract was void, in consequence of the failure of the patent; and also that there was no value received.

The trial was before Mr. Justice Orne, and was managed by Mr. Morse, for the plaintiff, and Mr. Merrill, for the defendant. On this trial, as on all others in which I have been engaged, there seemed to be the same fixed prejudice against me and my system of practice. The defendant's lawyer opened the defence with all the old slang about quackery, alluding to the report of my trial for murder, and that he was going to make out one of the greatest cases of deception and fraud ever known; but when he came to hear the evidence in support of my claim, and the great credit given to my medicine and practice, by many respectable witnesses, he altered his tone very much, and I hope became convinced of his erroneous impressions; and seemed to abandon this part of the defence, placing his dependence on the question of law, as to the failure of the patent. This question the Judge seemed not willing to decide alone, and the case was continued for argument before the full court, on this point.

The case was argued before the three Judges, who all agreed in the opinion, that the decision of the Circuit Court did not affect the patent right; but was a mere suspension, in consequence of an informality in the specifications, which did not debar me from recovering according to the contract. After this decision, another hearing was had, and another attempt made to prove that the defendant had not been furnished by me with the necessary information to enable him to practise with safety; but in this he failed altogether; for it was proved that he had the privilege of being a member of the

Friendly Botanic Society, and had also all the advantages that others had, and that if he did not improve it, it was his own fault. It was also proved that he had been in the constant practice of using the medicine in his family, and prepared and offered it for sale to others. In the course of the examination, Elias Smith was brought forward by the defendant, to prove, as I presume, that I was not capable of giving information on my own system of practice; but his testimony was so contradictory, to say the least of it, that jt did more harm than good to the defendant's cause. There was also a doctor of the regular order introduced in the defence; but he seemed to know nothing about the practice or the case before the court, and of course his evidence amounted to very little, as his opinion upon a subject that he knew nothing about, was not of much value, and was very properly objected to by the plaintiff's counsel.

In the course of the trial, a great number of gentlemen of undoubted veracity, were brought forward to prove the utility of my system of practice, who gave the most perfect testimony in its favour. Several stated, that they were so well convinced of its superiority over all others, and they were so well satisfied with the benefits they had derived from its use, that no sum of money whatever would induce them to be deprived of a knowledge of it. Among the witnesses, an eminent physician of Boston, who has on all occasions been very friendly, and shown a warm interest in support of my system of practice, voluntarily came forward and gave a very fair and candid statement in favour of its utility, the value of my discoveries, and the important additions I had made to the Materia Medica.

The Judge took several days to make up his judgment, and finally decided in my favour, giving me the full amount of my claim; thus settling the principle, that obligations given for family rights were good in law. This was the first time I have ever had a chance to prove the utility of my medicine and system of practice, before a court of law; having always before been prevented by some management of the court.

A knowledge of the vegetable medicine that I have brought into use in curing the diseases incident to this country, and what the faculty call, my "*novel mode of practice*," is fast gaining ground in all parts of the United States; but in no part of it of late, has it been more completely successful, than in the State of New York, notwithstanding the virulent opposition the doctors in that State have made to its progress. They have succeeded in getting a law passed by their Legislature, to put a stop to quackery, as they call all practice, except by those who get a diploma from some medical society established by law; depriving all others the right of collecting their demands for medical practice; and they have also gone one step further than any other State, by making it penal for any one who is not of the regular order, to sell medicine to the sick; imposing a fine of twenty-five dollars on all who offend; thus taking away from those who are so unfortunate as to be sick, all the right of determining for themselves, who they shall employ to cure them, or what medicine they shall make use of. The Medical Society of Pennsylvania, made an attempt to get a similar law passed in that State; but the good sense of Gov. Shultz, put a stop to it, for which he is entitled to great praise. After they had managed to get it through the Legislature, he refused to sign it, and returned the bill with his reasons; the principal of which was, that he considered it altogether unconstitutional; and it is to be hoped that the enlightened statesman and scholar, now Governor of New York,* will use his influence to stop the interested and monopolizing schemes of the medical faculty in that important and enterprising State.

The remarkable extension of the practice in the State of New York, was in a great measure owing to accident; and proves what I have found to be the case in many other places, that where it has met with the greatest opposition from the faculty, the spread of a knowledge of its utility, has been the most rapid and permanent. In the year 1821, my son, Cyrus Thomson, who had settled in Ohio, was passing through the State of New York, on a visit to his friends; while in Manlius, he stopped to see a man whom I had authorized to practise, and while

* The late Governor Clinton.

15.

there, was requested by him to go and see two patients
he had been requested to attend ; both of them had been
given over by the doctors, as incurable.   One of them
was found to be past help, very little was done for her,
and she soon after died.   The other was cured by the
use of the medicine.   The death of the above person
was taken advantage of by the doctors, who circulated a
report that she was murdered by the medicine that had
been given her.   This produced a strong excitement
among the people, who knew nothing about the facts;
a warrant was obtained, through the influence of the
doctors, and my son and the other man were arrested.   My son was thrown into prison, and the other
was put under bonds of a thousand dollars, to appear
at the next court.   The first, however, after laying in
jail three days, was enabled to give bonds, also, for his
appearance.

Being thus prevented from pursuing his journey, he
set himself down in the town where the above occur-
rence took place, and went into practice.   The persecutions of the faculty gave him friends, as it led the people
to inquire into their conduct, and being satisfied of their
motives, did all they could to protect him and increase
his practice.   His success has been greater than in any
other part of the country, the practice having spread
over a country of more than two hundred miles in extent; and his success in curing disease has been very
great, having lost but six patients out of about fifteen
hundred.   This has caused the faculty to follow up their
persecutions, in order to drive him out of the country ;
but he is too firmly established in the good opinion of
the people, for them to effect their object.   I have
another son established in the practice at Albany, who
has been very successful in introducing the knowledge
of it there ; and a number of gentlemen of the first
respectability, are taking a strong interest in promoting
its success.

A writer has lately come forward and published a
series of numbers in the Boston Patriot, under the title
of "Eclectic," who appears well qualified, and seems
disposed to do me and my system of practice justice,
by laying before the people a correct view of my case.

I shall now bring this narrative of those events and circumstances that have taken place in my life, in which the public are interested, to a close; having stated every particular that I thought worthy of being recorded, in as concise and plain a manner as I was capable ; and am not without a hope that my endeavours to promote the public good, will be duly appreciated. Some certificates and statements of cases that have been attended under my system of practice, from those who have been my agents, or who have purchased family rights, and have had long experience in the effects produced by a use of my medicine, are subjoined.* They furnish much useful information on the subject, and will convey a more correct view of the success which has attended the administering my medicine, and following the mode of treatment recommended by my system of practice, than could be given in any other manner. Reference has been made to some of them in the course of the foregoing narrative, and their publication in the work seemed necessary, to convey a correct knowledge of many statements therein given, to show the safety and success with which various diseases have been cured by others, who have had no other knowledge of medicine than the instructions received from me ; and will, I trust, be sufficient to satisfy every reasonable person how easy it would be for every one to become possessed with the means of curing themselves of disease, without being under the necessity of calling the aid of a physician.

Our Family Doctor.

Few families, particularly in cities, and villages, think they can do without a family doctor. But of what use is a family, other than his own, to a doctor, unless there be sickness? Hence it is for the interest of the doctor, if the family are not sick, to make them so. The family doctor has too often an opportunity of doing this with impunity; without detection, and without even exciting suspicion. Even contagion is often spread abroad which might have been cured by an old, or even a young woman at home.

* These certificates are now very much condensed.

" Behold, how great a matter, a little fire kindleth!"
James iii. 5.   For example.   A child is taken with the
belly-ache.   The family doctor is sent for, who pronounces its disorder to be worms, gives calomel and
jalap to destroy them, which reduces the child very much.
The next visit, bleeds it, to lay the fever, then gives it a
fever powder composed of nitre, opium and camphor,
once in two hours.   The patient now lays in a stupid,
senseless posture, with crimson spots on the cheeks, de-
noting putrefaction.   The doctor is again sent for in
haste, who now pronounces it to be the putrid fever.
The bleeding is repeated, and the fever powders continued.   The nerves become convulsed, and the doctor is
again sent for, who pronounces the disorder to be the
putrid nervous fever, and that it has become contagious;
the child dies, the family; worn out with fatigue, and
being much alarmed, begin to become sick, and by the
time the corpse of the child is interred, are all down
with the disorder.   The doctor now has much employ,
the neighbours are called in to watch, the putrefaction
runs high ; the neighbours, one after another, take the
disorder, and return home sick ; the doctor is called,
business gains rapidly in consequence of the same treatment, until the fever has gone through the whole village.
All thank the doctor for his incessant attention and kindness ; and he boasts of wonderful success, having lost
but *fifty* out of *one hundred and fifty!*   His bill is paid
with the greatest satisfaction.   By this time the doctor
can build his house without sitting down " to count the
cost."   [Pause.]

What is the cause of all this village sickness? Remember the text.   " Behold how great a matter a little
fire kindleth."   A child was taken with the belly-ache ;
and had no doctor been known, the mother, with one
gill of pepper and milk, could have cured the child, and
saved all this slaughter of the scourge of a family doctor.

Is not this the cause of the spread of so many contagious disorders which prevail unaccounted for ?   If so,
learn wisdom by the evils which others endure ; study
the nature of disease and how to remove it, and never
trust your own life, nor that of a child, in the hands of
what is called a family physician.

ADDITIONS

To the Third Edition....August, 1831.

In the year 1825, " The Friendly Botanical Society in Boston," being destitute of a practitioner, wished me to appoint an agent, whom I thought competent, to take the lead in practice, and sell my medicine. I recommended Mr. John Locke, of Portsmouth, as has been before related, in whom I had put the utmost confidence. He was sent for by the committee, and moved here in the summer of that same year. I gave him twenty dollars, and others of the committee, and members gave him something handsome for his encouragement. I agreed to furnish him with all the medicine, either used or sold by him, at stipulated prices, to give advice when needed, to furnish him with books for the sale of family rights, and to give him ten dollars for every right sold ; and for the medicine, I was to wait one year before demanding payment. At the end of the year, my principal agent, Col. House, and the three committee, looked over Mr. Locke's account, in my absence, and reported to me, that in their opinion, Mr. Locke had not made as much as he ought, and proposed for me to give him the privilege of making the medicine used in his practice. I indulged them in this proposal, and granted their request for one year. But, availing himself of this inch of indulgence, he took the liberty to prepare and sell for his own profit to all that should call on him for medicine. At the end of this year, in my absence, my principal agent, as committee, gave him liberty to proceed in the manner he had done. I continued to give advice as usual through this year, frequently calling on the committee to revoke the liberty they had given Mr. Locke, to prepare and sell my medicine for his own profit, without rendering me any account. In these two years, by my assistance, and that of my agent and committee, Mr. Locke seemed to be well established in the business, and boasted of his great success, not having lost a patient in two years.   But at the same time he seemed to lose sight that I had been any benefit to him, and rather paid his whole attention to the committee.

In all this time, I had never thought or mistrusted that there was a plot laid against me, either by him, my agent, or the committee, or with all combined, nor until about the end of the second year, which now seems but too obvious.   Having recently returned from the West, I was at Mr. Locke's house, and showed him a newspaper which contained an account of the masonic outrage at Batavia.   After reading it, he flew into a great passion, and accosted me as though I had made the story. I tried to argue the case with him; but in vain.   He called me by as many hard names as he could well think of, and occasionally, the words " lie" and " fool" were in the compound.   I did not think that I had merited such treatment, having rendered him my service and advice gratuitously, for two years.   He seemed to be so independent, that he said that he wanted nothing of me, nor cared any thing for me.   I retorted that I wanted nothing of him except an honourable settlement.   This settlement never came to a close until the fall of the year 1830, and then only in part.   He rendered an account of upwards of forty rights which he had sold, and for which he settled by my deducting about one quarter of my share; but as for the medicine which he has prepared and sold for his own benefit, he refuses to give me any account thereof.   So much for this inch of indulgence.   Such conduct appears to me to be rather hard, especially after all I and the society had done for him, to enable him to assist me in my old age.   But instead of this, with the assistance of the committee, and my principal agent, they have taken the lead of the business out of my hands as far as they were able to do it.

I have tried repeatedly to get a settlement with Col. House, my principal agent, but cannot effect it.   He has paid me nothing for the large number of rights sold in about ten years, nor will he render any account.   I know not how many books he has sold, as he took them when-

ever he wanted, in my absence. When I called on him
last to settle, he said he had lost his account of credit.
Here is the result of ten years agency! Besides which,
I lent him and his partner, ten years ago, two hundred
dollars, one of which he has paid in printing, the other
he refuses to pay. I might mention many other circumstances which would go to show a decided hostility
against me, and a determination to raise Mr. Locke, if
possible, at my expense ; but I forbear, for they have
neither built him up, nor put me down. I have paid no
attention to all this opposition ; but have kept on in a
straight forward course, attending to the preparing of
good medicine and supplying all those who wished
for it.

I have thought much on the opposition and abuse I
have met with here from those whom I considered my
best friends, and what I could have done to merit it in
their estimation. I will not undertake to say how far
masonry has been concerned in these transactions, but
certain I am that it commenced with Mr. Locke, on my
innocently showing him a newspaper which contained
an account of a masonic outrage. I thought no more
harm in this than as though I had showed him a paper
which contained an account of the murder of Mr. White.
Did Mr. Locke resent this because he was a mason ?
And why did my agent and committee from this time
possess such sympathy for him, and conspire against me,
insomuch that when an Infirmary was talked of, they
would not subscribe a cent unless Mr. Locke could be
at the head of it ? I think that my agent and two of
the committee are masons, and that Mr. Locke is a
mason, if so, four out of five against me were masons,
and whether masonry has had any effect on the mind
and conduct of these gentlemen, I shall leave the reader and the public to draw their own conclusions. It is
to be hoped that the good people who belonged to the
society, which the president and committee have suffered to be broken up by not calling the annual meeting,
for the choice of officers agreeably to the constitution ;
the good people who took no part in the above transactions, and who have had no part in the destruction of
the society, will make every effort for its resuscitation,

hoping that it will die no more; but that it will live to be
useful to the sick and infirm, and be an ornament to
generations yet unborn.

It is expected that arrangements will be made for the
delivery of Botanic lectures, when the society will revive and put on strength until the learned, as well as the
unlearned, shall join to revolutionize the medical world.

I shall not go into any further particular details of
agents, but only take a general view in the western parts
of the United States.

Since my last edition was printed in Boston, I have
been six times in and through the State of Ohio. In
the year 1825, I appointed Charles Miles, as agent in
Ohio, and furnished him with seventy-two books for
family rights. On his way home he purchased a number
of counterfeit books, of David Rogers, of Geneva, I understood about one hundred, more or less. He went
down into the central part of the State, and in the course
of eighteen months, sold about ten thousand dollars
worth of rights, and imposed on the inhabitants at a
great rate. Some he sold for seventy-five dollars, some
twenty-five, others twelve, and he would leave but one
book for four rights. When he came round again, he
would borrow my book and leave the other; and sell my
book again to another set of four or five; and so continued until he had sold all mine, and nearly all the others.
In the fall of 1826, Horton Howard caused a letter to
be sent to me, giving an account of Miles' conduct, and
requesting me to come on to see about it. I arrived in
January, 1827, and, following after Miles, I found his
conduct to be as had been stated. I published handbills, and otherwise showing that he had no authority
from me to do as he had done. I revoked his agency,
and pacified the rage of the people as well as I could, by
restoring the family right to those to whom he had so
improperly sold it, and besides this, I lost a great part
of what he owed me.

In January of the same year, I made Horton Howard
agent for the Western country, with authority to print
my book, and in three and a half years he had printed
about six thousand copies, and sold about four thousand
rights, with the assistance of his sub-agents, amounting

in all to about eighty thousand dollars. I tried at several different times to come to an honourable settlement with him, until August, 1830, at which time he utterly refused to give me an account from the beginning. I then had but one alternative, either to bring an action against him in the court of chancery, or else take what he was willing to give. I chose the latter, by which I sacrificed about seven-eighths of what should have been coming to me. I took his notes for four thousand dollars, in two annual payments, two thousand dollars each year. I revoked his agency in two days afterwards, August 9, 1830, and appointed four other agents in his stead, and took about two thousand copies of books, and left them with my other agents.

The practice has spread rapidly in the southern and western States, which has so much alarmed the doctors, that they have succeeded in getting laws passed, in almost all the States, to prevent the spread of my practice. This has caused me a great deal of trouble and expense, and has been of no great benefit to them. It has been like whipping fire among the leaves, which only tends to spread it the faster. The law is most severe in South Carolina, where a suit was attended two years ago. The fine is five hundred dollars for each offence, besides imprisonment. This violent outrage roused the patriotic spirit of the people, insomuch that the doctor who brought the complaint dared not come before the court to support it, and requested of the court leave of absence, which was granted him. The defence was made on the ground of the patent, and by proving the utility of the medicine; and the case was decided in favour of the defendant: If persecutions must take place, let persecutors go the whole extent of their power, as in the present case, and the rights of the people will be defended. Had I not obtained a patent, the people could not have defended their rights; but must have bowed down to the power of the doctors, they having the law on their side, as to a dagon.

But the dernier resort of the doctors will be to get my practice into their own hands, and under their own management, if possible. Finding that I should succeed in my Botanic practice, certain individuals of them have

16

set up what they call a reformed college, in New York,
where they have adopted my practice as far as they
could obtain a knowledge of it from those who had
bought the right of me, and would forfeit their word and
honour to give them instruction.   And finding that the
Botanic practice gained very fast at the West, they have
established a branch of their reformed college in Worthington, Ohio.   I saw Dr. Steel, last winter, who is the
President of that Institution, I was introduced to him
by Mr. Sealy, a member of the Senate, and Dr. Steel
was introduced to me as President of said college.   I
asked him if he was President of that reform which was
stolen from Thomson, in New York.   This seemed to
strike him dumb on the subject.   At the same place, a
few evenings after, I was introduced to one of the practitioners under this reform, who studied and was educated at the college in New York, and was one of the in-
structers at Worthington.   I asked him if he ever saw
any of my books in the college in New York.   He said
he had accidentally seen one there.   I replied, then
you accidentally confess that my books were studied in
that college.   I then asked him whether they used the
lobelia.   He said they did.   I then named the cayenne,
rheumatic drops, bayberry and nerve powders.   He confessed they used them all in manner and form, as I had
laid down in my books.   I am therefore, satisfied that if
my medicine were taken from them, their Institution
would not be worth one cent.   But, to have bought the
right, would have been too mean for such dignitaries;
but, to steal it from a *quack*, was, perhaps, in their estimation, much more honourable ! ! !   Every honest man
who hears any of the doctors speak of those colleges
with approbation, ought to upbraid them with these facts.

   In 1827, while instructing H. Howard, of whom mention has been made above, I was introduced to Governor
Trimble, and gave him a right.   He had a consumptive
wife, whom the doctors could not help.   I gave him a
sample of medicine, and what instruction I could.   He
went home, and finding her worse, and no person understanding the medicine within fifty miles, he took the
book and carried her through a course, and repeated it;
and she soon got well.   His wife and nurse cured two

other women with the same sample of medicine I gave him. The enemies of the practice, said that they should advertise him as a *steam doctor.* He said they need not take that trouble, for he would do it himself.

The practice has gained a respectable standing in nearly all the States in the Union, and also in Canada. A man by the name of Henry S. Lawson, has published my Guide to Health, in Buffalo, and sold them in Canada; and thus made a great speculation from my discoveries.

In 1829, Mr. Samuel Robinson, delivered before the members of the Friendly Botanical Society, in Cincinnati, Ohio, a series of fifteen lectures on "Medical Botany," denominated the Thomsonian system of practice. He is entitled to much credit for this service done to the system. Those lectures were delivered without my knowledge, being at the time a thousand miles from that place. Horton Howard obtained them, while acting as my agent, paid for them out of my money, secured the copy right in his own name, and printed an edition of them, which he sold for his own benefit. This book gave a great spread to the sale of rights. I have since secured the copy right in Boston, and printed an edition of two thousand copies, which are selling from fifty to sixty-two and a half cents a copy. They contain much information, relative to the practice of medicine, as taught in medical colleges, and found in medical authors; not to be found elsewhere in so small and so cheap a work.

During the agency of Horton Howard, to wit, in July, 1829, while I was at Columbus, he returned from the South, and was so unwell that he wrote to his wife at Tiffin, about eighty-four miles, that if she ever wished to see him alive, to come without delay. I attended him the next day through a thorough course of medicine, and relieved him, insomuch that I have not heard of his being sick since. His wife arrived in about four days, when, finding him about house, and well, she took him around the neck and burst into tears. I retorted in her behalf, saying, "you are not half so bad as I hoped you would be." This tended to dry her tears, and it passed off with a laugh. The next day we all calculated to go North, towards the lake. The day before

we were to start, about twelve o'clock, he had word that
his son-in-law, Samuel Forrow, was at the point of death,
and requested that some of the family would come as
soon as possible.   Mr. Howard and wife concluded to
go, and insisted on my going with them.   I with much
reluctance consented,   We started at three o'clock, on
Friday, with two horses and a wagon, and arrived there
on Saturday, about sun-set, a distance of eighty-six
miles.   Mr. Horton drove all the way, night and day,
notwithstanding he was calculating to die about five or
six days before.   We found Mr. Forrow very sick ; but
one of the patent doctors was there.   I gave him but
little that night, merely a pinch of cayenne, as snuff, as
he had the catarrh, and was much stuffed on the lungs.
In the morning, Sunday, I carried him through a course
of medicine, which roused the opium, that remained in
his system, into action, as though it had been but just
taken.   He tumbled and thrashed about in his frenzy
for about four hours, when he became composed.   He
was then steamed, when the medicine operated, which,
together with the heat, roused the physic into action,
which run him hard with a relax.   I tried to restore the
digestive powers, but could not on account of his not
being clear.   I was obliged to carry him through a second
course in thirty-six hours, instead of going forty-eight,
as I had calculated.   We began with him at dark.   But
as soon as the medicine took hold of the opium, it renewed its operation, which continued eight hours.   His
relatives stood on their feet, about ten in number, expecting to see him die before morning.   I lay down on
the floor until the flounce began to abate.   During six
hours there was not one second that he was still.   He
continually called for water, and drank about ten quarts
in the course of the night.   About three o'clock in the
morning, he began to be a little stiller, resting two or
three seconds at a time.   He began to inquire who those
black people were, which he fancied were there, and
what they were there for, and many other similar ex-
pressions, which showed that his senses were returning,
but were not yet regular.   I then told Mr. Howard and
the family, that they had better go to bed, and I would
attend him, with one of his sisters, the remainder of the

night. The medicine then began to operate, after the opium had all distilled off. He vomited powerfully about eight times, when he appeared to be clear of disorder. I filled him well with milk-porridge, and was in readiness to steam him when the family arose. He was steamed, ate breakfast, and rode out in the course of the day. I prepared a syrup for his relax, of the black cherry root bark, made into a strong tea, as strong as the same quantity of bark pounded would make; I then added peach or cherry stone meats pounded, then added one pound of loaf sugar, and one pint of brandy, which made two junk bottles of syrup, to drink on the way. On Wednesday, about ten o'clock, Mr. Howard and wife, Mr. Forrow and wife, and myself, started for Columbus, and staid at Wanesville that night, about fourteen miles. He stood the ride well, as air and exercise, when the disorder is removed, are as necessary for patients as their food. He was persuaded to stay on Thursday. On Friday we travelled to Charlestown, about thirty miles, and arrived at Columbus on Sunday about noon. In the afternoon, Gov. Trimble, paid him a visit, taking great interest in his welfare. Mr. Forrow was a noted man in the State, being a surveyor and superintendant of the Dayton Canal. The governor seemed highly pleased at the unexpected recovery of the man, and the more particularly when I told him that it was just one week that day since I administered to him on a supposed dying bed, and that he had since been conveyed eighty-six miles in a wagon, and was able to walk about, and was clear of disease. He staid at Columbus but two days, when he went on with Mr. Howard to Tiffin, about as much further, and arrived safe in four days, his health still gaining. I staid there with him about four days, and then started across the woods to New Haven. He paid me twenty-five dollars; but I would not have taken the risk again for five hundred. In fact it was risking my own life to save his.

Thus I have given a few prominent items, though but a small proportion of my experience, sufferings, perplexities and difficulties, since the second edition of this work was published. But much of that which operated to my disadvantage, as an individual, served to extend

16*

the knowledge and practice of the system. This gives me consolation in the midst of all my trials; and considering the Botanical practice as being now well established, I think it is time for me to retire from the field of contest and war with either learned ignorance or legal opposition.

I have collected about three hundred weight of the golden seal the year past, and a large quantity of cayenne from the island of Madagascar ; nearly three tons. I have sent to the southern States nearly twenty barrels, floured, which is a great help in the agues of that country.

And here it is proper to remark, that great impositions are practised on what is called the American cayenne. The doctors have declared it to be poison, and destructive to health, and I think they have made it as bad as they have represented it to be. It appears to be mixed with some red paint or mineral. When burnt, it leaves about two-thirds of the quantity, of the blackest substance. When taken inwardly, it produces violent vomiting, and ought to be shunned as a mad dog. There is but little or none sold at the groceries for ordinary purposes but of this kind. The only safe way to detect the poison, is to try it by burning. If it be pure, there will be a proportion of ashes as of other vegetables, and of a light colour ; if it be bad, the ashes will not only be black, but there will be double, and perhaps tribble or quadruple the quantity there should be for the quantity burnt.

A brief summary of the Certificates and Statements which accompanied the two former editions.

The system and practice of Dr. SAMUEL THOMSON having been so long before the public, and the numerous certificates given in the two first editions of his Narrative being so well known and understood, it is thought not expedient to give them here in full; but only the substance of them abridged, and in lieu thereof, to add some new and more recent cases.—*Ed. 3d ed.*

Of the cases already published, it is proper to mention that of the *Dysentery*, in Jericho, Vermont, in October, 1807, where but two out of twenty-two, lived, that were under the care of the regular physicians. Dr. *Thomson* was sent for, 130 miles; he arrived in five days; in three days, thirty were committed to his care, and in eight days, by the use of his medicine, the town was cleared of the disease, with the loss of two only, who were past cure before he saw them. Testified by JOHN PORTER. A case of Salt Rheum, of thirty years standing, cured in Portsmouth, May, 1813. Certified by ELIZABETH MARSHALL. The case of Spotted Fever, in Eastham, county of Barnstable, Mass. where upwards of forty had died by the 1st of May, and but few lived who had the fever. Dr. Thomson was called on for assistance; sold the right of using his medicine to several individuals, who, in one month, relieved upwards of thirty who were seized with this violent disease, with the loss of but one. At the same time and place, those who were attended by the regular physicians, eleven out of twelve died. Testified by PHILANDER SHAW, *Minister of Eastham;* OBED KNOWLES, *one of the Selectmen;* SAMUEL FREEMAN, *Do.;* HARDING KNOWLES, *Justice of the Peace,* and JOSEPH MAYO, *Agent for the Society, and Post Master.* A case of Rheumatism, of long standing, and many others, more than twelve of a consumption, one of mortification, one of a dropsy, one of numb-palsy, and others of divers diseases, testified by ALEXANDER RICE, *Kittery, Nov.* 20, 1821.

Five cases of consumption, supposed to be desperate, were relieved in the course of three weeks, and all of them restored to health. A case of the dropsy, considered hopeless, was cured in one week. Testified by JOHN BURGIN, JERRY BURGIN, and SOLOMON RICE, *Eastport, July* 20, 1821. The character and respectability of the above witnesses are confirmed by J. R. CHADBOURNE, *Justice of Peace.* The case of Seth Mason, Portland, whose case was truly a desperate one, and his recovery exceeded all expectation. Also, the case of Mrs. Sally Keating, of the same place, who, after being doctored a whole year by the first physician in Portland, had been given over as incurable. She was recovered to an excellent state of health. Testified by S. Sewell, *Scarborough, Jan.* 1, 1822. Several other similar cases are testified by S. Sewell, not necessary to be here particularized. A number of cases, several of which, the patients were given over as incurable by the regular physicians, were all relieved and cured by Dr. Thomson, as testified by Jabez True, *Elder of the Baptist Church in Salisbury, Dec.* 5, 1821.

The case of Elder Bolles was a very extraordinary one.   He was supposed to be in the very last stage of a consumption, and was cured.   John Lemmon was also cured of a consumption; Isaac Perkins' wife was cured of a dropsy of a desperate nature; all of which cures are testified by William Raymond, who says, "all these cures I was well knowing to, having been done at that time;" which statement is also confirmed by Rev. E. Williams, not only as it regards Elder Bolles, but also as it regards Ezra Lovett, on account of whose death, Dr. Thomson was indicted for murder, and tried for his life, about a year afterwards; but he was honourably acquitted, without having an occasion, or even an opportunity of making his defence.   Mr. Lovett was first relieved, then experienced a relapse of his disorder, in consequence of taking cold, by walking out some distance on a very cold day, in the month of December. Dr. Thomson was sent for; but on seeing him, he immediately expressed doubts of his being able to help him.   He gave him medicine which had no effect; and two respectable physicians were sent for, and came, under whose care he was twelve hours before he died. Yet such was the malice and prejudice of the doctors, that they seized upon this case, and tried to make it out murder, in order to destroy both Dr. Thomson and his practice.

Next follows a long statement of the diseases and manner of treatment, by Dr. Thomson's system and directions, and the benefit received under the administration of his medicine ; by Stephen Neal, Esq. *of Eliot, Maine.*   A similar statement by John Raitt, of the same place, *Eliot, Nov.* 28, 1821.

The case of Mary Eaton, which was a dropsy, had been pronounced hopeless by a consultation of four doc-

tors.   She continued, however, under the care of Dr.
Sheppard, until he said her complaint was beyond the
reach of medicine, and that she could not continue over
three weeks.   At this time, May, 1808, she says, "I
went to see Dr. Thomson, and in three weeks I was reduced about fifteen inches in bigness.   I returned home
and have gained until this day; and am now enjoying
a better state of health than I had before enjoyed for
sixteen years."   (Signed) MARY EATON, *Exeter, Nov.*
20, 1821.

An extraordidary case of Asthma, of Mrs. Hannah
Coleman, who had applied to six physicians without receiving any beneficial effect, by using Dr. Thomson's
medicine, she was enabled to lay in bed and rest comfortably for twelve years, as testified by her husband,
EPHRAIM COLEMAN, *Newington, Dec.* 3, 1821.

A young man in Roxbury, who from some cause unknown, had taken ratsbane with the intention of destroying himself, was so relieved that the next morning
he was quite comfortable.   Dr. P. who had been called,
said there was no more chance for him to live than there
would be if his head were cut off.   After he was relieved, Dr. P. called to see him and expressed great astonishment that he was alive, saying that there was not one
case in a thousand that a man could live under similar
circumstances.   Testified by ELIJAH SIMONS, who administered the medicine that gave relief, and who says,
"I attended him three or four days, and he is now so
far recovered as to walk about the room."   *Roxbury,*
Feb. 23, 1821.

Additional Testimony.

Although there is no real occasion to add any more
testimony, by way of certificates, yet as my case is more
recent, and my name may have some weight, I feel it a
duty I owe to the public, as well as to Dr. Thomson, to
state it, which I do as editor of the present edition of
Dr. Thomson's works, 1831.

I have for many years been opposed to, and latterly
very much prejudiced against, every thing which savor-
ed of *quackery*, which prejudices were greatly strengthened by having once been egregiously imposed upon by
a *quack doctor*, (I forbear giving his name for his rela-

tions sake, though he is now not living,) of whom I bought the skill, as he said, of curing cancers; but which proved to be nothing but a gross imposition on the public; hence, after trying the experiment on several, without effect, though it would effectually remove tumours not cancerous, I declined the practice altogether, lost my trouble, together with what I had paid for the skill, besides experiencing the mortification of having been thus duped by a man void of principle and moral honesty.

It was under these feelings, that the Thomsonian system was first recommended for my daughter who had what had been first called a white swelling, then a fever sore, but lastly, by Dr. Thomson, a *mercury sore*, on her arm, in the elbow joint, for nearly four years. The best encouragement she could get from the regular physicians was, either to have it amputated to save life, or (which was the advice of Dr. Warren) to lay by entirely and not to use it. She thought she should be in a manner useless herself, without her arm; for it was her right arm, and if she was not to use it, she might lose it almost as well as not. Under these impressions she was induced to try the Thomsonian system, under the direction of Mrs. Holman. It was soon found to have a salutary effect. In a very few weeks it was better than it had been before for more than three years. A great part of the time her arm had been so stiff that she could not raise her hand to her head. It is now entirely well, and her general health much improved; better than it has been for a number of years; for she has been sick every few years with fevers, or with what was called the liver complaint, ever since she had the typhus fever in 1812, when she was but a child. The favourable result the medicine had on her, softened the prejudices very much, which I had, till then, entertained against it; though they were not entirely removed, nor was she entirely well, when I was attacked with the fever and ague, which I considered but a presage to the return of the fever I had last fall, which I caught in travelling on the Erie Canal, and from which I did but just recover. After the second attack with the ague, I was taken down with the bilious fever, and was more violently seized

than I was last fall ; and had I received the same treatment which I did then, I have no idea that I could have
recovered, as my fever at that time run twelve days before it formed a crisis ; and then it was three weeks after
that, before I was able to be about.   But under the
Thomsonian system, the crisis was formed in just about
forty hours from the time I commenced taking the medicine ; at which time, I lay, as I have been informed, for
I could not measure the time, seven or eight hours in an
entirely unconscious state ; after which I fell into a
sweet sleep, and awoke in the morning free from all
fever, and have had none since.

After about ten days, however, the chills returned ;
but without any fever, which I had regularly every other
day for four or five weeks.   To wear out these, I pursued the regular courses of medicine, every few days, not
omitting injections, as often as I felt any occasion for
them, till the chills left me entirely, and I am now happy
to say that I am not aware that I have any disease about
me, or that I ever enjoyed better health.   All, therefore,
that my life is now worth to me, and all that I am now
enjoying, or shall hereafter enjoy, I must impute, in the
first instance, to the Thomsonian system, together with
the skill and faithfulness with which it was applied ;
which, it is but justice to say, in the most critical mo-
ment, the medicine that apparently saved my life, was
applied by Mrs. Holman ; for although Dr. Thomson
had been sent for in the night, yet before he arrived the
danger was in a manner over.

Whether the relapse I took was in consequence of
taking cold, or in consequence of the mercury and other
poisons which I had formerly taken, and from which my
system was not entirely cleansed, I shall not undertake
to say ; the doctor says, the latter ; I have only stated
the facts as I felt and experienced them ; and should it
be the means of giving others confidence to try the system in the most difficult cases, it will answer the object
I have in view in thus making them more publicly known.
It is true, the pain of the disease, or of the operation of
the medicine, or of both, was at first most excruciating ;
but this did not discourage me from trying it again, when
I took a relapse ; and the operation became more and

more mild, as the disease went off, till it was attended with but very little inconvenience.

ABNER KNEELAND.

NOTICE.

I hereby appoint ABNER KNEELAND, editor of the Boston Investigator, Agent, generally, but not exclusively, throughout the United States, to receive and answer my letters, to sell the Rights to my Botanical System of Practice in Medicine, and my Books containing a Narrative of my Life and System of Practice, and to attend to all matters and things expressed or implied in the above agency, especially during my absence, the same as I should or could do if present, and the agencies of E: G. House and John Locke, are hereby revoked.

SAMUEL THOMSON.

TO THE PUBLIC.

THE Subscriber, having been appointed Agent for Dr. SAMUEL THOMSON, as above stated, all letters intended for the Doctor, may be addressed either to him or to the Subscriber, as all the Doctor's letters come into the box of the Investigator, and of course into the hands of the Subscriber, who will keep family Rights, with the Books containing the System of Practice constantly for sale at the Investigator Office, Merchants' Hall, Congress Street; and who will appoint sub-agents, with the advice and consent of the Doctor, when, and wherever they shall be thought necessary, and as soon as he can make arrangements for the purpose, will also keep the Medicine for sale at the same prices, and as low as it can be bought of the Patentee, and the patronage in this line, which the public are disposed to give, will be gratefully received by the public's obedient servant,

ABNER KNEELAND.

PATENT BOTANICAL MEDICINE.

Prepared and sold by the Patentee, and MARY GOODRICH, No. 4, Clark Street; also by JOHN MARSH & CO. Nos. 96 & 98, State Street; AMOS B. PARKER, No. 18, Dock Square, and ELIAKIM DARLING, No. 52, Salem Street.

Thomson's **Wine Bitters,**
      "   **Composition Powders,**
      "   **Rheumatic Drops,**
      "   **Vegetable Pills,** &c.
Best of Cayenne,
Also, Books and Family Rights.

taken either by themselves or their children, for four generations, the people, I think, would improve in stature and vigour, and become "mighty men of renown;" such as we read of in olden times, before the poison doctors had destroyed the natural senses of our race; or at least, so perverted them that they cease to be subservient to their natural use. But, on the contrary, should the hood-winking system be continued, and the people continue to degenerate, in every sense of the word, so far as their health and bodily faculties are concerned, for four generations to come, as they have for two generations past, they will become more like a race of monkeys than like human beings.

From this source of poisons may be traced those hereditary and family consumptions we hear so often mentioned. If traced back, it will be found that the family consumption began with the family doctor; and so it will continue as long as you employ one. A treatise on the family doctor may be found on page 175, of this work. The family consumption was made with those families to whom the doctor gave the fever when he spread it through the village. Those who did not die, were left worse than dead. The poison left in the system caused them to linger out a miserable life in pain and torment; and the doctor gets clear by stating that they have all died with the family consumption. If you wish to keep clear of a family consumption, keep clear of a family doctor.

The priest is equally guilty of knocking down the sentinels of the mind and understanding, as the doctor is of knocking down the external and internal sentinels of the body. Death, in many instances is the effect of both. Bleeding and poison on the one hand, and insanity and suicide on the other. Both of them cause a grievous tax on the people; and the lawyer sweeps the board in collecting their bills and his fees.

Thus I have shown in part, the evils arising from giving up the guards and sentinels of the labouring class of the community, and substituting the three crafts to watch over them, and to "eat them that are fed, and clothe themselves with their wool; but they feed not the flock." They call themselves "shepherds;" but they are "wolves in sheep's clothing."

18

Why Meat will not Putrefy in very hot, or very cold climates.

Meat will not putrefy in Arabia, nor in South America, nor at the North or South Poles. Where the climate is so hot as almost to roast meat, it will not putrefy, as in Africa or South America. Where the sand will roast an egg in fifteen minutes, there the carcases dry up, and do not rot. So, on the North or South Poles, where every thing is frozen, there is no putrefaction. But half way between freezing and roasting, there is putrefaction. Much beef is dried on the sand in Brazils, without any salt, and used at sea as fresh beef. The cause why meat will not putrefy in either very hot, or very cold climates, as I apprehend, is, the water evaporates in the one case, and congeals to ice in the other, so suddenly, that the meat has no chance to decompose, as in either case it becomes hard.

The myrrh from Africa, is better than from Turkey or Russia, as the climate is steadily hot, and the myrrh is of a more spicy smell, and is much more powerful against all mortifications and putrid sores than that from the Straits; and is of a much higher price. There being no trade up the rivers, to the interior part of the country, all that is to be had, is brought by the Arabs to Mora or Madagascar. The cayenne from Madagascar is better than that from the West Indies, as it is more steady in its operation, and better against putrefaction; and is not fluctuating from a calm to a hurricane, as is that from the West Indies. The latter, often so frightens the people who take it, especially in a cold state of the body, that they never dare to take any more. It is seldom the case with that from Africa.

Beware of the American, which is manufactured, and coloured. It is poisoned, as I have remarked elsewhere.

Proposals for a Revolution in the practice of Medicine.

People have paid doctors for being sick, for about four thousand years. Let them now turn about, and pay for their health, which is much more reasonable. Let the doctor enter into contract with the head of a family, to

keep the family in health, for a certain sum, for each
member of the family, for one year; conditioned that
for each day's sickness in the family, by any member
thereof, the doctor, shall forfeit twenty-five cents, to be
deducted from the sum agreed upon. Hence all the account there is to be kept, is, the number of days of sickness there is in the family, in order to know what amount
there is to be deducted from the sum agreed upon. And
to prevent any imposition on the doctor, by the family,
any one saying, "I am sick," to save twenty-five cents;
the doctor must be called, and they must go through a
regular course of medicine, or else not have any allow-
ance made for their sickness. But if they comply, the
doctor must not only attend them for nothing, finding his
own medicine, but also pay them twenty-five cents for
every day they are sick; to be deducted at the end of
the year, from his salary. Were this plan generally
adopted, it would save nine-tenths of all the sickness of
our country.

Numbpalsy.

In looking over my Narrative and Guide to Health, I
find that this disease has been overlooked, and not treated upon. I carried the view in my mind, that I had recorded the case of my daughter, which happened about
twenty years ago; and the omission was not discovered
till it was too late to insert it in its proper place. I
shall, therefore, give it a place here.

While I was at Portsmouth, I do not recollect now exactly the year, I received a letter from home, that my
daughter, then about twenty years of age, was sick, and
her life despaired of. I obtained and took with me a
bottle of the best pepper-sauce. When I arrived, she
appeared to be dying, and had so appeared, as they said,
for some days. Her eyes were set; and she breathed
like one in the last struggles of life. I was advised to
do nothing for her. I thought it would do no harm to
try the pepper-vinegar. I therefore poured a spoonful
of it in her mouth, as it was open. In about two minutes she opened and moved her eyes. I then gave her
another spoonful, which was swallowed. In about the

space of ten minutes, she spoke, and said she had had a
shock of the numbpalsy.   This was the first idea we
had of the kind.   After awaking like a person from
sleep, or nearly dead, she gave a history of its beginning and progress to the then present time.   She said
the shock struck one half of the body and limbs, and
half of the tongue, insensible of feeling; like that caused by a knock of the elbow.   All one side was full of a
prickling sensation, attended at first with heavy and severe pain; the pain relaxed, however, as the side dead-
ened, and entirely ceased with the feelings; and all that
side remained dead, as to sensation, till the pepper-sauce
was given.   This brought back the pain and prickling
as at the commencement, until all parts had become
equalized.   I think I carried her through several courses
of medicine in usual form, until the system became clear
of obstruction, and the digestive powers restored.   She
soon recovered, with no other disadvantage than that of
the side which received the shock continuing weaker
and more subject to cold than the other.   She has had
two or three of those shocks since.   But by having the
medicine in the family, and by the assistance of the
neighbours who have the right, she has been always soon
relieved, so as not to be confined but a few days.   I saw
her last fall.   She has now no trouble from the complaint, except that above mentioned.   She has a family
of six children, and has done the greatest part towards
their support by practising abroad, under my system, and
by my finding her with medicine and rights to sell.   She
has relieved many of the same complaint.

I have given a history of this case, only on account
of the name.   Had the same case appeared without any
name, the treatment under the head of fits, drowned
persons, and all suspended animation would have answered.   The third preparation is the first resort; then
a full course of medicine, rigourously pursued, in proportion to the deadliness or violence of the disease, until
life becomes equalized through the body.   The whole
of the directions above given, is simply this.   A thorough
course of medicine administered with the best articles;
emetic seed, cayenne, drops, nerve powder, and bayberry, or No. 3.

Fever must have its course.

How consoling must these words be from the health-restoring physician, to his suffering patient, who wishes to know how long he must undergo those torturing administrations of poisonous physic, salivation, loss of teeth, together with bleeding and blistering! The doctor tells him that he does not know; perhaps nine days; some fevers run longer than others; and it must have its course! I have known a rich man's fever run a hundred days, when a poor man's fever would turn in ten days. The inflammatory fever, or hot fever, will soon come to its height, unless checked with small doses of calomel, opium, nitre, &c. which tend to prolong it. With these applications, the fever may be continued longer or shorter, as the money of the patient holds out.

Some times, before one fever turns, another will set in, until they have the whole list, *thirty-seven* and upwards. But the patient will be likely to die before he has had half of the above number of fevers. By this you may see that the doctor does not pretend to know any thing how long you will be sick, or whether you will live or die. Who, I would ask, has not heard part, if not all, of the above statements, made by the doctor to his patients, and yet not feel insulted at all?

Suppose you went to a landlord to doctor your hunger, and the landlord should tell you that your hunger must run from nine to a hundred days, would you not be disposed to cuff his ears for the insult? But is it not as much of an insult for the doctor to tell you that your fever must have its run, as for the landlord to tell you that your hunger must have its run? It would be so considered, if the people only knew that a fever can be relieved as certainly, and almost as speedily as hunger. In either case, it would be, as it is with the doctor, a plain confession that they have no remedy. Then why should the doctor continue his visits for a fee, any more than the landlord when he has no food? One is as much entitled to pick the pockets of his employers as the other. How long must custom and superstition become a law to ignorance and credulity?

18*

A remarkable Vision, seen in the Nineteenth Century, and published for the benefit of all who believe it a reality.

While in silent repose upon my bed, my mind was greatly agitated by a voice, which, in my dream, I heard saying, "Poor wretched inhabitants of a free country!" And I thought myself awake, and said, what is the cause of their wretchedness? As I spake, turning my eyes, I saw by my bed-side, a man clothed in a long white garment. I thought I said to him, who are you? He replied, "I am *Deception.*" I then said, why do you give yourself this odious name? He replied, "White denotes Purity, Innocence, and a Promoter of Health."

I then asked him what he was in reality; his reply was, "I am *Death* under the name of *Life;* or *Evil,* under the name of *Good.*" I then asked him to appear to me without any cover or disguise; this he did, by throwing off his white robe; all was blackness and darkness. I then asked him what he represented; he said "Death! and many of my victims you have known, and others you have lately heard of, and will continue to hear of them, until this mineral practice is changed. Many have I destroyed with my deadly weapons, some within a few days or hours."

After hearing all this, I asked him if he was a reality or not. He replied, "I am only the representative of many." This led me to inquire what he represented; to which he replied, "I shall call no names," and then showed me two pill bags, and said, "These, and what is inscribed on them, will teach you why I am *Death* under the name of *Life,* and why I kill under the name of preserving life." I then asked him what he meant by that inscription; he replied, "I mean those deadly weapons contained in the bags; the names of which are, according to the best of my recollection, *Arsenic, Mercury, Quinine, Opium, Nitre, Lancet,* and *Knife.*"

He then added, "These instruments of death are used under the pretence of curing diseases, or promoting life; and the men who use them, you know have been the cause of those who were so suddenly taken from their friends and all they held dear on earth:"

Having heard all this, I asked why he revealed this secret to me and not to another? He replied, "because I know you are able to write the particulars which are related to you." He added, "do not fail to publish what I have related; not only in this town, but in every direction; for this business of killing, under the name of healing, has gone far, and is going farther; for many have great wrath, because they think their time is short. Every thing which has been done here, and in other places, adapted to relieve the sick with the medicine of our country, which nature has so bountifully furnished, all these things have been despised, and those who kill others, cry, *Poison! Poison! Kill! Kill!*"

I asked him why they cried out in this manner, when so few died who used the medicine of our own country, and when so many fell under their deadly weapons? He replied, "you remember what I first stated; they will talk of pity, if one is likely to be cured, that they may kill him themselves. It is not strange for the eagle to cry death to birds, when the dove is among them, though he would gladly devour the dove with the other birds, were it in his power."

In my dream, I thought the one who spake to me, said, "I enjoin it on you to direct the people of the country, to keep in their libraries and reading rooms, three books* in use among those who use deadly weapons, viz. The New American Dispensatory, The Medical Dictionary, and The Medical Pocketbook."

"Lest you or any other may not happen to find what is said in the Dispensatory, concerning these deadly weapons, I now repeat a few words written there." He then handed me the following, page 285. Of *Nitre*, it is said, *This powerful salt, when inadvertantly taken in too large quantities, is one of the most fatal poisons.* Page 288, *Oxid of arsenic is one of the most sudden and violent poisons we are acquainted with.* The lancet we know the use of, and also mercury, which is called medicine, though poisonous.

* The first book shows how to prepare medicine; the second explains the dead languages; the third directs how much medicine or poison to give.

As these are so, how can people expect to be profited
by such articles as are acknowledged the most deadly
poison, though used as medicine, in the most difficult
cases ? After quoting these things from the Dispensatory, and making the above remarks, I thought that he
said, "do not fail to put them in mind of this important
question ; *What will become of your souls another day ?*
You must die as well as other men, and how can you
answer for the lives of those poor people who have died
in consequence of taking poison from your hands, under
the name of healing medicine ; while you have despised
the medicines which might have relieved them ; and especially when you did it for filthy lucre ?" When he had
said these words, he vanished, and I awoke, and behold
it was a dream.

Fearing I might forget these things, I arose immediately, and wrote down the vision according to my recollection ; and, as soon as possible, found the books mentioned, and to my great astonishment, found every word
in the Dispensatory, which had been related to me.

The dream, and what I found in the Dispensatory,
caused some serious reflections in my mind. I said thus
to myself ; If *arsenic, mercury*, and *nitre*, are in their
nature poison, can they in the hands of a physician, be
medicine ? If, when taken by accident, these things
kill, will they cure when given designedly ? Does not
mercury go to the same part of a man when taken by
accident, as when given by the doctor ? Surely it does ;
of course it will be poison, and be injurious whenever
it is taken.

These things are communicated to the public, that
they may judge of them according to the evidence given
of their being true or not.

CONCLUSION.

Dr. Thomson having gone into the State of New Hampshire, for a few weeks, and consequently left me, his Agent, to see to the completion of his work; and finding room in the Supplement to his Narrative, I embrace the opportunity to say a few words.

To the Public.

Friends of Humanity! You have seen by the foregoing Narrative, the labours, the trials, the persecutions, as well as the anxieties and vexations which the author has experienced in bringing his System of Medical Practice to the state of perfection to which it has arrived; and also in laying it fairly before the public; trials that would have broken down many hearts, and worn out, long before this, many constitutions.

You have seen the system growing into practice in spite of all opposition; not only against the inveterate hate of the doctors, but also against legal enactments; and that it is calculated to put to silence, and even to the blush, every species of opposition with all those who shall give it a fair trial. You have also seen those, after having tested the virtues of the system, and proved its value, who have been not only ready to rob Dr. Thomson of his hard earned reputation, and fair mead of praise, but also to build themselves up at his expense. All this you have seen, and much more. And it now remains to be seen whether either you, or the public, will any longer patronize, any longer uphold, any longer countenance, either directly or indirectly, such iniquity, such ingratitude, such shame-faced hypocrisy! How much better a person must feel to act in an open and honourable way! And were you sure that you could purchase the same thing, or nearly the same thing, of those who have no right to sell it, and might even use it with impunity, would you, for the sake of a few dollars, obtain it clandestinely, and thus rob the patentee of his just rights? It may be thought, perhaps, that Dr. Thomson has already become rich by his patent, and therefore can well afford to sustain these losses. Were this the fact, it is no good reason why he should be robbed. But you must consider the immense expense he has been at, and is still liable to bear, to defend his system of practice against legal enactments, and unfounded complaints; together with the losses he has sustained by unfaithful agents. This is a constant drawback upon his income. The defence of his legal prosecutions, and those of his agents, in far distant and remote states, as well as in almost every state in the Union, as in South Carolina, not long since; his answers to various slanders by hand-bills, the only way, at one time, that he could obtain any thing from the press in his favour, even for pay; and his various travels from the Eastern to the Western States, and from the North to the South; all, all these, and much more, are constant out-goes upon what should, and did the public duly appreciate the value of his system, other-wise would be his fair and honest gains. But he has one consolation.* His system will live to bless mankind, and his *name* will live with it, yea, be hailed with gratitude, when Dr. THOMSON shall be no more. Cold comfort this; when the subject or object of their gratitude shall be in his grave! Yet even this is better than nothing: and to know now, or to be firmly persuaded that such will be the fact, must afford some present peace, yea, a heart felt satisfaction. But I hope that it is not too late to do the subject of this Narrative justice, even in some measure, at least, now while he lives; to make the eve of his life as comfortable and happy as human nature, in a person of his years, is susceptible of being; and I can assure him and the public, that whatever I can do to bring about an event so just, and at the same time so desirable, shall be faithfully and cheerfully performed; for all that my life is now worth, either to myself, my family, or the public, I consider that both I and they are wholly indebted to the THOMSONIAN System of practice. And it is with much pleasure that I here once more have the opportunity of acknowledging the gratitude, and pledging the faithfulness of his and the public's humble servant,   ABNER KNEELAND,

General Agent for DR. SAMUEL THOMSON.

CONTENTS

To the Narrative of Samuel Thomson.

216   *Contents to the Narrative, &c.*

SUPPLEMENT

To the Third Edition of Thomson's Narrative,

Containing some new remarks which may be pleasing, if not profitable, to the reader; and add to the bigness of the book, if not to the stock of knowledge.

Cultivation of Bees.

As honey adds to the quality of medicine, as well as to enrich our food, I think a short treatise on this subject may add one particle to the stock of useful knowledge.

About twenty years of my life, from the age of from thirty to fifty years, I attended to the keeping of bees. I had a good farm, and used to calculate that the profits of a swarm of bees was as much as that of a cow.

After about fifteen years, I found that there was some lack on my part to enable them to be as industrious as was their nature and disposition; as it is obvious to every person who has paid any attention to the subject, as well as my own observation, that during the heat of the summer, and at a time when the white clover is mostly in bloom, from which more honey is obtained than all the other flowers of the field, that a great part of the bees are on the outside of the hive, and are idle. I then took the matter into consideration, to ascertain the cause why so industrious an insect as the bee should be idle in the best part of the season for making honey; and I found the fault to be in their owner, not in the bees. I had made their hive much too small, being only large enough for a quart of bees, when I had put in a swarm of nearly half a bushel; so that their hive was nearly one third full of bees, and thereby prevented them from having room to work. The space which was small at first, was soon filled with honey, and the bees that had no room were crowded on the outside, to give room for the rest. Hence the cause of all this idleness.

1

In the fall of the year, the owner of bees will try the weight of his hives, and if in any one he thinks there is not honey enough to winter the bees, he will take them up, and thus save from five to ten pounds of honey ; when at the same time, if the owner had made the hive large enough, so that all would have had room to work, they would have made from fifty to a hundred pounds of honey ; would have had enough to live on through the winter, or, if taken up, would have been a valuable prize to the owner.   This mode of raising bees is too much like the labour of mankind.   A few industrious ones labour, and many lazy or idle ones help eat up all the profits ; and if any starve, or are taken up, the industrious ones suffer as much as any ; with mankind, generally, more.   But to remedy this evil with bees, is much easier than to remedy it with mankind.

A few of the last years of my keeping bees, I made some improvement, in order to aid and assist this profitable insect in the making of honey.   I did it in the following manner.   Instead of making my hives to hold from a bushel to a bushel and a half, I made the first to hold three bushels, and put in a swarm from one of my small hives, and made my observations.   I noticed in the summer, that there were no idle bees.   In the fall, I found it heavy, but not full.   They wintered well. The next season, they worked well; but did not swarm. This hive did so well, I put a swarm into a four bushel hive this season.   They worked well until fall, at which time I found the other large hive, which had the work of two seasons, full.   I had previously learned that one good hog of eighteen months old, was worth more than three shoats at six months old.   I concluded to try the same rule with the bees.   I took up the old hive, and took out 160 pounds weight of the handsomest comb I ever saw.   I followed the same plan with the other large hive, and at eighteen months old, I found that full also. I then took it up, and took out two hundred weight of honey, equal to the other.   In this way I was satisfied that by putting a swarm into a large hive every year, and have one to take up, was as much better than to make small hives, as to have one good hog instead of two or three shoats.

I did not try the experiment long enough to know to what extent this mode of cultivating bees might be carried. But I am satisfied that if I had kept either of those swarms over, after they were full, that I should not only have had a swarm from that hive, but that they would have filled one of equal size the first season. Then by increasing the size of the hive to that of the swarm, and keeping but a few swarms, they may be all equally good. But be careful not to overstock; for bees may be starved in this way as well as other stock.

I will here relate an anecdote, which may be of use to some. At the time of my taking up my first large hive, we asked some neighbours in, to eat honey. I gave away about one hundred weight of honey, with biscuit and butter answerable. Before the season came round, I bought a few pounds in presence of one of the men who partook most liberally of the bounty. He asked, "Have you got rid of all your honey?" I replied, "Yes." "Why," said he, "you should not have been such a fool as to have given it all away." Here I made a notch in my memory. The next fall I took up my bees, and carried honey enough to Walpole, to fetch ten dollars. This I thought better than to be twitted for giving it away. However, in the course of the fall, I was in company with the same man; he asked, "Have you taken up your bees?" "Yes," was the answer. He rejoined, "And did you ask in the neighbours to eat honey?" My answer was, "No; I carried it to Walpole and sold it." He replied, "Why, they say you are a *hog* for not asking them." I replied, "You have learned me a lesson, which I had not thought of; when I gave my honey all away, I was a *fool*; and when I kept it, I was a *hog*; therefore, unless I am a hog at least half of the time, I cannot live." The conclusion is this. When a man begins the world, if he means to escape censure, he must observe a proper medium between being a *hog* and a *fool*, in the estimation of his neighbours, but if he has any thing which to them will be as sweet as honey, he must not keep all, nor give all away.

Question. Why is an industrious man in old age, like a hive well filled with honey, in the fall of the year?

Answer. Because all the drone bees who have been idle all summer, in time of harvest wish to eat as much honey in winter as those who laid it up. The old man, when he comes to be past labour, sees his children and grand-children hover round him, to suck the honey the old man has earned; and they are very apt to inquire of each other how much the old man is worth; begin to try the weight of his iron chest, or wherever he keeps his money, as the owner does his bee hives, and say, in a low voice, "Don't you think he has about done gaining? I fear he will begin to spend on the interest, if not on the capital. Now would be a good time to take him up, if it could be done and not expose ourselves." But the lesson of Mr. White, in Salem, who was taken up for the same purpose, will be a hard lesson to all such, during the present generation at least. What then is best to be done? I know of no better way than to let old people live as long as they can, and let them be as comfortable as they can, while they live; for notwithstanding the natural disposition of men, generally, is nearly the same, the risk in taking up old men prematurely, like taking up bees for the sake of their honey, is much greater than the risk that they will live, naturally, to spend all their earnings.

Every thing is in motion; all our hopes are in prospect, moving onward, nothing backward. The inquiry is, "How much will father leave for us?" not "what shall we do for our parents?" Hence it is wisdom, if a man has it, to keep enough in his own hands, for his own wants, and not to rely too much on the goodness of any one, even his own children.

When to set Fruit Trees, and lose no growth.

About the middle of October, trees have generally done growing for that season; yet they are still green and full of leaves. Taken up at this time, which is the most proper time, they will become well rooted before spring. It will be necessary to cut round and take up as much dirt as you conveniently can, and set the root well down in the ground, and pack it close, so that the wind will not shake them. A stake may be useful until they become well rooted. If the weather is dry, they should be watered often, for a few days. As soon as they will stand all day, without wilting, they are out of danger. They will get so rooted before spring, as to lose no growth; but will grow just as well as though they had not been moved. They are the most sure, if set when small.

Bad consequences of Stoves in Tight Rooms.

I visited a friend in Vermont, whose daughter was unwell; her bed was near a large stove in the kitchen, where the work of the house was done. While the doors were frequently opened, during the day, there appeared no bad effects from the dry air; but at evening, when the house was shut, the young woman grew much distressed, and about ten o'clock, she had a violent convulsion fit, and continued at intervals through the night. I was satisfied that the stove was the cause, or the dry air from it; but I could not convince the family that such was the fact. I tried to have her removed out of the room, and I succeeded in the course of the day. Her senses were gone, and her recollection did not return for some days. The cause I attribute to the water being dried out of the air, and her glands grew dry by inhaling the dry gas. In a healthy state we throw off moisture with the breath, and inhale as much more from the atmosphere. This keeps the lungs refreshed with moisture. When they grow dry, it causes fits.

I will here name another case, for further illustration or proof of this supposition. Mr. John M. Williams, of Baltimore, had a child taken sick about three o'clock in the morning. They got up, made a fire in the stove in the kitchen, and after administering to the child, put it in the cradle near the stove. They then proceeded to prepare their breakfast, and when it was ready, I came into the room, in which I could scarcely get my breath, it was so warm. All set round the table. The child in the cradle began to groan at every breath, and after continuing so for a short space, went into a convulsion fit.

1*

The family were much alarmed. I told them the fit was caused by the stove. I opened the door, the child was carried to it, the cry was, *what shall we do?* I told them to give it some of the 3d preparation. They tried to give it; but they spilled it in the bosom, as the jaws of the child were set. I told them to give me a spoon. I put my finger between the cheek and teeth, and poured in the liquid, and crowded it back to the throat, which let the jaws loose, and the child swallowed enough to make it vomit. The fit was off, and I ordered it into my chamber, where was a fire. It had no more fits. I followed it with medicine, and carried it through that forenoon. The senses of the child did not return till noon. The next day, it was well. So efficacious was the course pursued. One of the neighbours said, that he was glad the case happened; not on account of the child, but for the benefit of all present; for if I had not been there, they would not have known the cause of the fit. Had the child remained in the room, the probability is, it would not have lived till noon. And the cause being unknown, no remedy would have been known for others in a similar predicament.

There are similar cases from burning charcoal in a tight room, in which case, it sometimes happens that no sensible effect is experienced, till the senses of the person affected is gone. Others coming into the room, persons have been often found dead or senseless. As this is most generally the effect, it makes these cases the more alarming; and people ought to be more careful against such exposures. Men who work in furnaces in cold weather, and who often drink too much ardent spirits, and then crawl away under the roof, to find a warm place, have often suffered the same consequences by stupor or death.

Not many years ago, I was informed that in the hospital, the doctors had kept the rooms for the sick, to a certain warmth, by stoves, regulated by the thermometer, so that one sick person should have the same heat as another. This would not answer for all, even in a state of health. This plan, as I understand did not succeed. The patients died very fast, insomuch that the disorder was called the plague. They might have truly said, perhaps, the plague of the doctors! I understand that they have pulled down all their stoves, and substituted fire places, from which time the plague, of the stoves if you please, " was stayed." And should the plague of the poisons, and the bleeding, be stayed also, the people would have a greater cause for rejoicing than the Russians had at the defeat of Bonaparte, at the burning of Moscow. And should the fatal practice of bleeding and poison cease, and the people die with old age, the only cause of death, casualties excepted, naturally incident to man, then would death have a greater respit than it has had since the time the great butcher, Sydenham, first introduced the murderous practice of bleeding into the world. A certain writer says, " During the course of one hundred years, more died by the lancet alone, than all who perished by war in the same period." Another writer says, " The lancet has slain more than the sword, and mercury, more than powder and ball."

Value of Guards and Sentinels in War or Peace, and the danger of their Signals being neglected.

Guards and sentinels have been the principals of safety ever since human beings learned the art of war; and it is to this art of safety we are probably indebted for our independence. By this means was the treachery of Arnold detected, and the plots of our enemies defeated. And even in time of peace, when the enemy is either conquered or driven out, forts and breast works are still necessary, that they may be in readiness in time of war.

One of the greatest sentinels who have been set to guard the welfare of this nation, Thomas Jefferson, erected a permanent fort in the constitution, against the clergy, and the church and state party, who, were they not sufficiently guarded, would bring the people of this, as they have of other countries, under religious bondage. Another sentinel has recently distinguished himself, in defending the fort of Jefferson, against the church and state party, armed with their Sunday mail petitions; but they have been defeated by the watchful eye of Col. R. M. Johnson, armed with the constitution of equal rights.

Many useful lessons may be learned from the Scriptures; not excepting the Apocrypha; where we find some, to say the least, which are as useful as any other parts.   For this purpose I would refer the reader to the 13th chapter of Judith.

In this chapter may be found the result of silencing the guard, and sentinels, whereby through the deceit and influence of one woman, the destruction of a whole army, of about 160,000 soldiers, was effected.   No other possible means could have subdued them.   See the account.

I have referred to this chapter, to show what incalculable mischief may arise from such neglect; with a view at the same time to awaken the people from their drowsiness, and to arouse them to double their diligence in placing their guards and sentinels, or else stand themselves, to guard their rights and liberties, which are in as much danger of being destroyed ultimately, if not so speedily, as the great army under Holofernes, was, but a short time previous to their destruction.   And yet the people seem to rest as safely as did the army to which I have just alluded.

There is a power and influence as much to be guarded against now, as there was then, and the vigilance of all our guards will not be more than sufficient to protect the people.   Let them watch the secret workings of our enemies; especially those who appear as friends to our faces, and see what they are about in the dark.   Remember the light sayings and dark doings of Judith. While the army thought they were in safety, sudden destruction came upon them.

Look! See the rapid strides of the clergy!!   Behold all their secret working among the women and children of our land!!!   And the men have no sentinels to guard themselves.   I think we never had more need to be on our guard than at the present time.   As with the priest, so with the doctor; the people are crammed with the poison doctrines of the one, and the poison drugs of the other, without giving them any chance to examine and taste for themselves.   The priest crams them with his own ignorance and superstition; and the effects are delirium and suicide.   The doctor crams them with his

poison ; and the effects are pains, lingering sickness, and
death. When dead, the doctor often takes the whole,
or nearly the whole, of the little property remaining ;
and the widow and orphans become subjects of the poor-
house, or go out as servants. The question is, who is
to be blamed ? All, all are to be blamed. The priest,
the doctor, and the lawyer, for deceiving the people ;
and the people, for being deceived by them. But what
must *now* be the remedy ? Where it is not too late, the
remedy must be the same as it should have been in the
first place. But see.

Let us inquire, in the first place, what are the sentinels, both external and internal, which nature has placed
to guard the body from injury ? And how are these sentinels displayed ? We will suppose the danger is first
perceived by a certain sound, or some trifling noise.
This, of course, is first perceived by the ear, which says,
"Eyes, look !" The call is instantly obeyed ; and if
there appears to be danger, and flight is thought to be the
best mode of escape, the whole body is summoned, and
says, "Legs, carry me off as fast as you can." These
orders are obeyed as regularly as though a general gave
the command. The senses of seeing, hearing, tasting
and smelling, are the sentinels ; which, with the nerves
and muscles, constitute the whole army, either for defence or retreat ; and they are subject to the command
of each other.

The sentinels of the internal structure, or those which
are to judge of what is be swallowed, begin with the
eye ; and if it be pleasant to the eye, it passes to the
nose, the next sentinel ; if the *pass* be right, that is, if
the flavour be agreeable, it goes to the taste ; where, if
nothing disagreeable is perceived, it is carried from the
tongue to the swallow. Here are two roads, the one to
convey the food to the stomach, the other to convey the
air to the lungs ; the business of the sentinel here, is,
to prevent either from taking the wrong road ; for should
either, and especially the food, take the wrong road, it
is thrown back with a great explosion. When the food
is received into the stomach, it undergoes a general inspection. If any thing *treasonous*, that is, uncongenial
to health, is found in it, an uneasiness is almost the im-

mediate consequence, perhaps pain and sickness, and it is often sent back without consulting any of the guards or sentinels; for it is general orders. And if the general gives orders for any to pass or re-pass, without being hailed by the sentinels, such orders must be obeyed. And if the general loses his head, and thereby his whole army is defeated, it is no fault of the guards and sentinels, as in the case of Judith and Holofernes.

Nature has placed all the guards and sentinels in the body, which are necessary for its safety and protection; and the mind is so constituted, that it is capable of judging of all the signals which these sentinels give; but the devil, which is only another name for imposture and fraud, that is, learned ignorance, falsehood and art, are always at variance with simple and natural principles; the same as honesty and dishonesty are opposed to each other. Now, of what use is such reasoning to the people? None, until they can be brought back to a simple state of nature. Here the devil, or false learning, under the name of doctor, with his elegant cloak and powdered head, comes in and upsets the whole system of plain simple truth, and introduces his learned falsehood. Tells the people that those sentinels which nature has set in the body are all false; learning is the only true guide; and urges them to throw by all their natural ideas, and hear to learning, popular customs and fashions; and then they will be respected by the popular classes; that is, by the doctor, minister and lawyer, and the great dons around whom those learned professions fawn, and whom they like to flatter. Pay us, and we will attend to your most important concerns. Attend to your labour in building our houses, and making our rich clothing and furniture; cultivate the soil; raise the fatted calf, the poultry, and the flour, to feed us; and we will pray for your souls, doctor your bodies, and make your wills. You must not attempt to do any of these things for yourselves, for you have not sufficient learning.

Now, look, fellow labourers, and see to what a condition these three learned crafts have brought you at the present day. The learned doctor has knocked down all your natural sentinels, and has passed the poison down your throats as though it was as innocent as breast-milk is for the infant, until you are dying off like swarms of rats, and with the same poison. Then, in addition to the poison, he draws out your blood, to cure, as does the butcher the blood of the beast, to kill; and which often produces the same effect. This is what you have gained by suffering the doctors to knock down all your natural sentinels, and to substitute learned fools whose senses are below the grade of the beast. When the beast tries his food, by the sentinels of the eye and nose, he is never deceived. Nature always tells the truth. And when wild beasts go according to the dictates of nature, they are more successful in raising their offspring than are mankind in raising theirs by art. For the beast will neither eat poison themselves, nor force it down the throats of their offspring. But mankind, by the prejudice of false learning, will both eat poison themselves, and force it down the throats of their children till they by this means execute death upon them in their own arms. This is done by giving wine poisoned with antimony, or the tartrite of antimony, called tartar-emetic. So much is mankind reduced below the grade of the beast by the force of education. Were parents to take a lesson from a child two years old, and abide by it, it would be of greater use to the rising generation than all that ever came from the college by the three crafts I have named. It will be remembered that a child of two years old is troubled and makes a mournful complaint at the sight of blood, from the slightest wound, even if he feels no smart from it; or when taken by a doctor from another. His senses tell him that there is something wrong in it, and applies to those whom he thinks his friends, to remedy the evil. The child is not only afraid of the blood, but also of the doctor who takes it. Should parents from this lesson, learn to keep the doctor away, and to keep the blood in the body, where it belongs, for the preservation of life and health, for the space of twenty years, then visit the grave-yard, and examine the monuments of the dead, and see if three-fourths of the inhabitants died under thirty years of age, this, I think, would strike conviction to the deluded world.

I return to my text. The sentinels of life and preservation, as before mentioned, in the brute animals, never
deceive them. There is none found dead by poison,
either accidental or done on purpose. Their sentinels
have been true to them. Not so among the dupes of
learned ignorance, where they allow their sentinels to
be knocked down by the doctor, and poison to be crammed down their throats; for unless the general government of the stomach should so condemn his prescriptions as to throw the poison back in spite of him, the
patient must suffer; his sufferings may be long, but generally fatal; and his body will be carried out by the sex-
ton, in a coffin, as was the head of Holofernes, in the
bag, by Judith. Neither is this the greatest evil, caused
by these artificial monsters in human shape. How often
do we see our children sacrificed by being born artifi-
cially, instead of naturally? aided by the pincers of the
assassin, instead of the skilful hand of the midwife. All
their art, is to force nature, instead of assisting her.
These are some of the effects of learning, which termi-
nate in death. But there are others never to be forgotten. Cripples and invalids, dragging out a miserable
life, reduced almost to a state of starvation, for those
who survive their unnatural practice. Besides a tribute
of twenty dollars for destroying the comfort of a wife
and the life of a child! Yet the eyes of the people are
blinded by the sound of the word *learning*, and *learned
doctor;* and doubly blinded by the priest, or the parson,
who will clear the doctor from all blame, by saying, "the
Lord gave, and the Lord," not the doctor, "hath taken
away, and blessed" not cursed, "be the name of the Lord."
Had the priest declared, as often as it was really the
case, that in all probability the poison, bleeding and
blistering, had killed the patient, the doctor craft would
have been dead more than a thousand years ago.

Were it possible for mankind to be brought back to
his proper grade, that of other animals, and at the same
time to exercise all their natural faculties, and have their
sentinels which have been knocked down by the doctor
restored, so as to be as good as those of the beasts, so
that the sentinel of the eye and nose would regulate
their food and medicine, and prevent any poison being

NEW

GUIDE TO HEALTH;

OR,

BOTANIC FAMILY PHYSICIAN,

CONTAINING

A COMPLETE SYSTEM OF PRACTICE,

On a Plan entirely New;

WITH A DESCRIPTION OF THE VEGETABLES MADE USE
OF, AND DIRECTIONS FOR PREPARING AND ADMIN-
ISTERING THEM, TO CURE DISEASE.

TO WHICH IS ADDED,

A DESCRIPTION OF SEVERAL CASES OF DISEASE
ATTENDED BY THE AUTHOR, WITH THE MODE
OF TREATMENT AND CURE.

Third Edition.

———————

BY SAMUEL THOMSON.

———————

Boston:
PRINTED FOR THE AUTHOR, BY J. HOWE.
1831..

TO THE PUBLIC.

The preparing the following work for the press has been a task of much difficulty and labour; for to comprise in a short compass, and to convey a correct understanding of the subject, from such a mass of materials as I have been enabled to collect by thirty years practice, is a business of no small magnitude. The plan that has been adopted I thought the best to give a correct knowledge of my system of practice; and am confident that the descriptions and directions are sufficiently explained to be understood by all those who take an interest in this important subject. Much more might have been written; but the main object has been to confine it to the practice, and nothing more is stated of the theory, than what was necessary to give a general knowledge of the system. If any errors should be discovered, it is hoped that they will be viewed with candour; for in first publishing a work, such things are to be expected; but much care has been taken that there should be no error, which would cause any mistake in the practice, or preparing the medicine.

Many persons are practising by my system, who are in the habit of pretending that they have made great improvements, and in some instances, it is well known that poisonous drugs have been made use of under the name of my medicine, which has counteracted its operation, and thereby tended to destroy the confidence of the public in my system of practice; this has never been authorized by me. The public are therefore cautioned

against such conduct, and all those who are well disposed towards my system, are desired to lend their aid in
exposing all such dishonest practices, in order that justice may be done.   Those who possess this work, may,
by examining it, be able to detect any improper deviations therefrom; and they are assured that any practice
which is not conformable to the directions given, and
does not agree with the principles herein laid down, is
unauthorized by me.

AGREEMENT.

THE Subscriber, who is the discoverer and proprietor
of the system of medical practice contained in this work,
agrees to give, whenever applied to, any information,
that shall be necessary to give a complete understanding of the obtaining, preparing and using all such vegetables as are made use of in said system, to all those
who purchase the right; and the purchasers, in consideration of the above information, and also what is
contained in this book, agree in the spirit of mutual interest and honour not to reveal any part of said information, to any person, except those who purchase the right,
to the injury of the proprietor, under the penalty of for-
feiting their word and honour, and all right to the use
of the medicine.   And every person who purchases the
right, is to be considered a member of the Friendly
Botanic Society, and entitled to a free intercourse with
the members for information and friendly assistance.

SAMUEL THOMSON.

NEW GUIDE TO HEALTH;

OR,

BOTANIC FAMILY PHYSICIAN.

INTRODUCTION.

THERE are three things which have in a greater or
less degree, called the attention of men, viz. Religion,
Government, and Medicine.   In ages past, these things
were thought by millions to belong to three classes of
men, Priests, Lawyers, and Physicians.   The Priests held
the things of religion in their own hands, and brought
the people to their terms ; kept the Scriptures in the
dead languages, so that the common people could not
read them.   Those days of darkness are done away ;
the Scriptures are translated into our own language, and
each one is taught to read for himself.   Government was
once considered as belonging to a few, who thought
themselves "born only to rule:"   The common people
have now become acquainted. with the great secret of
government, and know that "all men are born free and
equal," and that Magistrates are put in authority, or
out, by the voice of the people, who choose them for
their public servants.
While these, and many other things are brought where
"common people" can understand them ; the knowledge and use of medicine, is in a great measure conceal-
ed in a dead language, and a sick man is often obliged
to risk his life, where he would not risk a dollar ; and
should the apothecary or his apprentice make a mistake,

1*

the sick man cannot correct it, and thus is exposed to receive an instrument of death, instead of that which would restore him to health had he known good medicine.

" It may be alleged," said Dr. Buchan, " that laying medicine more open to mankind, would lessen their faith in it. This indeed would be the case with regard to some; but it would have a quite contrary effect upon others. I know many people who have the utmost dread and horror of every thing prescribed by a physician, who will nevertheless, very readily take a medicine which they know, and whose qualities they are in some measure acquainted with."

"Nothing ever can, or will inspire mankind with an absolute confidence in physicians but by their being open, frank, and undisguised in their behaviour."

" The most effectual way to destroy quackery in any art or science, is to diffuse the knowledge of it among mankind. Did physicians write their prescriptions in the common language of the country, and explain their intentions to the patient, as far as he could understand them, it would enable them to know when the medicine had the desired effect; would inspire him with absolute confidence in the physician; and would make him dread and detest every man who pretended to cram a secret medicine or poison down his throat."

It is true that much of what is at this day called medicine, is deadly poison; and were people to know what is offered them of this kind, they would absolutely refuse ever to receive it as a medicine. This I have long seen and known to be true; and have laboured hard for many years to convince them of the evils that attend such a mode of procedure with the sick; and have turned my attention to those medicines that grow in our own country, which Nature has prepared for the benefit of mankind. Long has a general medicine been sought for, and I am confident I have found such as are universally applicable in all cases of disease, and which may be used with safety and success, in the hands of the people.

After thirty years study, and repeated successful trials of the medicinal vegetables of our own country, in all the diseases incident to our climate: I can with well grounded assurance, recommend my system of practice and medicines to the public, as salutary and efficacious.

Great discoveries and improvements have been made in various arts and sciences since the first settlement of our country, while its medicines have been very much neglected. As these medicines, suited to every disease, grow spontaneously upon our own soil; as they are better adapted to the constitution; as the price of imported drugs is very high; it follows, whether we consult health which is of primary importance, or expense, a decided preference should be given to the former, as an object of such magnitude as no longer to be neglected. Yet in the introduction of those medicines I have been violently opposed, and my theory and practice condemned, notwithstanding the demonstrative proofs in their favour. But those who thus condemn have taken no pains to throw off prejudice, and examine the subject with candour and impartiality. Such as have, are thoroughly satisfied of their utility and superior excellence.

From those who measure a man's understanding and ability to be beneficial to his fellow men only from the acquisition he has made in literature from books; from such as are governed by outward appearance, and who will not stoop to examine a system on the ground of its intrinsic merit, I expect not encouragement, but opposition. But this will not discourage me. I consider the discovery I have made, of inestimable value to mankind, and intended for the great benefit of those who are willing to receive it.

. Being born in a new country, at that time almost a howling wilderness, my advantages for an education were very small; but possessing a natural gift for examining the things of Nature, my mind was left entirely free to follow that inclination, by inquiring into the meaning of the great variety of objects around me.

Possessing a body like other men, I was led to inquire into the nature of the component parts of what man is made. I found him composed of the four elements—Earth, Water, Air and Fire. The earth and water I found were the solids; the air and fire the fluids. The two first I found to be the component parts; the two last kept him in motion. Heat, I found, was life; and

Cold, death.   Each one who examines into it will find
that all constitutions are alike.   I shall now describe the
fuel which continues the fire, or life of man.   This is contained in two things, food and medicines; which are in
harmony with each other; often grow in the same field,
to be used by the same people.   People who are capable
of raising their food, and preparing the same, may as
easily learn to collect and prepare all their medicines
and administer the same when it is needed.   Our life
depends on heat; food is the fuel that kindles and continues that heat.   The digestive powers being correct,
causes the food to consume; this continues the warmth
of the body, by continually supporting the fire.

The stomach is the deposit from which the whole body
is supported.   The heat is maintained in the stomach
by consuming the food; and all the body and limbs receive their proportion of nourishment and heat from that
source; as the whole room is warmed by the fuel which
is consumed in the fire place.   The greater the quantity
of wood consumed in the fire place, the greater the heat
in the room.   So in the body; the more food, well digested, the more heat and support through the whole
man.   By constantly receiving food into the stomach,
which is sometimes not suitable for the best nourishment,
the stomach becomes foul, so that the food is not well
digested.   This causes the body to lose its heat; then
the appetite fails; the bones ache, and the man is sick
in every part of the whole frame.

This situation of the body shows the need of medicine, and the kind needed; which is such as will clear
the stomach and bowels, and restore the digestive powers.
When this is done, the food will raise the heat again, and
nourish the whole man.   All the art required to do this
is, to know what medicine will do it, and how to administer it, as a person knows how to clear a stove and the
pipe when clogged with soot, that the fire may burn free,
and the whole room be warmed as before.

The body, after being cleared of whatever clogs it,
will consume double the food, and the food will afford
double the nourishment and heat, that it did before.   We
know that our life depends on food, and the stomach being in a situation to receive and digest it.   When the

stomach and bowels are clogged, all that is needed, is, the most suitable medicine to remove the obstructions in the system. All disease is caused by clogging the system; and all disease is removed by restoring the digestive powers, so that food may keep up that heat on which life depends.

I have found by experience, that the learned doctors are wrong in considering fever a disease or enemy; the fever is a friend, and cold the enemy. This I found by their practice in my family, until they had five times given them over to die. Exercising my own judgment, I followed after them, and relieved my family every time. After finding a general principle respecting fevers, and reducing that to practice, I found it sure in all disease, where there was any nature left to build on, and in three years constant practice, I never lost one patient.

I attended on all the fevers peculiar to our country, and always used it as a friend, and that returned the gratitude to the patient. I soon began to give this information to the people, and convinced many that they might as certainly relieve themselves of their disease, as of their hunger. The expense to them to be always able to relieve themselves and families, would be but small; and the medicine they may procure and prepare themselves.

This greatly disturbed the learned doctors, and some of them undertook to destroy me, by reporting that I used poison; though they made no mention of my using their instruments of death, Mercury, Opium, Ratsbane, Nitre, and the lancet. I considered it my duty to withstand them, though I found my overthrow was what they aimed at. A plan was once laid to take me in the night, but I escaped. Next I was indicted as though I had given poison, and a bill brought against me for wilful murder. I was bound in irons and thrust into prison, to be kept there through the winter, without being allowed bail. I petitioned for and obtained a special court to try the cause, and was honourably acquitted, after forty days imprisonment. I maintained my integrity in the place where my persecution began. In five years, while vindicating this new and useful discovery, I lost five thousand dollars, besides all the persecution, trouble, loss of health, and reproach which has been in connection with the losses.

It has been acknowledged, even by those who are un-
friendly to me and my practice, that my medicine may
be good in some particular cases, but not in all.   But
this is an error.   For there are but two great principles
in the constitution of things, whether applied to the mind
or body ; the principle of life and the principle of death.
That which contains the principle of life, may be perverted, by a misapplication, into an administration of
death ; as the stomach may be overloaded, and injured,
even by wholesome food; but nothing that is wholesome
in any case, unless abused, can be even tortured into an
administration of death.   If, then, a medicine is good in
any case, it is because it is agreeable to nature, or this
principle of life, the very opposite of disease.   If it is
agreeable in one case, it must be absolutely so in all.
By the active operation of nature, the whole animal
economy is carried on ; and the father of the healing
art, Hippocrates, tells us, what is an obvious truth, that
Nature is heat.   The principle is the same in all, differing only in degree.   When disease invades the frame,
it resists in proportion to its force, till overpowered into
submission, and when extinguished, death follows, and
it ceases to operate alike in all.   If then, heat is life,
and its extinction death, a diminution of this vital flame
in every instance, constitutes disease, and is an ap-
proximation to death.   All then, that medicine can do
in the expulsion of disorder, is to kindle up the decaying spark, and restore its energy till it glows in all its
wonted vigour.   If a direct administration can be made
to produce this effect, and it can, it is evidently immaterial what is the name, or colour of the disease, whether
bilious, yellow, scarlet or spotted ; whether it is simple
or complicated; or whether nature has one enemy or
more.   Names are arbitrary things, the knowledge of
a name is but the cummin and annis, but in the knowledge of the origin of a malady, and its antidote, lies
the weightier matters of this science.   This knowledge makes the genuine physician ; all without it is real
quackery.

It has been a general opinion that extensive study and
great erudition, are necessary to form the eminent physician.   But all this may be as Paul saith, but science,

falsely so called.   A man may have a scientific knowledge of the human frame, he may know the names in every language of every medicine, mineral and vegetable, as well as every disease, and yet be a miserable physician.   But there have been men without this to boast of, from the earliest ages of the world, who have " arisen, blest with the sublimer powers of genius, who have as it were, with one look pierced creation, and with one comprehensive view, grasped the whole circle of science, and left learning itself, toiling after them in vain."   A man never can be great without intellect, and he never can more than fill the measure of his capacity. There is a power beyond the reach of art, and there are gifts that study and learning can never rival.

The practice of the regular physicians, that is those who get a diploma, at the present time, is not to use those means which would be most likely to cure disease ; but to try experiments upon what they have read in books, and to see how much a patient can bear without producing death.   After pursuing this plan during their lives, they know just about as much as they did when they began to practice, of what is really useful to mankind.   If a patient dies under their hands, why, it is the will of God, and they are sure to get extravagantly paid for their trouble, and nothing more is said about it ; but if one out of hundreds of my patients die, and where the doctors have given them over as incurable, they at once cry out, that it is quackery, that I gave them poison, &c. for the purpose of running me and my medicine down, and to prevent its being used by the people.   The fact is well known to thousands who have used my medicine, and to which they are ready to attest, that it is perfectly harmless, and I defy the faculty to produce one instance wherein it has had any bad effects.

It is true that the study of anatomy, or structure of the human body, and of the whole animal economy is pleasing and useful ; nor is there any objection to this, however minute and critical, if it is not to the neglect of first great principles, and the weightier matters of knowledge. But it is no more necessary to mankind at large, to qualify them to administer relief from pain and sickness, than to a cook in preparing food to satisfy hunger and nourish-

ing the body.   There is one general cause of hunger
and one general supply of food; one general cause of
disease, and one general remedy.   One can be satisfied,
and the other removed, by an infinite variety of articles,
best adapted to those different purposes.   That medicine,
therefore, that will open obstruction, promote perspiration, and restore digestion, is suited to every patient,
whatever form the disease assumes, and is universally
applicable.   And acute disorders, such as fevers, colicks,
and dysentery, may be relieved thereby, in twenty-four
or forty-eight hours, at most.

REMARKS ON FEVERS.

Much has been said and written upon fevers, by the
professedly learned Doctors of Medicine, without throwing the most profitable light on the subject, or greatly
benefiting mankind.   They have been abundantly fruit-
ful in inventing names for disease, and with great care
and accuracy distinguished the different symptoms; but
they appear quite barren as to the knowledge of their
origin and remedy.   To the first, but little importance,
comparatively speaking, can be attached; the latter is of
the highest importance to all classes of people.

According to the writings of learned Physicians, there
are a great variety of fevers, some more and some less
dangerous.   But to begin with a definition of the NAME.
What is fever?   Heat, undoubtedly, though a disturbed
operation of it.   But is there in the human frame, more
than one kind of heat?   Yes, says the physician, strange
as it may appear, there is the pleuritic heat, the slow
nervous heat, the putrid heat, the hectic heat, the yellow
heat, the spotted or cold heat, the typhus or ignorant
heat, and many other heats; and sometimes, calamitous
to tell, one poor patient has the most, or the whole of
these fevers, and dies at last for want of heat!

Is fever or heat a disease?   Hippocrates, the acknowledged father of physicians, maintained that nature is
heat; and he is correct.   Is nature a disease?   Surely
it is not.   What is commonly called fever, is the effect,
and not the cause of disease.   It is the struggle of nature to throw off disease.   The cold causes an obstruc-

tion, and fever arises in consequence of that obstruction
to throw it off. This is universally the case. Remove
the cause, the effect will cease. No person ever yet
died of a fever! for as death approaches, the patient
grows cold, until in death, the last spark of heat is extinguished. This the learned doctors cannot deny; and
as this is true, they ought, in justice, to acknowledge that
their whole train of depletive remedies, such as bleeding, blistering, physicking, starving, with all their refrig-
eratives; their opium, mercury, arsenic, antimony, nitre,
&c. are so many deadly engines, combined with the disease, against the constitution and life of the patient. If
cold, which is the commonly received opinion, and which
is true, is the cause of fever, to repeatedly bleed the patient, and administer mercury, opium, nitre, and other
refrigerents to restore him to health, is as though a man
should, to increase a fire in his room, throw a part of it
out of the house, and to increase the remainder, put on
water, snow and ice!

As it is a fact, that cannot be denied, that fever takes
its rise from one great cause or origin, it follows of
course, that one method of removing that cause, will
answer in all cases; and the great principle is to assist
nature, which is heat.

At the commencement of a fever, by direct and proper
application of suitable medicine, it can be easily and
speedily removed, and the patient need not be confined
long. Twenty-four or forty-eight hours, to the extent,
are sufficient, and often short of that time, the fever may
be removed, or that which is the cause of it. But where
the patient is left unassisted, to struggle with the disease,
until his strength is exhausted, and more especially, when
the most unnatural and injurious administrations are
made if a recovery is possible, it must of necessity take
a longer time. These declarations are true, and have
been often proved, and can be again, to the satisfaction
of every candid person, at the hazard of any forfeiture
the faculty may challenge.

Notwithstanding all these things, how true are the
words of the intelligent Dr. Hervey, who says, "By what
unaccountable perversity in our frame does it appear,
that we set ourselves so much against any thing that is

new? Can any one behold, without scorn, such drones
of physicians, and after the space of so many hundred
years experience and practice of their predecessors, not
one single medicine has been detected, that has the least
force directly to prevent, to oppose, and expel a continued fever? Should any, by a more sedulous observation,
pretend to make the least step towards the discovery of
such remedies, their hatred and envy would swell against
him, as a legion of devils against virtue; the whole
society will dart their malice at him, and torture him
with all the calumnies imaginable, without sticking at
any thing that should destroy him root and branch. For
he who professes to be a reformer of the art of physic,
must resolve to run the hazard of the martyrdom of his
reputation, life and estate."

The treatment which the writer has received from
some of the learned physicians, since his discovery of
the remedy for the fever, and various other diseases, is
a proof of the truth of this last saying of Dr. Hervey.
They have imprisoned him, and charged him with every
thing cruel and unjust; though upon a fair trial, their
violent dealings have come down upon their heads;
while he has not only been proved innocent before the
court, but useful; having relieved many which the other
physicians had given over to die.

I will now take notice of the yellow fever. The cause
of this fatal disease is similar to the spotted fever. The
cause of death in the latter, is in consequence of its
producing a balance by cold, outward and inward; and
in the former there is a balance of heat outward and inward; both produce the same thing, that is a total cessa-
tion of motion, which is death. The colour of the skin
has given name to both these diseases. The yellow is
caused by the obstruction of the gall; instead of being
discharged through its proper vessels, it is forced and
diffused through the pores of the skin. The same effects that are produced by these two fevers may be observed in the motion of the sea; when the tide is done
running up, there is what is called slack water, or a
balance of power, and the same thing takes place when
it is done running down; when the fountain is raised,
the water runs from it; but when it is lowered the water

runs towards it. The same cause produces the same effects in the spotted and yellow fevers; for when a balance of power between the outward and inward heat takes place, death follows.

Having described the two kinds of fever which are the most alarming, they being most fatal, I shall pass over those of a less alarming nature, and merely observe, that there is no other difference in all cases of fever, than what is caused by the different degrees of cold, or loss of inward heat, which are two adverse parties in one body, contending for power. If the heat gains the victory, the cold will be disinherited, and health will be restored; but on the other hand, if cold gains the ascendency, heat will be dispossessed of its empire, and death will follow of course. As soon as life ceases, the body becomes cold, which is conclusive evidence that its gaining the victory is the cause of death. When the power of cold is nearly equal to that of heat, the fever or strife between the two parties, may continue for a longer or shorter time, according to circumstances; this is what is called a long fever, or fever and ague. The battle between cold and heat will take place periodically, sometimes every day, at other times, every other day, and they will leave off about equal, heat keeping a little the upper hand. In attempting to cure a case of this kind, we must consider whether the fever is a friend or an enemy; if it is a friend, which I hold to be the fact, when the fever fit is on, increase the power of heat; in order to drive off the cold, and life will bear the rule; but, on the contrary, should cold be considered a friend, when the cold fit is on, by increasing its power, you drive off the heat, and death must ensue. Thus you may promote life or death, by tempering cold and heat.

Much has been said by the doctors concerning the turn of a fever, and how long a time it will run. When it is said that a fever will turn at such a time, I presume it must mean that it has been gone; this is true, for it is then gone on the outside, and is trying to turn again and go inside, where it belongs. Instead of following the dictates of nature and aiding it to subdue the cold; the doctor uses all his skill to kill the fever. How, I would ask, in the name of common sense, can any thing turn when killed? Support the fever and it will return in-side; the cold, which is the cause of disease, will be driven out, and health will be restored. In all cases called fever, the cause is the same in a greater or less de-gree, and may be relieved by one general remedy. The cold causes canker, and before the canker is seated, the strife will take place between cold and heat; and while the hot flashes and cold chills remain, it is evidence that the canker is not settled, and the hot medicine alone, oc-casionally assisted by steam, will throw it off; but as the contest ceases, the heat is steady on the outside; then canker assumes the power inside; this is called a settled fever. The truth is, the canker is fixed on the inside and will ripen and come off in a short time, if the fever is kept up so as to overpower the cold. This idea is new and never was known till my discovery. By raising the fever with Nos. 1 and 2, and taking off the canker with No. 3, and the same given by injections, we may turn a fever when we please; but if this is not understood, the canker will ripen and come off itself, when the fever will turn and go inside and the cold will be driven out; there-fore they will do much better without any aid, than with a doctor. The higher the fever runs, the sooner the cold will be subdued; and if you contend against the heat, the longer will be the run of the fever, and when killed, death follows.

When a patient is bled, it lessens the heat and gives double power to the cold; like taking out of one side of the scale, and putting it in the other, which doubles the weight, and turns the scale in favor of the disease. By giving opium it deadens the feelings; the small doses of nitre and calomel tend to destroy what heat remains, and plants new crops of canker, which will stand in different stages in the body, the same as corn planted in the field every week, will keep some in all stages; so is the dif-ferent degrees in canker. This is the reason why there are so many different fevers as are named; when one fever turns another sets in and so continues one after another un-til the harvest is all ripe, if the season is long enough; if not, the cold and frost takes them off—then it is said they died of a fever. It might with as much propriety be said that the corn killed with frost, died with the heat. The question, whether the heat or cold killed the patient, is easily decided, for that power which bears rule in the body after death is what killed the patient, which is cold; as much as that which bears rule when he is alive is heat. When a person is taken sick, it is common to say I have got a cold, and am afraid I am going to have a fever; but no fears are expressed of the cold he has taken; neither is it mentioned when the cold left him. The fashionable practice is to fight the remains of heat till the patient dies, by giving cold the victory; in which case is it not a fact that the doctor assists the cold to kill the patient? Would it not have been more reasonable, or likely to have cured them, when the fever arose to throw off the cold, to have helped the fever and give nature the victory over its enemy, when the health would be restored the same as before they took the cold.

We frequently see in the newspapers accounts of people dying in consequence of drinking cold water when very warm. Some fall dead instantly, and others linger for several hours, the doctors have not been able to afford any relief when called. The principal symptoms are chills, and shivering with cold, which is viewed with astonishment by those who witness it. Proper caution should always be observed by persons when very warm and thirsty, who go to a pump to drink, by swallowing something hot before drinking the water, and swallowing a little at a time, which will prevent any fatal effects.

This strange circumstance of being cold on a hot day, and which has never been accounted for in a satisfactory manner to the public, I shall endeavour to explain in as comprehensive and plain language as I am capable. The component parts of animal bodies are earth and water, and life and motion are caused by fire and air. The inward heat is the fountain of life, and as much as that has the power above the outward heat, so much we have of life and strength, and when we lose this power of heat, our strength and faculties decay in proportion; and it is immaterial whether we lose this power by losing the inward heat or raising the outward heat above it, as the effect is the same. If you raise the stream level with the fountain, it stops the current, and all motion will cease,

2*

and the same effects will follow by lowering the fountain
to a level with the stream. When the outward heat becomes equal with the inward, either by the ones being
raised, or the others being lowered, cold assumes the
power, and death takes place.

The cause of the fatal effects by drinking cold water,
is because the fountain of life is lost by the stream being raised above the fountain, or the inward heat lowered by throwing into the stomach so large a quantity of
cold water as to give the outward heat the power of bal-
ancing the inward, and in proportion as the one approaches to an equality with the other, so the strength is
diminished, and when equal, they die.

I shall now make some further remarks on this and
other subjects, with a hope that it may be beneficial to
mankind. The reason why these extraordinary cases
appear so wonderful to the people, is because they are
unacquainted with the cause. Why should we wonder
at a person being cold on a hot day, when we are not,
any more than we should wonder at another being hun-
gry, when we have just been eating; or that others
can be in pain, when we are enjoying good health?
The one is as plain and simple as the other, when understood. The want of inward heat is the cause of their
being cold, just as much as the want of food is the
cause of hunger, or the want of health is the cause of
pain. One person may have lost the natural power of
heat, by an effect which others in similar situations may
not have experienced, and will suffer the consequences
of cold in proportion to the loss of inward heat; this is
manifest in the different degrees of sickness. If the
inward heat loses its balance of power suddenly, death
is immediate; which is the case in spotted fever, and in
drowned persons. When the inward and outward cold
is balanced, life ceases, and the blood being stopped in
its motion, settles in spots, which appearance has given
name to what is called spotted fever. The same appearances take place on drowned persons, and from the
same cause.

The practice of bleeding for the purpose of curing
disease, I consider most unnatural and injurious. Nature never furnishes the body with more blood than is

necessary for the maintenance of health; to take away part of the blood, therefore, is taking away just so much of their life, and is as contrary to nature, as it would be to cut away part of their flesh. Many experiments have been tried by the use of the lancet in fevers; but I believe it will be allowed by all, that most of them have proved fatal; and several eminent physicians have died in consequence of trying the experiment on themselves. If the system is diseased, the blood becomes as much diseased as any other part; remove the cause of the disorder, and the blood will recover and become healthy as soon as any other part; but how taking part of it away can help to cure what remains, can never be reconciled with common sense.

There is no practice used by the physicians that I consider more inconsistent with common sense, and at the same time more inhuman than blistering, to remove disease; particularly insane persons, or what the doctors call dropsy on the brain; in which cases they shave the head and draw a blister on it. Very few patients, if any, ever survive this application. What would be thought if a scald should be caused by boiling water to remove disease? Yet there is no difference between this and a blister made by flies. I have witnessed many instances where great distress and very bad effects have been caused by the use of blisters; and believe I can truly say that I never knew any benefit derived from their use. It very frequently causes stranguary, when the attempted remedy becomes much worse than the disease.

In support of my opinions on the subject, I will give the following extract from the writings of Dr. Hillary, an eminent physician of London.

" I have long observed that blisters are too frequently, and too often improperly used, as they are now so much in fashion. It is very probable, that we have no one remedy, in all the *Materia Medica*, that is so frequently, and so often improperly applied, not only in too many cases, where they cannot possibly give any relief, but too often where they must unavoidably increase the very evil, which they are intended to remove or relieve. How often do we see them applied, and sometimes several of them, by pretended dabblers in physic, not only where

there are no indications for applying them, but where
the true indication are against their application ; as,
in the beginning of most fevers, and especially those
of the inflammatory, and of the putrid kind, where, in
the first, the stimulous of the acrid salts of the *cantharides*, which pass into the blood, must unavoidably increase, both the stimulous, and the momentum of the
blood, which were too great before, and so render the
fever inflammatory, and all its symptoms worse.

"And it is well known that the *cantharides* contain
a great quantity of alkaline semi-volatile salts, which
pass into the blood, though they are applied externally ;
and attenuate, dissolve, and hasten, and increase its putrefaction, which is also confirmed by the putrid alkaline acrimony which they produce in the urine, with
the heat and stranguary, which it gives to the urinary
passage."

ON STEAMING.

Steaming is a very important branch of my system of
practice, which would in many cases without it, be insufficient to effect a cure.   It is of great importance in
many cases, but considered by the medical faculty as
desperate ; and they would be so under my mode of
treatment, if it was not for this manner of applying heat
to the body, for the purpose of reanimating the system
and aiding nature in restoring health.   I had but little
knowledge of medicine, when through necessity, I discovered the use of steaming, to add heat or life to the
decaying spark ; and with it I was enabled by administering such vegetable preparations as I then had a knowledge of, to effect a cure in cases where the regular practitioners had given them over.

In all cases where the heat of the body is so far exhausted as not to be rekindled by using the medicine
and being shielded from the surrounding air by a blanket,
or being in bed, and chills or stupor attend the patient,
then applied heat by steaming, becomes indispensably
necessary ; and heat caused by steam in the manner
that I use it, is more natural in producing perspiration,

than any dry heat that can be applied to the body in
any other manner, which will only serve to dry the air
and prevent perspiration in many cases of disease, where
a steam by water or vinegar would promote it and add
a natural warmth to the body, and thereby increase the
life and motion, which has laid silent in consequence
of the cold.

Dr. Jennings has contrived a plan to apply heat to the
body by a dry vapour, caused by burning spirit, which
he calls a vapour bath, the idea of which was, I have no
doubt, taken from hearing of my steaming to raise the
heat of the body. It may answer in some cases and
stages of disease ; but in a settled fever and other cases
where there is a dry inflammation on the surface of the
body, it will not answer any good purpose, and I think
would be dangerous without the use of my medicine to
first raise a free perspiration ; for when the surface of the
body is dry the patient cannot bear it, as it will crowd to
the head and cause distress, the same as is produced by
burning charcoal, or from hot stoves in a tight room, and
will bring on a difficulty in breathing, which is not the
case in steaming in my way. This machine can only
be used in bed, where the vapour cannot be applied to
the body equally at the same time, therefore is no better
than a hot dry stone put on each side and to the feet of
the patient, for he can turn himself and get heat from
them as well as to have all the trouble of burning spirit
and turning to the vapour of it, to get warm by this dry
heat. When the patient stands over a steam raised by
putting a hot stone in water, which gives a more equal
heat all over the body than can be done in any other
manner, it can be raised higher, and may be tempered
at pleasure by wetting the face and stomach with cold
water as occasion requires.

The method adopted by me, and which has always
answered the desired object, is as follows : Take several
stones of different sizes and put them in the fire till red
hot, then take the smallest first, and put one of them into
a pan or kettle of hot water, with the stone about half
immersed ; the patient must be undressed and a blanket
put around him so as to shield his whole body from the
air, and then place him over the steam. Change the

stones as often as they grow cool, so as to keep up a
lively steam, and keep them over it; if they are faint,
throw a little cold water on the face and stomach, which
will let down the outward heat and restore the strength;
after they have been over the steam long enough, which
will generally be about fifteen or twenty minutes, they
must be washed all over with cold water or spirit, and
be put in bed, or may be dressed, as the circumstances of
the case shall permit. Before they are placed over the
steam, give a dose of No. 2 and 3, or composition, to
raise the inward heat. When the patient is too weak to
stand over the steam, it may be done in bed, by heating
three stones, and put them in water till done hissing, then
wrap them in a number of thicknesses of cloths wet
with water, and put one on each side and one at the
feet, occasionally wetting the face and stomach with cold
water, when faint.

Many other plans may be contrived in steaming, which
would make less trouble and be more agreeable to the
patient, especially where they are unable to stand over
the steam. An open worked chair may be made, in
which they might sit and be steamed very conveniently;
or a settee might be made in the same manner, in which
they might be laid and covered with blankets so as to
shield them from the surrounding air. Such contrivances
as these would be very convenient in cases where the
patient would have to be carried through a course of
medicine and steamed a number of times, as is frequently necessary, particularly in complaints that have been
of long standing.-

As I have frequently mentioned a regular course of
medicine, I will here state what is meant by it, and the
most proper way in which it is performed. Firstly, give
No. 2 and 3, or composition, adding a tea spoonful of
No. 6; then steam, and when in bed repeat it, adding
No. 1, which will cleanse the stomach and assist in keeping up a perspiration; when this has done operating, give
an injection made with the same articles. Where there
are symptoms of nervous affection, or spasms, put half a
tea spoonful of the nerve powder into each dose given,
and into the injection. In violent cases, where immediate relief is needed, Nos. 1; 2, 3, and 6, may be given

together. Injections may be administered at all times, and in all cases of disease to advantage; it can never do harm, and in many cases, they are indispensably necessary, especially where there is canker and inflammation in the bowels, and there is danger of mortification, in which case, add a tea spoonful of No. 6. In cases of this kind, the injection should be given first, or at the same time of giving the composition or No. 3. The latter is preferable.

The use of steaming is good in preventing sickness as well as curing it. When a person has been exposed to the cold, and is threatened with disease, it may be prevented, and long sickness and expense saved by a very little trouble, by standing over a steam - and following the directions before given, till the cold is thoroughly thrown off, and a lively perspiration takes place; then go to bed, taking the stone from the kettle, and wrap it in wet cloths, and put it to the feet. This may be done without the medicine, when it cannot be had; but is much better to take something to raise the inward heat at the same time. A tea made of mayweed or summer-savory, or ginger and hot water sweetened, may be given, or any thing that is warming. This advice is for the poor, and those who have not a knowledge of the medicine; and will many times save them much trouble and long sickness.

Steaming is of the utmost importance in cases of suspended animation, such as drowned persons; in which case, place the body over a moderate steam, shielded by a blanket, from the weight of the external air, and rarifying the air immediately around them with the steam. Pour into the mouth some of the tincture of Nos. 1, 2, and 6; and if there is any internal heat remains, there will be muscular motion about the eyes, and in the extremities. If this symptom appears, repeat the dose several times, and renew the hot stones, raising the heat by degrees; if the outward heat is raised too sudden, so as to balance the inward, you will fail of the desired object, even after life appears. This is the only danger of any difficulty taking place; always bear in mind to keep the fountain above the stream, or the inward heat above the outward, and all will be safe. After life is restored, put them in bed and keep the perspiration free for twelve hours, by hot stones wrapped in cloths wet with water, and occasionally giving the tincture as before mentioned, when the coldness and obstructions are thrown off, and the patient will be in the enjoyment of his natural strength. Beware of bleeding, or blowing in the mouth with a bellows, as either will generally prove fatal.

In many cases of spotted fever, steaming is as necessary as in drowned persons; such as when they fall apparently dead; then the same treatment is necessary to lighten the surrounding air till you can raise the inward heat so as to get the determining power to the surface. Begin with a small stone, and as life gains, increase the steam as the patient can bear it; if the distress is great, give more hot medicine inside, and as soon as an equilibrium takes place the pain will cease. In all cases of this kind, the difficulty cannot be removed without applied heat to the body, and is more natural by steam than by any other means that can be made use of. In cases of long standing, where the patient has been run down with mercury, and left in a cold and obstructed state, liable to rheumatism and other similar complaints, they cannot be cured with medicine without applied heat by steam, as nothing will remove mercury but heat.

When a patient is carried through a course of my medicine and steamed, who has been long under mercurial treatment; and while under the operation of the steam, when the heat is at the highest, the face will swell, in consequence of the poisonous vapour being condensed by the air, the face being open to it. To relieve this, put them in bed, and take a hot stone wrapped in several thicknesses of cloth wet with water, pouring on a little vinegar, and making a lively steam; put it in the bed and cover the head with the clothes and let them breathe the steam as hot as can be borne, until the sweat covers the swelled part. This will in about fifteen or twenty minutes throw out the poison, and the swelling will abate. This method also is of great service in agues and teethache caused by cold; and many other cases of obstruction from the same cause, especially young children stuffed on the lungs.

To steam small children, the best way is to let them sit in the lap of a person, covering both with a blanket and set over the steam, pouring a little vinegar on the stone ; or it may be done in bed with a hot stone, wrapped in cloths wet with water, putting on a little vinegar ; and covering them with the bed clothes laid loosely over them ; but in this way you cannot exercise so good judgment in tempering the steam, as when you are steamed with them. If the child appears languid and faint, the outward heat is high enough ; put a little cold water on the face or breast, which will restore the strength, then rub them in a cloth wet with vinegar, spirit or cold water, put on clean clothes, and put them in bed, or let them sit up as their strength will permit. This is safe in all cases of cold and obstructed perspiration. It ought always to be borne strongly in mind, to give a child drink often, when under the operation of medicine, or while steaming ; if this is not done, they will suffer much, as they cannot ask for it.

In all cases of falls or bruises, steaming is almost infallible ; and is much better than bleeding, as is the common practice, which only tends to destroy life instead of promoting it. If the person is not able to stand over the steam, it must be done in bed, as has been described. Give the hottest medicine inside that you have, and keep the perspiration free till the pain and soreness abates, and the strength will be soon restored. If the advantages of this mode of treatment was generally known, bleeding in such cases, or any other, to remove disease, would never be resorted to by the wise and prudent.

The use of steaming is to apply heat to the body where it is deficient, and clear off obstructions caused by cold, which the operation of the medicine will not raise heat enough to do ; for as the natural heat of the body becomes thereby lower than the natural state of health, it must by art be raised as much above as it has been below ; and this must be repeated until the digestive powers are restored, sufficient to hold the heat by digesting the food, then the health of the patient will be restored by eating and drinking such things as the appetite shall require. In this way the medicine removes disease, and food, by being properly digested, supports nature and continues that heat on which life depends.

3

Some who practise according to my system, boast of carrying their patients through in a shorter time without the trouble of steaming; this is easily accounted for; steaming is the most laborious part of the practice for those who attend upon the sick, and the most useful to the patient; as one operation of steaming will be more effectual in removing disease, than four courses without it; and to omit it is throwing the labour upon the patient, with the expense of three or four operations more of the medicine, than would be needed, did the person who attends do his duty faithfully.

ON GIVING POISON AS MEDICINE.

The practice of giving poison as medicine, which is so common among the medical faculty at the present day, is of the utmost importance to the public; and is a subject that I wish to bring home to the serious consideration of the whole body of the people of this country, and enforce in the strongest manner on their minds, the pernicious consequences that have happened, and are daily taking place by reason of giving mercury, arsenic, nitre, opium and other deadly poisons to cure disease. It is admitted by those who make use of these things, that the introducing them into the system is very dangerous, and that they often prove fatal. During thirty years practice, I have had opportunity to gain much experience on this subject, and am ready to declare that I am perfectly and decidedly convinced, beyond all doubt, that there can be no possible good derived from using in any manner or form whatever, those poisons; but on the other hand, there is a great deal of hurt done. More than nine-tenths of the chronic cases that have come under my care, have been such as had been run down with some one or the whole of the above named medical poisons; and the greatest difficulty I have had to encounter in removing the complaints which my patients laboured under, has been to clear the system of mercury, nitre, or opium, and bring them back to the same state they were in before taking them. It is a very easy thing to get them into the system, but very hard to get them out again.

Those who make use of these things as medicine, seem to cloak the administering them under the specious pretence of great skill and art in preparing and using them; but this kind of covering will not blind the people, if they would examine it and think for themselves, instead of believing that every thing said or done by a learned man must be right; for poison given to the sick by a person of the greatest skill, will have exactly the same effect as it would if given by a fool. The fact is, the operation of it is diametrically opposed to nature, and every particle of it, that is taken into the system, will strengthen the power of the enemy to health.

If there should be doubts in the minds of any one of the truth of what I have said concerning the articles I have named being poisonous and destructive to the constitution and health of man, I will refer them to the works published by those who recommend their use; where they will find evidence enough to satisfy the most credulous, of the dangerous consequences and fatal effects, of giving them as medicine. To remove all doubts of their being poison I will make a few extracts from standard medical works, as the best testimony that can be given in the case.

"*Muriate of Mercury*, is one of the most violent poisons with which we are acquainted. Externally it acts as an escharotic or a caustic; and in solution, it is used for destroying fungous flesh, and for removing hepetic eruptions; but even externally, it must be used with very great caution." Yet, reader, this active poison is used as medicine, and by being prepared in a different form, and a new name given it, Calomel, its good qualities are said to be invaluable, and is a certain cure for almost every disease.

"*Oxyd of Arsenic*, is one of the most sudden and violent poisons we are acquainted with. In mines, it causes the destruction of numbers of those who explore them: and it is frequently the instrument by which victims are sacrificed, either by the hand of wickedness or imprudence. The fumes of Arsenic are so deleterious to the lungs, that the artist ought to be on his guard to prevent their exhalation by the mouth; for if they be mixed and swallowed with the saliva, effects will take place similar

to those which follow its introduction into the stomach
in a saline state; namely, a sensation of a piercing,
gnawing, and burning kind, accompanied with an acute
pain in the stomach and intestines, which last are violently contorted; convulsive vomiting; insatiable thirst,
from the parch'd and rough state of the tongue and throat:
hiccough, palpitation of the heart and a deadly oppres-
sion of the whole breast, succeed next; the matter eject-
ed by the mouth, as well as the stools, exhibit a black,
fœted, and putrid appearance; at length with the mortification of the bowels, the pain subsides, and death terminates the sufferings of the patient." "When the
quantity is so very small as not to prove fatal, tremors,
paralysis, and lingering hectics succeed."

Notwithstanding this terrible description of the fatal
effects of this article, the author says, "though the
most violent of mineral poisons, arsenic, according to
Murray, equals, when properly administered, the first
medicines in the class of tonics." "Of all the diseases, says Dr. Duncan, in which white Oxyd of Arsenic has been used internally, there is none in which it
has been so frequently and so successfully employed,
as in the cure of intermittent fevers. We have now
the most satisfactory information concerning this article
in the Medical Reports, of the effects of arsenic in the
cure of agues, remitting fevers, and periodical head-
aches, by Dr. Fowler, of Stafford." Such are the
powers of this medicine, that two grains of it are often
sufficient to cure an intermittent that has continued for
weeks! "As an external remedy, arsenic has long been
known as the basis of the celebrated *cancer powders;*
"Arsenic has ever been applied in substance, sprinkled
upon the ulcer; but this mode of using it is exceeding-
ly painful, and extremely dangerous. There have been
fatal effects produced from its absorption." No other
escharotic possesses equal powers in cancerous affections; it not unfrequently amends the discharge, causes
the sore to contract in size, and cases have been related
of its having effected a cure. But, says Dr. Willich,
"we are, on the combined testimony of many medical
practitioners, conspicious for their professional zeal and
integrity, irresistibly induced to declare our opinion,

at least, against the internal use of this active and dangerous medicine."

I shall leave it to the reader, to reconcile, if he can, the inconsistencies and absurdities of the above statements, of the effects of ratsbane; and ask himself the question, whether it can be possible, for an article, the use of which is attended with such consequences, to be in any shape or form, proper to be used as medicine; yet it is a well known fact, that this poison is in constant use among the faculty, and forms the principal ingredient in most of those nostrums sold throughout the country, under the names of drops, powders, washes, balsams, &c. and there can be no doubt that thousands either die, or become miserable invalids in consequence.

"*Antimony*, in the modern nomenclature, is the name given to a peculiar metal. The antimonial metal is a medicine of the greatest power of any known substance; a quantity too minute to be sensible in the most delicate balance, is capable of producing violent effects, if taken dissolved, or in a soluable state." "Sulphureted antimony was employed by the ancients in Collyria, against inflammation of the eyes, and for staining the eyebrows black. Its internal use does not seem to have been established till the end of the fifteenth century; and even at that time it was by many looked upon as poisonous." "All the metalic preparations are uncertain, as it entirely depends on the state of the stomach, whether they have no action at all, or operate with dangerous violence." "The principal general medicinal application of antimony has been for the use of febrile affections." "In the latter stage of fever, where debility prevails, its use is inadmissible." Of the propriety of using this metal as medicine, I shall leave it to the reader to judge for himself.

Nitre. Salt-Petre. This salt, consisting of nitric acid and potash, is found ready formed on the surface of the soil in warm climates." "Purified nitre is prescribed with advantage in numerous disorders. Its virtues are those of a refrigerent and diuretic. It is usually given in doses from two or three grains to a scruple, being a very cooling and resolvent medicine, which by relaxing the spasmodic rigidity of the vessels, pro-

3*

motes not only the secretion of urine, but at the same
time insensible perspiration, in febrile disorders; while
it allays thirst and abates heat; though in malignant
cases in which the pulse is low, and the patient's strength
exhausted, it produces contrary effects." "This powerful salt, when inadvertantly taken in too large quantities,
is one of the most fatal poisons." "For some interest-
ing observations relative to the deleterious properties of
salt-petre, the reader is referred to Dr. Mitchell's letter
to Dr. Priestly."

I have found from a series of practical experiments for
many years, that salt-petre has the most certain and
deadly effects upon the human system, of any drug that
is used as medicine. Although the effects produced by
it are not so immediately fatal as many others, yet its
whole tendency is to counteract the principles of life, and
destroy the operation of nature. Experience has taught
me that it is the most powerful enemy to health, and that
it is the most difficult opponent to encounter, with any
degree of success, that I have ever met with. Being in
its nature *cold*, there cannot be any other effects produced by it, than to increase the power of that enemy of
heat, and to lessen its necessary influence.

"*Opium*, when taken into the stomach, to such an extent as to have any sensible effect, gives rise to a pleasant serenity of the mind, in general proceeding to a certain degree of languor and drowsiness." "It excites
thirst and renders the mouth dry and parched." "Taken
into the stomach in a larger dose, gives rise to confusion
of the head and vertigo. The powers of all stimulating
causes of making impressions on the body are diminished; and even at times, and in situations, when a person
would naturally be awake, sleep is irresistably induced.
In still larger doses, it acts in the same manner as the
narcotic poisons, giving rise to vertigo, headache, tremors, delirium and convulsions; and these terminating
in a state of stupor, from which the person cannot be
roused. This stupor is accompanied with slowness of
the pulse, and with stertor in breathing, and the scene is
terminated in death, attended with the same appearances as take place in an appoplexy." "In intermit-
tents it is said to have been used with good effect." "It

is often of very great service in fevers of the typhoid type." "In small pox, when the convulsions before erruption are frequent and considerable, opium is liberally used." "In cholera and pyrosis, it is almost the only thing trusted to." "The administration of opium to the unaccustomed, is sometimes very difficult. The requisite quantity of opium is wonderfully different in different persons and in different states of the same person. A quarter of a grain will in one adult, produce effects which ten times the quantity will not do in another. The lowest fatal dose to the unaccustomed, as mentioned by authors, seems to be four grains; but a dangerous dose is so apt to puke, that it has seldom time to occasion death."

From the above extracts, it will readily be seen that the use of opium as medicine, is very dangerous, at least, if not destructive to health; its advocates, it will be observed, do not pretend that it will cure any disorder, but is used as a paliative for the purpose of easing pain, by destroying sensibility. Pain is caused by disease, and there can be no other way to relieve it, but by removing the cause. Sleep produced by opium is unnatural, and affords no relief to the patient, being nothing more than a suspension of his senses; and it might with as much propriety be said, that a state of delirium is beneficial, for a person in that situation is not sensible of pain. The fact is, opium is a poison, and when taken into the system, produces no other effect than to strengthen the power of the enemy to health, by deadening the sensible organs of the stomach and intestines, and preventing them from performing their natural functions so important to the maintaining of health and life. In all the cases that have come within my knowledge, where the patient has been long in the habit of taking opium, I have found it almost impossible, after removing the disease, to restore the digestive powers of the stomach.

I have made the foregoing extracts on the subject of poisons, for the purpose of giving a more plain and simple view of the pernicious consequences caused by their being given as medicine, than I could do in any other manner. In this short address, it is impossible to do

that justice to the subject that I could wish, and which its
importance demands; but I am not without hope, that
what is here given will satisfy every candid person who
reads it, of the truth of those principles which it has been
at all times my endeavour to inculcate, for the benefit of
mankind, and convince them, that what has a tendency
to destroy life, can never be useful in restoring health.

In support of what has been before said on the use
of mercury, I will here give a short extract from Dr.
Mann's Medical Sketches, which is but a trifle in com-
parison with the many cases that he has given of the
fatal effects of that poison. "Calomel should never be
administered, unless the patient is so situated that the
skin may be preserved in its natural warmth. If this is
not attended to during its administration, either the
bowels or the glands of the mouth suffered. To one of
these parts it frequently directed all its stimulating powers, and induced on one or the other high degrees of inflammation, which terminated in mortification of the intestines, or destruction of not only the muscles, but the
bones of the face.

"Four cases under these formidable effects of mercurial ptyalism, were admitted into the general hospital,
at Lewistown; three of whom died with their jaws and
faces dreadfully mutilated. The fourth recovered with
the loss of the inferior maxilla on one side, and the
teeth on the other. He lived a most wretched life, de-
formed in his features, when I last saw the patient, incapable of taking food, except through a small aperture
in place of his mouth."

There are several vegetables that grow common in
this country, which are poisons; and in order that the
public may be on their guard against using them as
medicine, I will here give a list of those within my
knowledge, viz. Garden Hemlock, Night Shade, Apple
Peru, Poppy, Henbane, Poke-root, Mandrake-root, Gar-
get-root, Wild Parsnip, Indigo-weed, Ivy, Dogwood,
Tobacco, and Laurel. In case either of these articles,
or any other poison should be taken through accident,
or otherwise, a strong preparation of No. 1, with a
small quantity of No. 2, will be found to be a sovereign
remedy.

Cases frequently occur in the country, of being poisoned externally, by some of the above vegetable poisons,
in which they swell very much.   When this happens, by
taking No. 2, or Composition, and washing with the
tincture, or the third preparation of No. 1, relief may be
speedily obtained.

It is a common thing with the doctors to make use of
many of the above mentioned vegetable poisons as medicine ; but I would caution the public against the use of
them in any way whatever, as they will have no other
effect than to increase the difficulty, and injure the constitution of the patient ; being deadly poisons, it is impossible that they can do any good.   No dumb beast will
ever touch them, and they are correct judges of what is
good for food or medicine.

Great use is made in many parts of the country of
garden hemlock, Scicuta, and is recommended by the
doctors for many complaints, to be taken or applied externally.   I have been credibly informed that large quantities of this article are collected and boiled down to a
thick substance, by the people in the country, and sold
by them to the doctors and apothecaries.   It is well
known to be the greatest poison of any vegetable, and
was used in ancient times to put criminals to death ; but
this was before it was ever thought of, that the same article that would cause immediate death when taken for
that purpose, would also cure disease.

Many persons that pretend to make use of my system
of practice, are in the habit of using some of the vegetables that I have mentioned as poisonous.   I wish the
public to understand that it is entirely unauthorized by
me, as there is nothing in my practice or writings, but
what is directly opposed to every thing of a poisonous
nature being used as a medicine ; for it has always been
my aim, to ascertain and avoid the use of every thing
except such articles as I knew by actual experience to
be agreeable to nature, and also free from all danger or
risk in using them to cure disease.   I therefore, caution
the public against putting any confidence in such as
make use of either vegetable or mineral poison.

There has been several cases of death published by
the doctors, which they say were caused by those who

practice by my system; and from the description they
have given of the treatment, I have good reason to suppose, if there is any truth at all in them, were attended
by such as I have before mentioned, pretending to practise by my system without having a correct knowledge
of it; and who are tampering with every kind of medicine they can find; for there is no such treatment of disease, as they describe, ever been recommended by me,
or that can be found in my writings or practice. It is
very convenient for them, and has become common, to
say, when they happen to be successful, it is their own
great improvements; but when the patient dies, it is then
laid to the Thomsonian system of practice. This is unjust,
and ought to be exposed; and I ask all those who have
a wish to promote the practice, to adopt some means to
ascertain the truth, and make it public.

THE DOCTORS WITHOUT A SYSTEM.

That the doctors have no system is a fact pretty generally acknowledged by themselves; or at least they
have none that has been fixed upon as a general rule for
their practice. Almost every great man among them
has had a system of his own, which has been followed
by their adherents till some other one is brought forward
more fashionable. This is undoubtedly a great evil,
for it makes every thing uncertain; where it is constantly changing, there can be no dependence on any
thing, and the practice must always be experimental; no
useful knowledge can be obtained by the young practitioners, as they will be constantly seeking after new theories. What should we say of a carpenter who should
undertake to repair a building without having any rule
to work by, and should for want of one, destroy the half
of all he undertook to repair. The employers would
soon lose all confidence in him, and dismiss him as an
ignorant blockhead. And is it not of infinitely more importance for those who undertake to repair the human
body, to have some correct rule to work by? Their
practice is founded on visionary theories, which are so
uncertain and contradictory, that it is impossible to form

any correct general rule as a guide to be depended upon. In order to show the opinions of others as well as my own, I shall make a few extracts from late writers on the subject. Speaking of the revolutions of medicines, one says :

"We have now noticed the principal revolutions of medicine; and we plainly perceive that the theory of medicine, not only has been, but is yet, in an unsettled state, that its practical application is wavering, fallacious, and extremely pernicious ; and taking a survey of the various fortunes of the art, we may well say with Bacon, that medicine is a science that hath been more professed than laboured, and yet more laboured than advanced, the labour having been in a circle, but not in progression."

"Theories are but the butterflies of the day; they buzz for a while and then expire. We can trace for many centuries past, one theory overturning another, yet each in its succession promising itself immortality."

"The application of the rules which the practitioner lays down to himself is direct, and in their choice, no one can err with impunity. The least erroneous view leads to some consequence. We must remember the lives of our fellow creatures are at stake. For how many cruel and premature deaths, how many impaired and debilitated constitutions have paid for the folly of theories ! Follies, which have proved almost always fascinating. The study of a system is more easy than an investigation of nature ; and in practice, it seems to smooth every difficulty."

"In my lectures on the art of physic, says Dr. Ring, both theoretical and practical, I have fully proved that there is no necessity for that bane of the profession, *conjecture* or *hypothesis ;* and if I were asked whether, if I myself were dangerously ill, I would suffer any hypothetical, however plausible physician, to prescribe for my malady, my answer would be *no,* assuredly *no,* unless I wished to risk the loss of my life. I could give a remarkable instance of this.

"Speculation and hypothesis are always at variance with *sound experience* and successful *practice.*"

The above extracts evince the pernicious effects of false theory and hypothesis, which at the present day, constitute nearly the whole art of physic.

The following just remarks are copied from the writings of the Rev. John Wesley.

" As theories increased, simple medicines were more and more disregarded and disused ; till, in a course of years, the greater part of them were forgotten, at least in the more polite nations. In the room of these, abundance of new ones were introduced, by reasoning, speculative men ; and those more and more difficult to be applied, as being more remote from common observation. Hence rules for the application of these, and medical books were immensely multiplied ; till at length physic became an abstruse science, quite out of the reach of ordinary men. Physicians now began to be held in admiration, as persons who were something more than human. And profit attended their employ, as well as honour. So that they had now two weighty reasons for keeping the bulk of mankind at a distance, that they might not pry into the mysteries of their profession. To this end they increased those difficulties, by design, which were in a manner by accident. They filled their writings with abundance of technical terms, utterly unintelligible to plain men. '

" Those who understood only how to restore the sick to health, they branded with the name of Empirics. They introduced into practice abundance of compound medicines, consisting of so many ingredients, that it was scarce possible for common people to know which it was that wrought a cure. Abundance of exotics, neither the nature nor names of which their own countrymen understood."

" The history of the art of medicine in all ages," says Dr. Blane, " so teems with the fanciful influence of superstitious observances, the imaginary virtues of medicines with nugatory, delusive, inefficient, and capricious practices, fallacious and sophistical reasonings, as to render it little more than a chaos of error, a tissue of deceit unworthy of admission among the useful arts and liberal pursuits of man."

DESCRIPTION

OF THE

Vegetable Medicine, used in my System of Practice.

———

IN describing those vegetables which I make use of in removing disease and restoring the health of the patient, agreeably to my system of practice, I shall mention those only which I have found most useful by a long series of practical knowledge; and in the use of which I have been successful in effecting the desired object. A much greater number of articles in the vegetable kingdom, that are useful as medicine, might have been described and their medical virtues pointed out, if I had thought it would be beneficial; in fact I am confident there are very few vegetable productions of our country, that I have not a tolerable good knowledge of, it having been my principal study for above thirty years; but to undertake to describe them all would be useless and unprofitable to my readers, and could lead to no good result. The plan that I have adopted in describing such articles as I have thought necessary to mention, and giving directions how to prepare and administer them, is to class them under the numbers which form my system of practice; this was thought to be the best way to give a correct and full understanding of the whole subject. Each number is calculated to effect a certain object, which is stated in the heading to each as they are introduced ; every article therefore, that is useful in promoting such objects will be described as applicable to the number under which it is classed. The three first are used to remove disease and the others as restoratives. There are a number of preparations and compounds, that I have made use of and found good in curing various complaints ; the directions for making them and a description of the articles of which

4

they are composed are given as far as was deemed necessary. The manner of applying them will be hereafter
more particularly stated, when I come to give an account
of the manner of treating some of the most important cases
of disease which have come under my care.

No: 1.—*To cleanse the Stomach, overpower the cold, and promote a free perspiration.*

EMETIC HERB. LOBELIA INFLATA OF LINÆUS.

In giving a description of this valuable herb, I shall be
more particular, because it is the most important article
made use of in my system of practice, without which it
would be incomplete, and the medical virtues of which
'and the administering it in curing disease, I claim as my
own discovery. The first knowledge I ever had of it,
was obtained by accident more than forty years ago, and
never had any infomation whatever concerning it, except what I have gained by my own experience. A
great deal has been said of late about this plant, both in
favour and against its utility as a medicine; but all that
the faculty have said or published concerning it, only
shows their ignorance on the subject; for there is very
little truth in what they have stated concerning its medical properties, except wherein they have admitted it to
be a certain cure for the asthma, one of the most distressing complaints that human nature is subject to. It
is a truth which cannot be disputed by any one, that all
they have known about this article, and the experiments
that have been made to ascertain its value, originated in
my making use of it in my practice.

In the course of my practice, a number of the doctors
discovered that the medicine I made use of, produced
effects which astonished them, and which they could not
account for; this induced them to conclude, that because
it was so powerful in removing disease, it must be
poison. This I think can be very satisfactorily accounted for; they have no knowledge of any thing in all
their medical science, which is capable of producing a
powerful effect upon the human system, except what is
poisonous, and therefore naturally form their opinions
agreeably to this erroneous theory. There is a power

to produce life and a power to produce death, which are of course directly opposed to each other; and whatever tends to promote life, cannot cause death, let its power be ever so great. In this consists all the difference between my system of practice and that of the learned doctors. In consequence of their thus forming an erroneous opinion of this herb, which they had no knowledge of, they undertook to represent it as a deadly poison; and in order to destroy my practice, they raised a hue-and-cry about my killing my patients by administering it to them. Some of the faculty even made oath, that it was poison, and when taken into the stomach, if it did not cause immediate vomiting it was certain death. It is unnecessary for me now to point out the falsity of this, for the fact is pretty well known, that there is no death in it; but on the contrary, that there is no vegetable that the earth produces, more harmless in its effects on the human system, and none more powerful in removing disease and promoting health.

There is no mention made of this herb, by any author, that I have been able to find, previous to my discovering it, excepting by Linæus, who has given a correct description of it under the name of Lobelia Inflata; but there is nothing said of its medical properties, it is therefore reasonable to conclude that they were not known till I discovered it, and proved it to be useful. When the faculty first made the discovery that I used the Emetic Herb in my practice, they declared it to be a deadly poison; and while persecuting me by every means in their power, and representing to the world that I killed my patients with it, they were very ready to call it my medicine, and allow it to be my own discovery; but since their ignorance of it has been exposed, and they find it is going to become an article of great value, an attempt seems to be making to rob me of all the credit for causing its value to be known, and the profits which belong to me for the discovery. In which some who have been instructed by me are ready to join, for the purpose of promoting their own interest at my expense.

Dr. Thacher, in his Dispensatory, has undertaken to give an account of this herb; but is very erroneous, except in the description of it, which is nearly correct.

It appears that all the knowledge he has on the subject, as to its virtues, is borrowed from others, and is probably derived from the ridiculous ideas entertained of its power by those doctors who knew nothing about it, except what they gained by my making use of it, as has been before stated. As to its being dangerous to administer it, and that if it does not puke, it frequently destroys the patient, and sometimes in five or six hours; and that even horses and cattle have been supposed to be killed by eating it accidentally, is as absurd as it is untrue, and only proves their ignorance of the article. He tells a melancholy story about the Lobelia Inflata being administered by the adventurous hand of a noted empiric, who he says frequently administered it in a dose of a tea spoonful of the powdered leaves, and often repeated; which he says furnishes alarming examples of its deleterious properties and fatal effects. This, there is no doubt, alludes to me, and took its rise from the false statements circulated about me at the time of my trial, to prejudice the public against my practice. It is true the dose that I usually prescribed is a tea-spoonful of the powder; but that it ever produced any fatal effect, is altogether incorrect, and is well known to be so by all who have any correct knowledge on the subject.

What is quoted in the Dispensatory, from the Rev. Dr. M. Cutler, concerning this herb, is, in general, correct, particularly as it regards its being a specific for the asthma; though he laboured under many mistaken notions about its effects when taken into the stomach; he says, "if the quantity be a little increased, it operates as an emetic, and then as a cathartic, its effects being much the same as those of the common emetics and cathartics." In this he is mistaken, for it is entirely different from any other emetic known; and as to its operating as a cathartic, I never knew it to have such an effect in all my practice. And I certainly ought to know something about it, after having made use of it for above twenty years, and administering it in every form and manner that it can be given, and for every disease that has come within my knowledge. It appears that all the knowledge he and other doctors have got of this herb's being useful in curing disease, particularly in the asthma, was obtained from me ; for when I was prosecuted, I was obliged to expose my discoveries to show the falsity of the indictment. Dr. Cutler was brought forward as a witness at my trial, to prove the virtues of this plant, by his evidence, that he cured himself of the asthma with it. He says the first information he had of its being good for that complaint, was from Dr. Drury, of Marblehead. In the fall of the year, 1807, I introduced the use of the Emetic Herb, tinctured in spirit, for the asthma and other complaints of the lungs, and cured several of the consumption. In 1808, I cured a woman in Newington, of the asthma, who had not laid in her bed for six months. I gathered some of the young plants not bigger than a dollar, bruised them, and tinctured them in spirits, gave her the tincture and she lay in bed the first night. I showed her what it was, and how to prepare and use it, and by taking this and other things according to my direction, she has enjoyed a comfortable state of health for twelve years, and has never been obliged to sit up one night since. The same fall I used it in Beverly and Salem ; and there can be no doubt but all the information concerning the value of this article was obtained from my practice.

After Dr. Cutler had given his testimony of the virtues of this herb, and the doctors having become convinced of its value, they come forward and say it is good medicine in skilful hands. Who, I would ask, is more skilful than he who discovered it, and taught them how to prepare and use it in curing one of the most distressing complaints known ? If it is a good medicine, it is mine, and I am entitled to the credit of introducing it into use, and have paid dear for it ; if it is poison, the doctors do not need it, as they have enough of that now. Dr. Thacher undertakes to make it appear that the fatal effects he tells about its producing, was owing to the quantity given ; and says I administered a tea-spoonful of the powder ; and when he comes to give directions for using it, says that from ten to twenty grains may be given with safety. It appears strange that different terms should produce such different

4*

effects in the operation of medicine. If a tea-spoonful
is given by an empiric, its effects are fatal; but if the
same quantity is administered by a learned doctor, and
called grains, it is a useful medicine.

This herb is described in Thacher's Dispensatory
under the names of Lobelia Inflata, Lobelia Emetica,
Emetic Weed, and Indian Tobacco; and several other
names have been given it, some by way of ridicule and
others for the purpose of creating a prejudice against
it; all of which has so confounded it with other articles
that there is a difficulty in ascertaining what they mean
to describe. I have been informed that there is a poisonous root grows in the Southern States, called Lobelia, which has been used as a medicine; the calling this
herb by that name, has probably been one reason of its
being thought to be poison. Why it has had the name
of Indian Tobacco given it, I know not; there is a
plant that is called by that name, which grows in this
country, but is entirely different from this herb both in
appearance and medical virtues. In the United States
Pharmacopoeia, there are directions given for preparing
the tincture of Indian Tobacco; whether they mean
this herb or the plant that has been always called by
that name, does not appear; but it is probable they
mean the emetic herb, and that all the knowledge they
have of it is from Dr. Cutler's description. It is said
by Thacher, that it was employed by the aborigines and
by those who deal in Indian remedies; and others who
are attempting to rob me of the discovery affect to believe the same thing; but this is founded altogether upon
conjecture, for they cannot produce a single instance of
its having been employed as a medicine till I made use
of it. The fact is, it is a new article, wholly unknown
to the medical faculty, till I introduced it into use, and
the best evidence of this is, that they are now ignorant
of its powers; and all the knowledge they have of it has
been obtained from my practice. It would be folly for
me to undertake to say, but that it may have been used
by the natives of this country; but one thing I am certain of, that I never had any knowledge of their using
it, nor ever received any information concerning it from
them, or any one else.

The Emetic Herb may be found in the first stages of its growth at all times through the summer, from the bigness of a six cent piece to that of a dollar, and larger, lying flat on the ground, in a round form, like a rose pressed flat, in order to bear the weight of snow which lays on it during the winter, and is subject to be winter-killed like wheat. In the spring it looks yellow and pale, like other things suffering from wet and cold; but when the returning sun spreads forth its enlivening rays upon it, it lifts up its leaves and shoots forth a stalk to the height of from twelve to fifteen inches, with a number of branches, carrying up its leaves with its growth. In July it puts forth small pointed pale blue blossoms, which is followed by small pods about the size of a white bean, containing numerous very small seeds. This pod is an exact resemblance of the human stomach, having an inlet and outlet higher than the middle; from the inlet it receives nourishment, and by the outlet discharges the seeds. It comes to maturity about the first of September, when the leaves and pods turn a little yellow; this is the best time to gather it. It is what is called by botanists, a bienneal plant, or of only two years existence.

This plant is common in all parts of this country. Wherever the land is fertile enough to yield support for its inhabitants it may be found. It is confined to no soil which is fit for cultivation, from the highest mountains to the lowest valleys. In hot and wet seasons it is most plenty on dry and warm lands; in hot and dry seasons on clayey and heavy lands. When the season is cold, either wet or dry, it rarely makes its appearance; and if the summer and fall is very dry the seed does not come up, and of course there will be very little to be found the next season. I have been in search of this herb from Boston to Canada, and was not able to collect more than two pounds; and in some seasons I have not been able to collect any. I mention this to show the uncertainty of its growth, and to put the people on their guard to be careful and lay up a good stock of it when plenty. In the year 1807, if I had offered a reward of a thousand dollars for a pound of this herb, I should not have been able to have obtained it. I have

seen the time that I would have given two dollars for an
ounce of the powder, but there was none to be had;
which necessity taught me to lay up all I could obtain
when it was plenty.

In seasons when this herb is plenty, it may be found
growing in highways and pastures, by the side of old
turnpikes, and in stubble land, particularly where it has
been laid down to grass the year before; when grass is
scarce, it is eaten by cattle, and is hard to be found
when full grown.   It is a wild plant, and a native of this
country ; but there is no doubt of its being common to
other countries.   It may be transplanted and cultivated
in gardens, and will be much larger and more vigourous
than when growing wild.   If some stalks are left, it
will sow itself, and probably may be produced from the
seed ; but how long the seeds remain in the ground before they come up, I do not know, never having made
any experiments to ascertain the fact.   It is certain that
it is produced from the seed, and there is no good reason
to suppose that it may not be cultivated in gardens from
the seed as well as other vegetables; I think it most
probable, however, from the nature of the plant, that it
will not come up till the seeds have laid at least one winter in the ground.

This plant is different in one very important particular, from all others that I have a knowledge of, that the
same quantity will produce the same effect in all stages
of its growth, from its first appearance till it comes to
maturity ; but the best time for gathering it, as has before been mentioned, is when the leaves and pods begin
to turn yellow, for then the seed is ripe, and you have all
there can be of it.   It should then be cut and kept clean,
and spread in a large chamber or loft, to dry, where
it is open to the air in the day time, and to be shut from
the damp air during the night.   When perfectly dry, shake
out the seed and sift it through a common meal sieve, and
preserve it by itself; then beat off the leaves and pods from
the stalks, and preserve them clean.   This herb may be
prepared for use in three different ways: viz. 1st. The
powdered leaves and pods.   2d.   A tincture made from
the green herb with spirit.   3d. The seeds reduced to a
fine powder and compounded with Nos. 2 and 6.

1. After the leaves and pods are separated from the stalks, pound or grind them in a mortar to fine powder, sift it through a fine sieve, and preserve it from the air. This is the most common preparation, and may be given in many different ways, either by itself or compounded with other articles. For a common dose, take a tea-spoonful of this powder with the same quantity of sugar in half a tea-cupful of warm water, or a tea of No. 3 may be used instead of the water ; this dose may be taken all at one time, or at three times, at intervals of ten minutes. For a young child strain off the liquor and give a part as circumstances shall require. There is but one way in which this herb can be prepared, that it will refuse its services, and that is when boiled or scalded; it is therefore important to bear in mind that there must never be any thing put to it warmer than a blood heat.

2. To prepare the tincture, take the green herb in any stage of its growth, if the small plants are used, take roots and all, put them into a mortar and pound them fine, then add the same quantity of good spirits ; when well pounded and worked together, strain it through a fine cloth and squeeze and press it hard to get out all the juice ; save the liquor in bottles, close stopped, for use. Good vinegar, or pepper-sauce may be used instead of the spirit. Prepared in this manner, it is an effectual counter-poison, either taken, or externally applied. It is also an excellent medicine for the asthma, and all complaints of the lungs. This is the only way in which the doctors have made use of the Emetic Herb ; and they acknowledge it to be one of the best remedies in many complaints, that has been found, though they know but little about it. For a dose, take from half to a tea-spoonful. Its effects will be more certain if about the same quantity of No. 2, is added, and in all cases where there are nervous symptoms, add half a tea-spoonful of nerve powder, Umbil, to the dose.

3. Reduce the seeds to a fine powder in a mortar, and take half an ounce of this powder, or about a large spoonful, with the same quantity of No. 2, made fine, and put them in a gill of No. 6, adding a tea-spoonful of Umbil; to be kept close stopped in a bottle for use ;

when taken, to be well shaken together.   This preparation is for the most violent attacks of disease, such as lock-jaw, bite of mad dog, drowned persons, fits, spasms, and in all cases of suspended animation, where the vital spark is nearly extinct.   It will go through the system like electricity, giving heat and life to every part.   In cases where the spasms are so violent that they are stiff, and the jaws become set, by pouring some of this liquid into the mouth between the cheek and teeth, as soon as it touches the glands at the roots of the tongue, the spasms will relax, and the jaws will become loosened so that the mouth will open; then give a dose of it, and as soon as the spasms have abated, repeat it, and afterwards give a tea of No. 3, for canker.   This course I never knew fail of giving relief.   It is good in less violent cases, to bring out the measles and small pox; and if applied to pimples, warts, &c. will remove them. I have cured three dogs with this preparation, who were under the most violent symptoms of hydrophobia; one of my agents cured a man with it who had been bitten by a mad dog; and I have not the least doubt of its being a specific for that disease.   For a dose, take a teaspoonful.

Much has been said of the power of the Emetic Herb, and some have expressed fears of it on that account; but I can assure the public, that there is not the least danger in using it; I have given it to children from one day old to persons of eighty years.   It is most powerful in removing disease, but innocent on nature.   Its operation in different persons, is according to their different tempers, moving with the natural current of the animal spirits.   There is two cases where this medicine will not operate, viz. when the patient is dying, and where there is no death; or in other words, when there is no disease.   There can be no war where there is no enemy. When there is no cold in the body there is nothing to contend against, and when there is no heat in the body there is nothing to kindle; in either case therefore this medicine is silent and harmless.   It is calculated to remove the cause and no more, as food removes hunger, and drink thirst.   It clears all obstructions to the extremities, without regard to the names of disease, until

it produces an equilibrium in the system, and will be felt
in the fingers and toes, producing a prickling feeling like
that caused by a knock of the elbow ; this symptom is
alarming to those unacquainted with its operation ; but is
always favourable, being a certain indication of the turn
of the disorder, and they generally gain from that time.

In regard to the quantity to be given as a dose, it is
matter of less consequence than is generally imagined.
The most important thing is to give enough to produce
the desired effect. If too little is given, it will worry
the patient, and do little good ; if more is given than
what is necessary, the surplus will be thrown off, and is
a waste of medicine. I have given directions what I
consider as a proper dose in common cases, of the different preparations, but still it must be left to the judgment of those who use it, how much to give. The most
safe way will be to give the smallest prescribed dose
first, then repeat it till it produce the wished operation.
In cases where the stomach is cold and very foul, its
operation will be slow and uncertain ; in which case
give No. 2, which will assist it in doing its work. See
also, page 90, § 11.

When this medicine is given to patients that are in
a decline, or are labouring under a disease of long standing, the symptoms indicating a crisis will not take place
till they have been carried through from three to eight
courses of the medicine ; and the lower they have been
the more alarming will be the symptoms. I have seen
some who would lay and sob like a child that had been
punished, for two hours, not able to speak or to raise
their hand to their head ; and the next day be about, and
soon get well. In cases where they have taken considerable opium, and this medicine is administered, it will
in its operation produce the same appearances and symptoms that is produced by opium when first given, which
having laid dormant, is roused into action by the enlivening qualities of this medicine, and they will be
thrown into a senseless state ; the whole system will be
one complete mass of confusion, tumbling in every direction ; will take two or three to hold them on the bed ;
they grow cold as though dying ; remaining in this way
from two to eight hours, and then awake, like one from

sleep after a good nights rest ; be entirely calm and sensible as though nothing had ailed them. It is seldom they ever have more than one of these turns ; as it is the last struggle of the disease, and they generally begin to recover from that time. I have been more particular in describing these effects of the medicine, as they are very alarming to those unacquainted with them, in order to show that there is no danger to be apprehended, as it is certain evidence of a favourable turn of the disease.

The Emetic Herb is of great value in preventing sickness as well as curing it; by taking a dose when first attacked by any complaint it will throw it off, and frequently prevent long sickness. It not only acts as an emetic, and throws off the stomach every thing that nature does not require for support of the system : but extends its effects to every part of the body. It is searching, enlivening, quickening and has a great power in removing all obstructions ; but it soon exhausts itself, and if not followed by some other medicine to hold the vital heat till nature is able to support itself by digesting the food, it will not be sufficient to remove a disease that has become seated. To effect this important object put me to much trouble and after trying many experiments to get something that would answer the purpose, I found that what is described under No. 2, was the best and only medicine I have a knowledge of, that would hold the heat in the stomach, and not evaporate ; and by giving No. 3 to remove the canker, which is the great cause of disease ; and then following with Nos. 4 and 5 to correct the bile, restore the digestion, and strengthen the system, I have had little trouble in effecting a cure. Directions for preparing &c.—see page 79.

No. 2.—*To retain the internal vital heat of the system and cause a free perspiration.*

CAYENNE.—Capsicum.

This article being so well known it will be unnecessary to be very particular in describing it. It has been a long time used for culinary purposes, and comes to us prepared for use by being ground to powder; and a proportion of salt mixed with it; this destroys in some degree its stimulating effects and makes it less pungent; but it is not so good for medicine as in the pure state. It is said to be a native of South America and is cultivated in many of the West India Islands; that which comes to this country is brought from Demarara and Jamaica. It also grows in other parts of the world. I once bought one hundred pounds of it in the pod, which was brought from the Coast of Guinea; had it ground at Portsmouth, and it was as good as any I ever used. There are several species that are described under the name of Capsicum; all of which are about the same, as to their stimulating qualities. The pods only are used; they are long and pointed, are of a green colour till ripe when they turn of a bright orange red. When the pods are green they are gathered and preserved in salt and water and brought to this country in bottles, when vinegar is put to them, which is sold under the name of Pepper-Sauce. The ripe pods ground to a powder is what is used for medicine and cooking; but the Pepper-Sauce is very good to be taken as medicine and applied externally; the green pods hold their attracting power till ripe, and therefore keep their strength much longer when put in vinegar; as the bottle may be filled up a number of times and the strength seems to be the same; but when the ripe pods are put in vinegar, the first time will take nearly all the strength.

I shall not undertake to dispute but that Cayenne has been used for medical purposes long before I had any knowledge of it; and that it is one of the safest and best articles ever discovered to remove disease, I know to be a fact, from long experience; but it is equally true that the medical faculty never considered it of much value, and the people had no knowledge of it as a medicine, till I introduced it, by making use of it in my practice. Mention is made of Cayenne in the Edinburgh Dispensatory, as chiefly employed for culinary purposes, but that of late it has been employed also in the practice of medicine. The author says that "there can be little doubt that it furnishes one of the purest and strongest stimulants which can be introduced into the stomach; while at the same time it has nothing of the narcotic effects of ardent spirits. It is said to have been

5

used with success in curing some cases of disease, that
had resisted all other remedies." All this I am satisfied is true, for if given as a medicine it always will be
found useful; but all the knowledge they had of it seems
to have been derived from a few experiments that had
been made, without fixing upon any particular manner
of preparing or administering it, or in what disease, as
is the case with all other articles that are introduced
into general practice. In Thacher's Dispensatory, the
same account is given of Cayenne, as in the Edinburgh,
and in almost the same words.

I never had any knowledge of Cayenne being useful
as a medicine, or that it had ever been used as such, till
I discovered it by accident, as has been the case with
most other articles used by me. After 1 had fixed upon
a system for my government in practice, I found much
difficulty in getting something that would not only produce a strong heat in the body, but would retain it till
the canker could be removed and the digestive powers
restored, so that the food, by being properly digested,
would maintain the natural heat. I tried a great number of articles that were of a hot nature; but could find
nothing that would hold the heat any length of time.
I made use of ginger, mustard, horse-radish, peppermint,
butternut bark, and many other hot things; but they
were all more or less volatile, and would not have the
desired effect. With these, however, and the Emetic
Herb, together with the aid of steam, I was enabled to
practice with pretty general success. In the fall of the
year 1805, 1 was out in search of Umbil, on a mountain,
in Walpole, N. H. I went into a house at the foot of
the mountain, to inquire for some rattlesnake oil;
while in the house I saw a large string of red peppers
hanging in the room, which put me in mind of what I
had been a long time in search of, to retain the internal
heat. I knew them to be very hot; but did not know of
what nature. I obtained these peppers, carried them
home, reduced them to powder, and took some of the
powder myself, and found it to answer the purpose better than any thing else I had made use of. I put it in
spirit with the Emetic Herb, and gave the tincture mixed in a tea of witch-hazel leaves, and found that it would

retain the heat in the stomach after puking; and preserve the strength of the patient in proportion. I made use of it in different ways for two years, and always with good success.

In the fall of 1807, I was in Newburyport, and saw a bottle of pepper-sauce, being the first I had ever seen; I bought it and carried it home; got some of the same kind of pepper that was dried, which I put into the bottle; this made it very hot. On my way home, was taken unwell, and was quite cold; I took a swallow from the bottle, which caused violent pain for a few minutes, when it produced perspiration, and I soon grew easy. I afterwards tried it and found that after it had expelled the cold, it would not cause pain. From these experiments, I became convinced that this kind of pepper was much stronger, and would be better for medical use than the common red pepper. Soon after this I was again in Newburyport, and made inquiry, and found some Cayenne; but it was prepared with salt for table use, which injured it for medical purposes. I tried it by tasting, and selected that which had the least salt in it. I afterwards made use of this article, and found it to answer all the purposes wished; and was the very thing I had long been in search of. The next year I went to Portsmouth, and made inquiries concerning Cayenne, and from those who dealt in the article, I learned that it was brought to this country from Demarara and Jamaica, prepared only for table use, and that salt was put with it to preserve it and make it more palatable. I became acquainted with a French gentleman who had a brother in Demarara; and made arrangements with him to send to his brother, and request him to procure some, and have it prepared without salt. He did so, and sent out a box containing about eighty pounds, in a pure state. I sent also by many others, that were going to the places where it grows, to procure all they could; in consequence of which, large quantities were imported into Portsmouth, much more than there was immediate demand for. I was not able to purchase but a small part of what was brought, and it was bought up by others on speculation, and sent to Boston; the consequence was, that the price was so much reduced,

that it would not bring the first cost, which put a
stop to its being imported, and it has since been very
scarce.

When I first began to use this article, it caused much
talk among the people in Portsmouth, and the adjoining
towns ; the doctors tried to frighten them by telling that
I made use of Cayenne Pepper as a medicine, and that
it would burn up the stomach and lungs as bad as vitriol.
The people generally, however, became convinced by
using it, that all the doctors said about it was false,
and it only proved their ignorance of its medicinal virtues and their malignity towards me.   It soon came
into general use, and the knowledge of its being useful
in curing disease was spread all through the country.   I
made use of it in curing the spotted fever, and where it
was known, was the only thing depended on for that
disease.   I have made use of Cayenne in all kinds of
disease, and have given it to patients of all ages and
under every circumstance that has come under my
practice ; and can assure the public, that it is perfectly harmless, never having known it to produce any bad
effects whatever.   It is no doubt the most powerful
stimulant known ; its power is entirely congenial to
nature, being powerful only in raising and maintaining that heat on which life depends.   It is extremely
pungent, and when taken sets the mouth as it were on
fire ; this lasts, however, but a few minutes, and I consider it essentially a benefit, for its effects on the glands
causes the saliva to flow freely and leaves the mouth
clean and moist.

The only preparation necessary, is to have it ground
or pounded to a fine powder.   For a dose, from half to
a tea-spoonful may be taken in hot water sweetened,
or the same quantity may be mixed with either of the
other numbers when taken.   It will produce a free
perspiration, which should be kept up by repeating the
dose, until the disease is removed.   A spoonful, with
an equal quantity of common salt, put into a gill of vinegar, makes a very good sauce, to be eaten on meat, and
will assist the appetite and strengthen the digesture.
One spoonful of this preparation may be taken to good
advantage, and will remove faint, sinking feelings, which

some are subject to, especially in the spring of the year. Pepper-sauce is good for the same purpose. A tea-spoonful of Cayenne may be taken in a tumbler of cider, and is much better than ardent spirits. There is scarce any preparation of medicine that I make use of in which I do not put some of this article. It will cure the ague in the face, by taking a dose, and tying a small quantity in fine cloth, and put it between the cheek and teeth, on the side that is affected, setting by the fire covered with a blanket. It is good to put on old sores.

RED PEPPERS.

These are very plenty in this country, being cultivated in gardens, and are principally made use of for pickling; for which purpose the pods are gathered when green, and preserved in vinegar. It is of the same nature as Cayenne pepper, but not so strong; and is the best substitute for that article, of any thing I have ever found. For medical use they should not be gathered till ripe, when they are of a bright red colour; should be reduced to a fine powder, and may be used instead of Cayenne, when that article cannot be obtained.

GINGER.

This is a root which is brought from foreign countries, and is too well known to need any further description. It is a very good article, having a warming and agreeable effect on the stomach. It is a powerful stimulant, and is not volatile like many other hot articles; and is the next best thing to raise the inward heat and promote perspiration; and may be used with good success for that purpose, as a substitute for Cayenne, when that or the red peppers cannot be had. It is sold in the shops ground, but is sometimes mixed with the other articles to increase the quantity, and is not so strong. The best way is to get the roots and grind or pound them to a fine powder. The dose must be regulated according to circumstances; if given to raise the internal heat and cause perspiration, it must be repeated till it has the desired effect. It makes an excellent poultice, mixed with pounded cracker, or slippery-elm bark, for which I make much use of it. To keep a

5*

piece of the root in the mouth and chew it like tobacco, swallowing the juice, is very good for a cough, and those of a consumptive habit; and this should be also done by all who are exposed to any contagion, or are attending on the sick, as it will guard the stomach against taking the disease. It may be taken in hot water sweetened, or in a tea of No. 3.

BLACK PEPPER.

This may be used to good advantage as a substitute for the foregoing articles, when they are not to be had, and may be prepared and administered in the same manner. These four that I have mentioned, are all the articles I have been able to find, that would hold the heat of the body for any length of time; all the others that I have tried, are so volatile, that they do little good. See Directions, page 80.

———

No. 3.—*To scour the Stomach and Bowels, and remove the Canker.*

Under this head I shall describe such vegetable productions as are good for Canker, and which I have found to be best in removing the thrush from the throat, stomach and bowels, caused by cold, and there will be more or less of it in all cases of disease; for when cold gets the power over the inward heat, the stomach and bowels become coated with canker, which prevents those numerous little vessels calculated to nourish the system from performing their duty. A cure, therefore, cannot be effected without removing this difficulty, which must be done by such things as are best calculated to scour off the canker and leave the juices flowing free. There are many articles which are good for this, but I shall mention only such as I have found to be the best. Several things that are used for canker, are too binding, and do more hurt than good, as they cause obstructions. I have adopted a rule to ascertain what is good for canker, which I have found very useful; and shall here give it as a guide for others; that is, to chew some of the article, and if it causes the saliva to flow freely, and leaves the mouth clean and moist, it is good; but on the other hand, if it dries up the juices, and leaves the mouth rough and dry, it is bad, and should be avoided.

BAYBERRY; or, CANDLEBERRY.

This is a species of the myrtle, from which wax is obtained from the berries, and grows common in many parts of this country. It is a shrub growing from two to four feet high, and is easily known by the berries which it produces annually, containing wax in abundance ; these grow on the branches close to them, similar to the juniper ; the leaves are of a deep green. The bark of the roots is what is used for medicine, and should be collected in the spring, before it puts forth its leaves, or in the fall, after done growing, as then the sap is in the roots; this should be attended to in gathering all kinds of medicinal roots ; but those things that the tops are used, should be collected in the summer when nearly full grown, as then the sap is in the top. The roots should be dug and cleaned from the dirt, and pounded with a mallet or club, when the bark is easily separated from the stalk, and may be obtained with little trouble. It should be dried in a chamber or loft, where it is not exposed to the weather ; and when perfectly dry, should be ground or pounded to a fine powder. It is an excellent medicine either taken by itself or compounded with other articles ; and is the best thing for canker of any article I have ever found. It is highly stimulating and very pungent, pricking the glands and causing the saliva and other juices to flow freely. Is good used as tooth powder, cleanses the teeth and gums, and removes the scurvy; taken as snuff, it clears the head and relieves the head-ache. It may be given to advantage in a relax, and all disorders of the bowels. When the stomach is very foul, it will frequently operate as an emetic. For a dose, take a tea-spoonful in hot water, sweetened.

WHITE POND LILY.—The Root.

This is well known from the beautiful flower which it bears, opening only to the sun, and closing again at night. It grows in fresh water ponds, and is common in

all parts of this country where I have been. The best
time to gather it, is in the fall of the year, when dry,
and the water in the ponds is low, as it may then be obtained with little difficulty. It has large roots, which
should be dug, washed clean, split into strips, and dried
as has been directed for the Bayberry root bark. When
perfectly dry, it should be pounded in a mortar, and preserved for use. This article is a very good medicine for
canker, and all complaints of the bowels, given in a tea
alone, or mixed with other articles.

HEMLOCK—the inner Bark.

This is the common Hemlock tree, and grows in all
parts of New England. The best for medicine is to
peel the bark from the young tree, and shave the ross
from the outside, and preserve only the inner rhine; dry
it carefully, and pound or grind it to a powder. A tea
made by putting boiling water to this bark, is a good
medicine for canker, and many other complaints. The
first of my using the Hemlock bark as medicine, was in
1814; being in want of something for canker, I tried
some of it by chewing, and found it to answer, made use
of it to good advantage. Since then, have been in constant use of it, and have always found it a very good medicine, both for canker and other complaints of the bowels
and stomach. A tea made of this bark, is very good and
may be used freely ; it is good to give the emetic and
No. 2, in, and may be used for drink in all cases of sickness, especially when going through a course of medicine
and steaming. This, with Bayberry bark and the Lily
root, forms No. 3, or what has been commonly called
coffee, though many other things may be added, or either
of them may be used to advantage alone. The boughs,
made into a tea, are very good for gravel and other obstructions of the urinary passages, and for rheumatism.

MARSH ROSEMARY—the Root.

This article is very well known in all parts of this
country, and has been made use of for canker and sore
mouth. I have made use of it with Bayberry bark as
No. 3, in my practice, for many years, with good success ; but after finding that the Lily root and Hemlock

bark were better, have mostly laid it aside. It is so
binding in its nature that it is not safe to use it without
a large proportion of the Bayberry bark.

SUMACH—the Bark, Leaves and Berries.

This appears to be a new article in medicine, entirely
unknown to the medical faculty, as no mention is made
of it by any author. The first of my knowledge that it
was good for canker, was when at Onion River in 1807,
attending the dysentery; being in want of something to
clear the stomach and bowels in that complaint, found
that the bark, leaves or berries answered the purpose
extremely well, and have made much use of it ever
since. It is well known, and is found in all parts of the
country; some of it grows from eight to twelve feet high,
and has large spreading branches; the berries grow in
large bunches, and when ripe, are a deep red colour,
of a pleasant sour taste; and are used by the country
people to dye with. The leaves and young sprouts are
made use of in tanning morocco leather. For medicine, the bark should be peeled when full of sap, the
leaves, when full grown, and the berries, when ripe;
they should be carefully dried, and when used as part of
No. 3, should be pounded, and may be used altogether,
or either separate. A tea made of either or altogether,
is very good, and may be given with safety in almost all
complaints, or put into the injections. It will scour the
stomach and bowels, and is good for stranguary, as it
promotes urine and relieves difficulties in the kidneys,
by removing obstructions and strengthening those parts.
I have been in the habit of late years, of making use of
this article with Bayberry bark and Lily root, or Hemlock bark, equal parts, for No. 3, or coffee, and it has
always answered a good purpose.

WITCH-HAZLE—the Leaves.

I found the use of this article as medicine, when I
was quite young; and have made much use of it in all
my practice. It is too well known in the country to
need any description; is a small tree or bush, and grows
very common, especially in new land. A tea made of
the leaves, is an excellent medicine in many complaints,

and may be freely used to advantage. It is the best thing for bleeding at the stomach of any article I have ever found, either by giving a tea made of the dry leaves, or chewing them when green ; have cured several with it. This complaint is caused by canker eating off the small blood-vessels, and this medicine will remove the canker and stop the bleeding. I have made much use of the tea, made strong for injections, and found it in all complaints of the bowels to be very serviceable. An injection made of this tea, with a little of No. 2, is good for the piles, and many complaints common to females ; and in bearing-down pains it will afford immediate relief, if properly administered. These leaves may be used in No. 3, to good advantage, as a substitute for either of the other articles, or alone for the same purpose.

RED-RASPBERRY—the Leaves.

This is an excellent article, and I believe was never made use of as medicine, till discovered by me. When at Eastport, I had no article with me good for canker and resorted to my old rule of tasting, and found that these leaves were good for that complaint ; made into a strong tea, it answered every purpose wished. I gathered a large quantity of the leaves, and dried them, and have been in constant use of it as a medicine ever since, and have found it an excellent article, both for canker and many other complaints ; for relax and other bowel complaints of children, it is the best thing that I have found ; by giving the tea and using it in the injections, it affords immediate relief. A tea made of the leaves sweetened, with milk in it, is very pleasant, and may be used freely. It is the best thing for women in travail, of any article I know of. Give a strong tea of it, with a little of No. 2, sweetened, and it will regulate every thing as nature requires. If the pains are untimely, it will make all quiet ; if timely and lingering, give more No. 2 and Umbil in the tea. When the child is born, give it some of the tea with sugar and milk in it ; this prevents sore mouth ; and the tea is good to wash sore nipples with. A poultice made with this tea and cracker, or slippery elm bark, is very good for burns or scalds; if the skin is off, by applying this poultice or washing with the tea, it will harden and stop smarting. It may be used in No. 3 as a substitute for other articles, or alone, to good effect.

SQUAW-WEED—Indian name Cocash.

This is known in the country by the name of frost-weed, or meadow scabish; it is a wild weed, and grows in wet land, by the sides of brooks; it has a stalk that grows four or five feet high, which is rough and woolly with a narrow leaf; and bears a blue blossom late in the fall, which remains till the frost kills it. The root lives through the winter, and in the spring puts forth a new stalk; the leaves at the bottom remains green through the winter. The roots and top are used for medicine; it has a fragrant taste and smell like lovage. It was the first thing I ever knew used for canker, and was given to me when I had the canker-rash, being considered then the best article known for canker; I have frequently used it for that complaint and found it very good. Take the green roots and leaves, bruise them, and pour on hot water; give this tea sweetened. It may be kept by adding a little spirit, and is good for rheumatism and nervous affections. It is perfectly harmless and may be used freely. It makes a very good bitter tinctured with hot water and spirit, and is good for dizziness and cold hands and feet. See Directions, &c. page 80.

No. 4.—*Bitters, to correct the Bile and restore Digestion.*

BITTER HERB, or BALMONY.

This herb grows in wet mowing land by the side of brooks; it is about the size of mint, the leaves some larger; the stalk is four square; the leaves are of a dark green, of a sweetish bitter taste. It bears a white blossom of singular form, resembling a snakes head with the mouth open. This herb is very good to correct the bile, and create an appetite. A tea of it may be used alone, or it may be added to the other articles described under this number, which are all calculated to restore the digestive powers.

POPLAR BARK.

There are several species of the poplar tree, that grow common in this country. One kind is called the white poplar and another stinking poplar; the bark of both these kinds are good for medicine; but the latter is the best, being the most bitter. It has tags hanging on the limbs, which remain on till it leaves out, which is about a week later than the other kind. It has short brittle twigs, which are extremely bitter to the taste. The inner bark given in tea is one of the best articles to regulate the bile and restore the digestive powers, of any thing I have ever used. The bark may be taken from the body of the tree, the limbs or the roots, and the outside shaved off and preserve the inner bark, which should be dried and carefully preserved for use. To make the bitters, No. 4, it should be pounded or ground fine, and mixed with the other articles, or it may be used alone for the same purpose. To make a tea, take a handful of the bark pounded or cut into small strips and put into a quart mug, and fill it with boiling water, which if taken freely will relieve a relax, head-ache, faintness at the stomach, and many other complaints caused by bad digestion. Is good for obstructions of the urine and weakness in the loins; and those of a consumptive habit will find great relief in using this tea freely.

BARBERRY—the Bark.

This is a well known shrub, producing red berries, of a pleasant sour taste, which are much used as a pickle, and are also preserved with sugar or molasses. The bark of the root or top is a good bitter and useful to correct the bile and assist the digesture. The bark should be collected at the proper season, carefully dried and pounded or ground to fine powder; and is used as a part of the bitters, No. 4. A tea made of this bark is very good for all cases of indigestion, and may be freely used.

BITTER-ROOT, or WANDERING MILK-WEED.

This valuable vegetable grows in meadows and in hedges, and in appearance is something like buckwheat, having similar white blossoms; when the stalk is broken it discharges a milky substance; it has two small pods about the size of the cabbage seed pods, with a silky substance. This herb is wandering, that is, the roots run about under ground to a considerable distance and produces many stalks, which grow up from different parts of the root to the height of about two feet. The kind that is commonly known by the name of wandering milk-weed, grows only on upland; there is another kind which grows near rivers and on islands, where high water flows over it, this differs some from the other in appearance; the roots run deep in the sand; it has leaves and pods like the first, and both are good for medicine. The bark of the root is used. The roots should be dug and dried; and when perfectly dry may be pounded in a mortar, when the bark is easily separated from the woody part. This root is very bitter and is one of the greatest correctors of the bile I know of; and is an excellent medicine to remove costiveness, as it will cause the bowels to move in a natural manner. A strong decoction of this root, made by steeping it in hot water, if drank freely will operate as a cathartic, and sometimes as an emetic; and is most sure to throw off a fever in its first stages. It should be used in all cases of costiveness.

GOLDEN SEAL; or, OHIO KERCUMA—the Root.

This article grows only in the Western country; I am not well enough acquainted with the herb, to give a description of it; but of the medical virtues of the root, I have had a sufficient experience, to recommend it as a very pleasant bitter, and in cases where the food in the stomach of weak patients causes distress, a teaspoonful of the powder given in hot water sweetened, will give immediate relief. It is an excellent corrector of the bile and may be used for that purpose alone, or

6

with the bitter root, or may be compounded with either
or all the articles described under this number, to restore
the digestive powers.   See Directions, &c. page 82.

———

The purposes for which the articles described under
this head are used, is to regulate the stomach, so that
the food taken into it, may be properly digested; and
I have mentioned enough to enable those who make use
of the practice to effect that object, if properly attended
to.   This is a very important part of the system of practice, for unless the food is digested, it is impossible to
keep up that heat upon which life depends.

———

No. 5.—*Syrup for the Dysentery, to strengthen the Stomach and Bowels, and restore weak patients.*

The articles used in this preparation, are the bark of
poplar and bayberry, which have been described, peach-
meats, or meats of cherry-stones, sugar and brandy.

PEACH-MEATS.

The meats that are in the peach stones have long been
used as medicine, and need but little to be said about
them, except that they are of great value to strengthen
the stomach and bowels, and restore the digesture;
for which purpose I have made much use of them, and
always to good advantage.   Made into a cordial, with
other articles, in the manner as will be hereafter directed, forms one of the best remedies I know of, to recover the natural tone of the stomach after long sickness; and to restore weak patients, particularly in dysentery.   A tea made of the leaves of the peach-tree is
very good for bowel complaints in children and young
people, and will remove cholic.

CHERRY-STONES.

The meats of the wild cherry-stones, are very good,
and may be used instead of the peach-meats, when they

cannot be had. Get these stones as clean as possible, when well dried, pound them in a mortar, and separate the meats from the stones, which is done with little trouble; take the same quantity as is directed, of the peach-meats, and it will answer equally as well. A tea made of the cherries, pounded with the stones, and steeped in hot water, sweetened with loaf sugar, to which add a little brandy, is good to restore the digestive powers, and create an appetite.

Bitter almonds may be used as a substitute for the peach-meats or cherry-stones, when they cannot be had. See Directions, &c. page 82.

No. 6.—*Rheumatic Drops, to remove pain, prevent mortification, and promote a natural heat.*

The principal articles used in this preparation, are high wines, or fourth proof brandy, gum myrrh and Cayenne; for external application, spirits of turpentine is added, and sometimes gum camphor. The manner of preparing will be hereafter given.

GUM MYRRH.

This is a gum obtained from a tree, which grows in the East Indies, and is brought to this country and sold by the apothecaries for medicinal uses; there is nothing sold by them that possesses more useful and medicinal properties than this article; though the Doctors seem to have but little knowledge of its virtues. All those whom I have heard express an opinion upon it, consider it of very little value. When I obtained my patent, Dr. Thornton, the clerk of the Patent Office, said it was good for nothing; all this, however, does not lessen its value. The first knowledge I had of it, was when I was laid up with my lame ancle, at Onion River, as has been before related in my narrative. An old man from Canada, passing that way, and hearing of my case, called to see me, and observing the putrid

state I was in, told my father that gum myrrh would
be good for me, as it was an excellent article to prevent mortification.   He immediately obtained some of
the tincture, and not having a syringe, he took some
in his mouth, and squirted it through a quill into the
wound; the smarting was severe for a short time.   By
tasting it himself and finding it a pleasant bitter, he
gave me some to take; by using it, there was a favourable alteration, both in my bodily health, and in the
state of my wound.   After this, I had great faith in
this article, and was seldom without it.   When I came
to have a family, I made much use of myrrh; it was
one of the principal articles used in restoring my wife,
when given over by the mid-wife, as related in my narrative.   In several cases of bad wounds and old sores,
it afforded great relief; and in what the doctors call
worm complaints in children, by giving the tincture,
when such symptoms appeared, it removed them.   I
used it at this time, by making a tincture with spirit;
but after having a knowledge of Cayenne, I put some
of this with it, which made it much better.   I found
out by accident, that boiling it would prevent the fumes
of the spirit from rising to the head, which would
otherwise, in some cases, produce bad effects, particularly in such as were subject to hysterical affection.
This was the origin of my rheumatic drops, a preparation which has proved more generally useful than any
one compound I make use of.   In selecting myrrh for
use, take that of a light brown colour, somewhat trans-
parent, and of a bitter taste, a little pungent.   It should
be reduced to a fine powder, by being pounded in a
mortar, before used.

SPIRIT OF TURPENTINE.

This article is too well known to need any description, being used by painters.   The only way in which
I use it, is in such preparations as are intended for external application, in which I have found it useful.   A
proportion of it should be added to the rheumatic drops,
when used for the itch or other bad humours.   It is a
powerful article, and should be used with caution.

GUM CAMPHOR.

I shall say but little about this article, as I never found any very great advantages from its use, though I never knew it to do any harm. It is made much use of, and I think there is more credit given to it than what it deserves. I have been in the habit of adding some of it to the rheumatic drops, when used for bad sprains, and in such cases have found it useful ; and I have no doubt but that it may be sometimes given to advantage to warm the stomach, and relieve pain ; but there are other articles which I make use of for that purpose, that are much better. See Directions, &c. page 83.

NERVE POWDER.

American Valerian, or Ladies' Slipper ; sometimes called Umbil, or Male and Female Nervine.

There are four species of this valuable vegetable, one male and three female ; the male is called yellow umbil, and grows in swamps and wet land ; has a large cluster of fibrous roots matted together, joined to a solid root, which puts forth several stalks that grow about two feet high ; it has leaves something resembling the poke leaf. The female kinds are distinguished by the colour of the blossoms, which are red, red and white, and white. The red has but two leaves, which grow out of the ground, and lean over to the right and left, between which a single stalk shoots up to the height of from eight to ten inches, bearing on its top a red blossom of a very singular form, that gives it the name of female umbil. This kind is found on high ledges and in swamps. The red and white, and white umbil, grows only in swamps, and is in larger clusters of roots, than the yellow, but in a similar form ; its top is similar to the red, except the colour of the blossom. The yellow and red are the best for medicine ; the roots should be dug in the fall, when done growing, or in the spring, be-

6*

fore the top puts forth. If dug when growing, the roots will nearly all dry up. When the roots are dug, they should be washed clean, carefully dried, and pounded or ground to a fine powder, sifted through a fine sieve, and preserved from the air for use.

This powder is the best nervine known; I have made great use of it, and have always found it to produce the most beneficial effects, in all cases of nervous affection, and in hysterical symptoms; in fact, it would be difficult to get along with my practice in many cases without this important article. It is perfectly harmless, and may be used in all cases of disease with safety; and is much better than opium, which is generally given in cases of spasmodic affection, and which only deadens the feelings, and relieves pain only by destroying sensibility, without doing any good. It has been supposed by the doctors to be of a narcotic nature; but this is a mistake. They have drawn this conclusion, I suppose, from its tendency to promote sleep; but this is altogether owing to its quieting the nerves, and leaving the patient at ease, when nature requires sleep to recover the natural tone of the system. Half a tea-spoonful may be given in hot water sweetened, and the dose repeated if necessary; or the same quantity may be mixed with a dose of either the other numbers, when given, and put into the injections; and where there is nervous symptoms, it should never be dispensed with. See Directions, &c. page 83.

I have thus far given a description of all the important vegetables made use of in my system of practice, with the manner of preparing and using them. I shall now proceed to describe a number of articles of less importance, all of which I have used and found good in various complaints. Some of them form a part of my medical preparations, and many others may be used as substitutes for some that have been mentioned. They are all of a warming nature, and may be used to advantage in throwing off disease in its first stages.

SPEARMINT.

This is a well known herb, and makes a very pleasant tea, which may be freely used in sickness. The most valuable property it possesses, is to stop vomiting. If the Emetic Herb, or any other cause should produce violent vomiting, by giving a strong tea made of this herb, it will stop it, and sit pleasantly on the stomach.

PEPPERMINT.

This article is very hot in its nature, and may be used to advantage to promote perspiration and overpower the cold. I have frequently used it for that purpose with success; but it is volatile, and will not retain the heat long in the stomach. In colds and slight attacks of disease, to drink freely of a tea made of this herb on going to bed, will throw it off. The essence, put in warm water, is good to give children, and will relieve pain in the stomach and bowels. A few drops of the oil, given in warm water, or on loaf sugar, is good for the same purpose.

PENNYROYAL.

This herb grows common in all parts of the country, and is too well known to need any description. It is an article of great value in medicine, and a tea of it may be freely used in all cases of sickness. It is good for the stomach, being warming and cleansing; if drank freely, will produce perspiration, and remove obstructions. In colds and slight attacks of disease, it will be likely to throw it off, and prevent sickness. It is very good for children, and will remove pain in the bowels and wind. In going through a course of medicine, a tea of this herb may be given for drink, and will cause the medicine to have a pleasant operation.

SUMMERSAVORY.

This herb grows in gardens, and is made use of to season meats in cooking; it is of a very pleasant flavour and of a hot nature. A tea of it is good for colds, and may be used freely in case of sickness.   There is an oil made from this herb, which will cure the tooth-ache, by putting a little on cotton wool, and applying it to the affected tooth.

HOARHOUND.

This plant grows common in this country, and is made much account of in removing cough. An infusion made of the leaves, sweetened with honey, is good for the asthma, and all complaints of the lungs. The syrup of this plant will loosen tough phlegm, and remove hoarseness caused by a bad cold.   The hoarhound candy is very useful for such as are troubled with cough, particularly old people, and those that are short winded.

ELECAMPANE.

The root of this plant made into syrup, is good for a cough ; and I have made use of it for that purpose with advantage in many cases, and can recommend it as a safe and useful remedy in complaints of that kind.

MAYWEED.

A tea made of this herb, to be drank hot when going to bed, is very good for a cold ; and in slight attacks of a fever, if used freely, and a hot stone put to the feet, will in most cases throw it off.   It grows common in old fields, and by the sides of roads.

WORMWOOD.

This herb is a very wholesome bitter, and may be taken to advantage in different ways.   It is of a hot nature and is good for the stomach, to create an appetite, and assist the digesture.   It may be taken in tea, or the green herb may be pounded and tinctured in spirit, which is good to apply to a bruise or sprain.

TANSY.

This is a hot bitter herb, grows common in highways, and is cultivated in gardens.   A tea made of this herb is good for hysterics and other female complaints; it will strengthen those that have weak reins and kidneys, and is good for the stranguary, or stoppage of urine.— The green leaves pounded, are good to put on bruises and sprains, and will allay the swelling.

CHAMOMILE.

This is a well known herb, the flowers are sold by the apothecaries and are made much use of in a tea for many complaints. It is good given in a tea for bowel complaints, and externally applied, will relieve sprains, bruises, and swellings, and remove callouses, corns, &c. and restore shrunk sinews.

BITTER-SWEET.

This herb has long been esteemed as a medicine of considerable value for many complaints. It grows common in this country, in hedges where the ground is moist, and the top runs along the ground or climbs on bushes. Its taste when chewed is first bitter and then sweet, which has given its name. It is said to be a good medicine for internal injuries and to remove obstructions, which I have no doubt is correct; but the only way I make use of it is for external application; the bark of the root with chamomile and wormwood makes an ointment of great value, which is an excellent thing for a bruise, sprain, calice, swelling, or for corns.

MULLEN.

The leaves of this plant are very good to bring down swelling and to restore contracted sinews, by pounding them and applying them warm to the part affected. For external use, they are an excellent article in many complaints. This herb is too well known to need any description. It is an important article in my strengthening plaster.

BURDOCK.

The leaves of this plant wilted by the fire and applied to an external injury, will allay the inflammation

and ease pain; and they are good pounded and put on
to a bruise or sprain, as it will give immediate relief.
It is made use of in the strengthening plaster. The
leaves are good applied to the feet in case of fever, to
keep them moist and promote perspiration.

SKUNK-CABBAGE.

This vegetable grows common in all parts of New-
England; it has large leaves something resembling cabbage, from which and its disagreeable smell, it takes its
name; it may be found in the meadows and wet land.
The root only is used for medicine, which should be
dug and split into strips and carefully dried; when dry
it should be pounded or ground to a powder. This
powder may be taken in tea sweetened, or made into a
syrup, or half a tea-spoonful may be mixed in honey
and taken in the morning, or at night when going to
bed. It is good for asthma, cough, difficulty of breathing, and all disorders of the lungs, and with other articles makes one of the best preparations for those complaints I have ever found.

WAKE ROBIN.

This plant grows wild in this country. It has three
triangular leaves, from between them it puts forth a na-
ked stalk, on the top of which, is a singular stem or
pistil enclosed in a sheath, resembling a flower, which is
followed by a bunch of reddish berries. The root is used
for medicine, and resembles a small turnip. This root
is extremely pungent and stimulating, and is often given
for cholic and pain in the bowels, and to expel wind.
I have mostly made use of it for cough and disorders of
the lungs, for which I have found it a very useful article,
and it forms part of my composition for coughs. The
root should be dried and reduced to a powder, and may
be given mixed with honey, or in a syrup.

THOROUGHWORT.

This herb is well known in the country, and is made
use of by the people in tea for many complaints. It is

of a warming nature, and is good for cough and other complaints of the lungs. It is used in my compound, prepared for coughs.

FEATHERFEW.

This herb is stimulating and is good for hysteric complaints, and many other disorders common to females. It promotes the passage of urine, and removes obstructions in those parts. It should be taken in tea alone, or may be added with chamomile, and used to advantage in all cases of obstructions.

CLIVERS.

This is a sort of joint grass and grows in mowing land, where the ground is wet. It has small leaves at each joint; the stalk is four square and the edges are rough like a sickle. This herb made into a strong tea and drank freely is very good for the stoppage of urine, and may be made use of for all obstructions in those parts to advantage.

BLACK BIRCH BARK.

A tea made of this bark is useful in curing all complaints of the bowels and to remove obstructions. I have made much use of it in dysentery. This tea with peachmeats or cherry stone meats, made into a syrup, is an excellent article to restore patients after having been reduced by that disease, and to promote the digesture. It is good for canker and all complaints of the bowels.

EVAN ROOT.

This is called by some people chocolate root, on account of its resembling that article in taste, and is made use of by some for common drink instead of tea or coffee. It is good for canker, and may be used in No. 3 as a substitute for other articles. It grows common in this country and is too well known to need describing.

SLIPPERY ELM BARK.

The inner bark of this tree is an article of much value, and may be used to advantage in many different ways. There are several species of the elm that grow common in this country; and there are two kinds of the slipperry elm, one the bark is rather hard and tough, and the other is very brittle;' the latter is the best for medicinal uses. The bark should be peeled, the outside ross shaved off, dried, and ground or pounded to a fine powder. If used internally, put a tea-spoonful of this powder into a tea-cup with as much sugar, mix them well together, then add a little cold water and stir it till perfectly mixed, and then put hot water to it and stir till it forms a jelly thick enough to be eaten with a spoon. A tea-spoonful may be taken at a time, and is an excellent medicine to heal soreness in the throat, stomach and bowels, caused by canker; or more hot water may be put to it and made into a drink, and freely taken for the same purpose. I have made much use of this bark for poultices, and have in all cases found it a most excellent article for that purpose. Mixed with pounded cracker and ginger it makes the best poultice I have ever found; for burns, scalds, felons, old sores, &c. it is the best thing I have met with, to allay the inflammation, ease the pain and heal them in a short time.

BALSAM FIR.

This balsam is obtained from a tree well known in many parts of this country; it is taken from small blisters which form in the bark. It is of a very healing nature, and is good to remove internal soreness. It forms an important article in my healing salve. When taken it may be dropped on loaf sugar.

GENTIAN.

This root grows wild in this country; and is found plentifully in Vermont. It was formerly collected for exportation, and large quantities of it were sent to China, where it brought a great price. It is said the peo-

ple of that country considered it of great value; but
for what purpose they use it, is, I believe, only known
to themselves. It is a nervine and may be used to
advantage in all cases of nervous affection, either alone
or mixed with other articles. The root should be dug
in the fall, dried and reduced to a fine powder; from
half to a tea-spoonful may be given for a dose, in hot
water sweetened.

SNAKEROOT.

This is a well known article, grows wild. and may
be found in most parts of this country. It is of a
hot nature, and is made much use of in tea, for measles and other eruptions, to keep the disorder out,
for which it is considered very good; this is owing
to its warming qualities, which keeps the determining powers to the surface, which effect may be produced by almost any strong stimulant; but No. 2, or the
composition powders, is much the best for that purpose.
A tea made of this root may be given to advantage
in many cases of disease; it has a tendency to promote perspiration, and is good to remove pain in the
stomach and bowels, and expel wind. The roots reduced to powder may be mixed with gentian or umbil
for all nervous complaints.

MUSTARD.

The seed of this herb is principally made use of for
culinary purposes, being eaten on meat; for which it is
ground to a fine powder and mixed with warm water.
It is very pungent and of a hot nature; but is volatile
and will not hold the heat long enough to do much good
in retaining the internal heat. It is good to create an
appetite and assist the digesture; and given in hot water sweetened, will remove pain in the bowels and
stomach. It is frequently used for rheumatism, both internally and externally; but Nos. 2 and 6, are much better for that purpose.

7

HORSERADISH.

The root of this plant is mostly used for culinary purposes, and it has some medicinal properties. It is of a hot nature, but very volatile; its warming qualities will mostly evaporate before it gets into the stomach. The roots may be given to promote the appetite and assist the digesture. The leaves are sometimes applied to remove external pain, but is apt to raise a blister.

BALM OF GILEAD.

This tree is of the species of the poplar and possesses some medicinal virtues. It resembles the kind of poplar that has been described, having similar tags; but the buds and leaves are larger. The buds bruised and tinctured in spirit, produces an effect something like the tincture of myrrh; and is good taken inwardly as a restorative, and for bathing sores. The bark scraped from the twigs and steeped in hot water, is a good corrector of the bile, and will operate both as an emetic and cathartic; it is more harsh than the other kind of poplar, but may be used to advantage in many cases of disease.

BUTTERNUT.

This tree grows common in this country, and is well known from the nut which it bears, of an oblong shape and nearly as large as an egg, in which is a meat containing much oil, and very good to eat. The bark of this tree is used by the country people to colour with. The bark taken from the body of the tree or roots and boiled down till thick, may be made into pills, and operates as a powerful emetic and cathartic; a syrup may be made by boiling the bark and adding one third molasses and a little spirit, which is good to give children for worm complaints. The buds and twigs may also be used for the same purpose, and are more mild. White ash bark and balm of gilead may be added, equal parts, and made into syrup or pills. Those who are fond of drastic purges may have their ends sufficiently answered by these preparations, and they are the most safe and harmless of any that I know of; and those who wish to be tortured with blisters, can have them cheap, by bruising the green shell of the nut, or the bark, and applying it where the blister is wanted, keeping the bandage wet, and in three hours they will be completely drawn, and the skin as black as that of an African. This is much quicker and safer than if done with flies, and will not cause stranguary. The bark of the butternut is the principal ingredient in Dr. Hawkes' rheumatic and cancer pills, and also of Chamberlain's bilious cordial, which have been so celebrated for many complaints. It is called by some people oilnut and lemon walnut.

BLUE AND WHITE VERVINE.

This is a well known herb, growing very common; it ranks next to the emetic herb, for a puke; and may be used for that purpose either alone or combined with thoroughwort. It is good to prevent a fever in its first stages. This herb has been used with considerable success in consumption, having cured several cases where the doctors had given them over. It may be used in a tea made of the dry herb, or prepared in powder like the emetic herb.

PIPSISWAY, or RHEUMATIC WEED.

This herb grows on mountainous land, and on pine plains, where the boxberry or checkerberry is found plenty. It is an ever-green, and grows from three to six inches high, has a number of dark green leaves, about half an inch wide and from one to two inches long, with a scolloped edge; bears several brown seeds resembling all-spice. The tops and roots are used for medicine. The roots when chewed are very pungent, which will be felt for several hours on the tongue, as though burnt. A strong tea made of this plant is good for cancers and all scrofulous humours, by drinking the tea and bathing with it the parts affected.

Another evergreen plant, called wild lettuce, grows on the same kind of land, which possesses much the same medical properties as the above. It has round leaves, from the size of a cent to that of a dollar, resembling a common lettuce. The roots of this plant and of the pipsisway, dried and powdered together, equal parts, is good to cure all bad humours. Take a tea-spoonful of the powder in a glass of hot water, and bathe the parts affected with the same. . It is also good to restore weak nerves.

GOLDENROD.

This herb may be found common on pine plains and in hedges; it grows about two or three feet high, has a long narrow leaf, very smooth and glossy, and a large cluster of yellow blossoms; it has a sweet spicy taste and smell, resembling fennel or annise. There is an oil obtained from this herb good for medicine; and also prepared in essence, is good for pain in the head, to be taken, or the outside bathed with it. The oil is good to scent the bayberry and bitter-root snuff, which is very good to be taken and snuffed up the nose. There are several herbs that resemble this in appearance, but are very different in smell and taste.

MEADOW FERN.

This is a shrub, and grows in meadows and by the side of stagnant water, sometimes growing in the water; it is found in thick bunches, and grows from two to three feet high. When the leaves are off it has a large bud, which is larger on some bushes than others; some of them bear a small bur, or cluster of seeds, which, when rubbed between the fingers, leaves an oily or balsamy substance, having a fragrant smell, something like spirits of turpentine.

These burs pounded fine and simmered in cream, hogs lard or fresh butter, is almost a sovereign remedy for the itch, or external poison, and all bad humour sores. When the burs cannot be had, take the bush and buds and make a strong decoction; drink of this and wash with the same. This liquor may be prepared in syrup, and by boiling it down may be made into ointment as has been described for the burs; the syrup should be taken and the ointment put on the affected parts. This ointment, or the wash, is good for salt-rheum, or canker sores, and may be used freely.

YELLOW DOCK.

The root of this plant is well known as being made into ointment for the itch. The roots should be bruised fine in a mortar and put in a pewter bason, add cream enough to make an ointment, keep it warm for twelve hours, be careful not to scald it. Rub it on at night when going to bed. Three times using it will generally effect a cure. The foregoing described ointments, together with No. 3, and the rheumatic drops prepared with the spirits of turpentine, will be sufficient to cure any case of this complaint.

PRICKLY ASH.

This is a shrub or bush that grows in the Western country, and is well known by the people there. It grows from eight to twelve feet high, and bears a berry that grows close to the limbs; it has leaves like the white-ash. The bark and the berries are used for medical purposes. The berries are very pungent, and are a powerful stimulant, as also the bark of the top and roots, though not so strong. It should be pounded to a powder and steeped in hot water, then put into wine or spirit, and it makes a very good hot bitter. Take half a glass two or three times a day; it is good for fever and ague, for which it is much used; and for lethargy, or sleepiness, and for cold feet and hands, and other complaints caused by cold.

BITTER THISTLE.

This herb is a species of the thistle, and is cultivated in gardens. It is of one years growth, the seed being sown in the spring and it comes to maturity in the fall. The stalk has a number of branches, and a great quan-

7*

tity of leaves. The leaf is some larger than the Canada
thistle, with prickles like it; and it bears seeds about
the size of the barley corn, with a beard on the end
nearly as long as the seed. The leaves are used for
medicine, which may be steeped in hot water, and drank
like other herb tea, or they may be reduced to a powder
and taken in molasses or warm water, or in wine or spirit.
It is an excellent corrector of the bile, and may be
safely used for that purpose. The Cardis Benedictus, or
beloved thistle, is cultivated in the same manner, and
may be used for the same purpose.

ARCHANGEL.

This herb grows wild in wet land, and may be often
found among the grass, and at the edges of plough fields.
It grows from four to twelve inches high; the leaves
are rather smaller than mint leaves; it bears a kind of
bur containing seed, which grows round the stalk at each
joint. There are two kinds which grow near each other;
they look very much alike, but are very different in
taste. One is very bitter and the other has no bitter
taste, but is very rough and of a balsamic taste. They
may be used together in a tea or syrup, and answer two
important purposes; the rough removes the canker and
the bitter is a corrector of the bile. By adding No. 2,
the compound contains the three great principles of the
healing art, viz. hot, rough and bitter.

DIRECTIONS

VEGETABLE MEDICINE.

No. 1.—*Emetic Herb.*

The preparation of this herb has been sufficiently described, for which see page 43. It is prepared and used in three different ways, viz:

1. The powdered leaves and pods. This is the most common form of using it; and from half to a tea-spoonful may be taken in warm water sweetened; or the same quantity may be put into either of the other numbers when taken; to cleanse the stomach, overpower the cold, and promote a free perspiration.

2. A tincture made from the green herb in spirit. This is used to counteract the effects of poison; to be either internally or externally used; and for asthma and other complaints of the lungs. For a dose take a tea-spoonful, adding about the same quantity of No. 2, in half a tea-cupful of warm water sweetened, and in all cases of nervous affection add half a tea-spoonful of nerve powder. For the external effects of poison, take the above dose, and bathe the parts affected with the tincture, repeating it till cured.

3. The seeds reduced to a fine powder and mixed with Nos. 2 and 6. This is for the most violent attacks of spasms and other complaints, such as lock-jaw, bite of a mad dog, fits, drowned persons, and all cases of suspended animation, where the vital spark is nearly extinct. For a dose give a tea-spoonful, and repeat it till relief is obtained; then follow with a tea of No. 3, for canker.

For children, the dose must be regulated according to their age. If very young, steep a dose of the powder

in half a tea-cupful of warm water, or tea of raspberry
leaves, and give a tea-spoonful at a time of the tea,
strained through a fine cloth, and sweetened, repeating
the dose every ten minutes, till it operates; and give
pennyroyal, or some other herb tea for drink.

No. 2.—*Cayenne.*

This is a medicine of great value in the practice, and
may be safely used in all cases of disease, to raise and
retain the internal vital heat of the system, cause a free
perspiration, and keep the determining powers to the
surface.   The only preparation is to have it reduced to
a fine powder.   For a dose, take from half to a tea-
spoonful, in hot water, or a tea of No. 3, sweetened; or
the same quantity may be mixed with a dose of either
the other numbers when taken.   The dose should be
repeated every ten or fifteen minutes till the desired object is effected, and continued occasionally till health is
restored.   When this number is given, the patient should
be kept warm, by sitting by the fire, covered with a
blanket, or in a warm bed.

No. 3.—*For Canker.*

Take Bayberry root bark, white pond Lily root, and
the inner bark of Hemlock, equal parts of each pounded and well mixed together; steep one ounce of the
powder in a pint of boiling water, and give for a dose, a
common wine glass full, sweetened.
.If the above cannot be had, take as a substitute,
sumach bark, leaves or berries, red-raspberry or witch-
hazle leaves, marsh rosemary, or either of the other
articles described under the head of No. 3; they are
all good for canker, and may be used together or separate.
When the violence of the disease requires a course of
medicine, steep one ounce of the above mentioned powder, No. 3, in a pint of boiling water, strain off a wine
glass full while hot, and add a tea-spoonful of No. 2,
and the same quantity of sugar; when cool enough to

take, add a tea-spoonful of No. 1, and half that quantity of nerve powder. Let this dose be given three times, at intervals of fifteen minutes; and let the same compound be given by injection, and if the case requires it again repeat it. If mortification is apprehended, a tea-spoonful of No. 6, may be added to each dose, and to the injections.

After the patient has recovered sufficiently from the operation of the medicine, which is usually in two or three hours, place them over the steam, as is directed in page 21.

This operation is sufficient for one time, and must be repeated each day, or every other day, as the circumstances of the case may require, till the disorder is removed. Three times will generally be sufficient, and sometimes once or twice will answer the purpose; but in bad chronic cases it may be necessary to continue to carry them through a regular course two or three times a week, for a considerable length of time.

Great care must be taken to keep up an internal heat, so as to produce perspiration, after they have been through the operation, by giving occasionally No. 2, or the composition powder, for if this is not attended to, the patient may have a relapse, in which case it will be very difficult to raise it again, as they will fall as much below a natural heat as they have been raised above it by artificial means.

During the operation give milk porridge, or gruel, well seasoned, with a little cayenne in it; and after it is over, the patients may eat any kind of nourishing food that the appetite may crave.

A tea-cupful of the tea of No. 3, should be taken night and morning, to prevent a relapse of the disease, and during the day drink frequently of a tea made of poplar bark; and if costive, use the bitter root.

As soon as the disorder is removed, use the bitters, No. 4, to correct the bile and restore the digesture; and half a wine glass full of the syrup, No. 5, may be taken two or three times a day, which will strengthen the stomach and assist in regulating the digestive powers,

The foregoing directions are calculated for the more
violent attacks of disease, and such as have become settled; but those of a less violent nature must be treated
according to circumstances. In the first stages of a
disease, it may be most generally thrown off by a dose
of the emetic herb, with No. 2, to raise a free perspiration, followed by a tea of No. 3, to remove the canker,
and the bitters or a tea of poplar bark, to regulate the
digesture. For a sudden cold, take a dose of the composition powder on going to bed, and put a hot stone,
wrapped in wet cloths, at the feet, which will in most
cases remove the complaint; but if these applications do
not answer the purpose, the patient should be carried
through a regular course as soon as possible. Steaming
is safe and will always do good, and the injections must
not be neglected, particularly where the bowels are disordered. In consumption, and all old lingering complaints, give the composition powder for two or three
days before going through a regular course.

No. 4.—*Bitters.*

Take the Bitter Herb, or Balmony, Barberry and
Poplar bark, equal parts, pulverized, one ounce of the
powder to a pint of hot water, and half a pint of spirit.
For a dose, take half a wine glass full. For hot bitters,
add a tea-spoonful of No. 2.

This preparation is calculated to correct the bile and
create an appetite, by restoring the digestive powers;
and may be freely used both as a restorative and to prevent disease.

When the above articles cannot be had, either of
those that have been before described under No. 4,
which are all good for the same purpose, may be used
as a substitute.

No. 5.—*Syrup.*

Take Poplar bark and bark of the root of Bayberry,
one pound each, and boil them in two gallons of water,
strain off and add seven pounds of good sugar; then

scald and skim it, and add half a pound of peachmeats;
or the same quantity of cherry-stone meats, pounded
fine.　When cool, add a gallon of good brandy; and,
keep it in bottles for use.　Take half a wine glass full
two or three times a day.

Any other quantity may be prepared, by observing the
same proportion of the different articles.

This syrup is very good to strengthen the stomach
and bowels, and to restore weak patients; and is
particularly useful in the dysentery, which leaves the
stomach and bowels in a sore state.　In a relax, or
the first stages of the dysentery, by using a tea of No.
3, freely, and giving this syrup, it will generally cure
it, and will also prevent those exposed, from taking the
disease.

No. 6.—*Rheumatic Drops.*

Take one gallon of good fourth proof brandy, or any
kind of high wines, one pound of gum Myrrh pounded fine, one ounce of No. 2, and put them into a stone
jug, and boil it a few minutes in a kettle of water, leaving the jug unstopped.　When settled, bottle it up for
use.　It may be prepared without boiling, by letting it
stand in the jug for five or six days, shaking it well
every day, when it will be fit for use.

These drops are to remove pain and prevent mortification, to be taken, or applied externally or to be put
into the injections　One or two tea-spoonfuls of these
drops may be given alone, or the same quantity may
be put into a dose of either of the medicines before
mentioned; and may be also used to bathe with in all
cases of external swellings or pains.　It is an excellent remedy for rheumatism, by taking a dose and
bathing the parts affected with it.　In the headache,
by taking a swallow, and bathing the head, and snuff-
ing a little up the nose, it will remove the pain.　It is
good for bruises, sprains, swelled joints, and old sores;
as it will allay the inflammation, bring down swelling,
ease pain, and produce a tendency to heal; in fact,
there is hardly a complaint, in which this useful medi-

cine cannot be used to advantage. It is the best preservative against mortification of any thing I have ever found.

For bathing, in rheumatism, itch, or other humours, or in any swelling or external pain, add one quarter part of spirits of turpentine; and for sprains and bruises, a little gum camphor may be added.

NERVE POWDER.

This is the American Valerian, or Umbil, and the preparation has been sufficiently described, for which see page 65. This powder is a valuable and safe medicine, and may be used in all cases without danger; and when there are nervous symptoms, it must never be dispensed with. For a dose, take half a tea-spoonful in hot water sweetened; or the same quantity should be put into a dose of either of the other medicine, and also into the injections, in all nervous cases.

COMPOSITION; or, VEGETABLE POWDER.

Take two pounds of the bayberry-root bark, one pound of the inner bark of Hemlock, one pound of ginger, two ounces of Cayenne, two ounces of cloves, all pounded fine, sifted through a fine sieve, and well mixed together. For a dose, take a tea-spoonful of this powder, with an equal quantity of sugar, and put to it half a tea-cupful of boiling water; to be taken as soon as sufficiently cool, the patient being in bed, or by the fire, covered with a blanket.

This composition is calculated for the first stages and in less violent attacks of disease. It is a medicine of much value, and may be safely used in all complaints of male or female, and for children. It is good for relax, dysentery, pain in the stomach and bowels, and to remove all obstructions caused by cold, or loss of inward heat; by taking a dose on going to bed, and putting a hot stone to the feet, wrapped in wet cloths, it will cure a bad cold, and will generally throw off a disease in its first stages, if repeated two or three times. If the symptoms are violent, with much pain, add to each dose a tea-spoonful of No. 6, and half a tea-spoonful of No. 1; and in nervous symptoms, add half a tea-spoonful of nerve powder; at the same time give an injection of the same. If these should not answer the purpose, the patient must be carried through a regular course of the medicine, as has been before described.

COUGH POWDER.

Take four tea-spoonfuls of Skunk Cabbage, two of Hoarhound, one of Wake-robin, one of No. 1, one of No. 2, one of Bayberry bark, one of Bitter root, and one of nerve powder, all made fine and well mixed together. When taken to be mixed with molasses. Take half a tea-spoonful of the powder on going to bed; keep warm, and continue taking it till relief is obtained, particularly on going to bed.

Where the cough has been of long standing, it will be best, while taking this prescription, to go through a regular course of the medicine, and repeat it if necessary.

CANCER PLASTER.

Take the heads of red clover, and fill a brass kettle, and boil them in water for one hour; then take them out, and fill the kettle again with fresh ones, and boil them as before in the same liquor. Strain it off and press the heads to get out all the juice; then simmer it over a slow fire till it is about the consistence of tar, when it will be fit for use. Be careful not to let it burn. When used it should be spread on a piece of bladder, split and made soft. It is good to cure cancers, sore lips, and all old sores.

SALVE.

Take one pound of Bees-wax, one do. of salt Butter, one and a half do. of Turpentine, twelve ounces of Balsam-fir; melt and simmer them together; then strain it off into a basin, and keep it for use. It may be used to heal fresh wounds, burns, scalds and all bad sores, after the inflammation is allayed, and the wound cleansed.

8

STRENGTHENING PLASTER.

Take Burdock leaves and Mullen leaves, bruise them and put them in a kettle, with a sufficient quantity of water, and boil them well ; then strain off the liquor, press or squeeze the leaves, and boil it down till about half as thick as molasses ; then add three parts of Rosin and one of Turpentine, and simmer well together, until the water is evaporated ; then pour it off into cold water, and work it with the hands like shoemaker's wax ; if too hard put in more turpentine, when it will be fit for use. It should be spread on soft leather and applied to the part affected ; and it is good to strengthen weakness in the back and other parts of the body.

VOLATILE SALTS.

Take crude Sal Amoniac, one ounce, Pearlash, two ounces, and pound each by itself, mix them well together, and keep it close stopped in a bottle for use. By damping it with spirit or essence, will increase the strength. This applied to the nose, is good for faintness, and to remove pain in the head ; and is much better than what is generally sold by the apothecaries.

NERVE OINTMENT.

Take the bark of the root of Bitter-sweet, two parts ; of wormwood and chamomile, each equal, one part, when green, or if dry, moisten it with hot water ; which put into horse or porpoise oil, or any kind of soft animal oil, and simmer them over a slow fire for twelve hours ; then strain it off, and add one ounce of spirits of Turpentine to each pound of ointment. To be used for a bruise, sprain, calice, swelling, or for corns.

POULTICE.

Make a strong tea of Raspberry leaves, or of No. 3 ; take a cracker pounded fine, and slippery-elm bark pulverized, with ginger, and make a poultice of the same. This is good for old sores, whitlows, felons, and for bad burns, scalds, and parts frozen. Apply this poultice and renew it, at least as often as every twelve or twenty-four hours, and wash with soap suds at every renewal ; wet-

ting it in the interim with cold water, or a tea of Raspberry leaves, till it discharges; then apply the salve till
a cure is effected.

INJECTIONS, or CLYSTERS.

This manner of administering medicine is of the
greatest importance to the sick; it will frequently give
relief when all other applications fail. It is supposed that
the use of them is of great antiquity; whether this be
true or not, the using them to relieve the sick, was certainly a very valuable discovery; and no doubt thousands
of lives have been saved by it. The doctors have long
been in the practice of directing injections to be given to
their patients, but they seem to have no other object in administering them, than to cause a movement in the bowels;
therefore it was immaterial what they were made of.

According to the plan which I have adopted, there
are certain important objects aimed at in the administration of medicine to remove disease, viz. to raise the
internal heat, promote perspiration, remove the canker,
guard against mortification, and restore the digestion.
To accomplish these objects, the medicine necessary to
remove the complaint, must be applied to that part
where the disease is seated; if in the stomach only, by
taking the medicine, it may be removed; but if in the
bowels, the same compound must be administered by
injection. Whatever is good to cure disease when taken into the stomach, is likewise good for the same
purpose if given by injection, as the grand object is to
warm the bowels, and remove the canker. In all cases
of dysentery, cholic, piles, and other complaints, where
the bowels are badly affected, injections should never
be dispensed with. They are perfectly safe in all cases,
and better that they be used ten times when not needed,
than once neglected when they are. In many violent
cases, particularly where there is danger of mortification, patients may be relieved by administering medicine
in this way, when there would be no chance in any
other. I do, therefore, most seriously advise that these
considerations be always borne in mind; and that
this important way of giving relief, be never neglected,
where there is any chance for it to do good. In many

complaints peculiar to females, they are of the greatest importance in giving relief, when properly attended to; for which purpose it is only necessary to repeat what has been before stated; let the remedy be applied with judgment and discretion to that part where the disease is seated.

The common preparation for an Injection or Clyster, is to take a tea-cupful of strong tea made of No. 3, strain it off when hot, and add half a tea-spoonful of No. 2, and a tea-spoonful of No. 6; when cool enough to give, add half a tea-spoonful of No. 1, and the same quantity of nerve powder. Let it be given with a large syringe made for that purpose, or where this cannot be had, a bladder and pipe may be used. They must be repeated as occasion may require, till relief is obtained.

Many other articles may be used to advantage in the injections; a tea of witch-hazle and red-raspberry leaves, either or both together, are very good in many cases. For canker, a tea of either the articles described under the head of No. 3, will answer a good purpose. When the canker is removed, the bowels will be left sore, in which case, give injections of witch-hazel or raspberry leaves tea, with slippery-elm bark. When injections are used to move the bowels only, No. 1, should be left out. It is always safe to add the nerve powder, and if there is nervous symptoms, it must never be omitted.

STOCK OF MEDICINE FOR A FAMILY.

1 ounce of the Emetic Herb,
2 ounces of Cayenne,
½ lb. Bayberry root bark, in powder,
1 lb. of Poplar Bark,
1 lb of Ginger,
1 pint of the Rheumatic Drops.

This stock will be sufficient for a family for one year, and with such articles as they can easily procure themselves, when wanted, will enable them to cure any disease, which a family of common size may be afflicted with during that time. The expense will be small, and much better than to employ a doctor, and have his extravagant bill to pay.

GENERAL DIRECTIONS

In Curing or Preventing Disease.

1. Be careful to always keep the determining powers to the surface, by keeping the inward heat above the outward, or the fountain above the stream, and all will be safe.

2. It must be recollected that heat is life, and cold death; or in other words, cold is disease; that fever is a friend and cold the enemy; it is therefore necessary to aid the friend and oppose the enemy, in order to restore health.

3. That the construction and organization of the human frame, is in all men essentially the same; being formed of the four elements. Earth and water constitute the solids of the body, which is made active by fire and air. Heat in a peculiar manner, gives life and motion to the whole; and when entirely overpowered from whatever cause by the other elements, death ensues.

4. A perfect state of health arises from a due balance of temperature of the elements; and when it is by any means destroyed, the body is more or less disordered. When this is the case, there is always a diminution of heat, or an increase of the power of cold, which is its opposite.

5. All disorders are caused by obstructed perspiration, which may be produced by a great variety of means; that medicine, therefore, must be administered, that is best calculated to remove obstructions and promote perspiration.

6. The food taken into the stomach, and being well digested, nourishes the system and keeps up that heat on which life depends; but by constantly taking food into the stomach, which is sometimes not suitable for nourishment, it becomes foul, so that the food is not well digested; this causes the body to lose its heat, and disease follows.

7. Canker is caused by cold, and there is always more or less of it in all cases of disease; continue to make use

8*

of such articles as are calculated to remove it, as long as there is any appearance of disorder.

8. When the disease is removed, make free use of those things that are good to restore the digestive powers, not forgetting to keep up the inward heat, by giving occasionally, No. 2.

9. Keep always in mind, that an ounce of prevention is better than a pound of cure ; and give medicine on the first appearance of disorder, before it becomes seated ; for it may be then easily thrown off, and much sickness and expense prevented.

10. In case of a fever, increase the internal heat by giving hot medicine, so as to overpower the cold, when the natural heat will return inwardly, and the cold will pervade the whole surface of the body, as the heat had done before ; this is what is called the turn of the fever.

11. If No. 1 should sicken and not puke, there may be two causes for it, viz. the coldness or acidity of the stomach ; for the first, give No. 2 more freely, and for the latter, dissolve a piece of pearlash about the size of a large pea, in a wine glass of water, and let them take it, which will counteract the acidity. If this fails, make use of the steam, which will open the pores, extract the cold, and set the medicine into operation.

12. In giving medicine to children, give about one half, a little more or less according to their age, of the quantity directed, for a grown person. Be particular to offer them drink often, especially young children who cannot ask for it.

13. Dysentery is caused by canker on the bowels, for which, make free use of the tea of No. 3, with No. 2, and give the same by injection, in the first of the disease, and afterwards give the syrup, No. 5, to strengthen the stomach and bowels, and restore the digestive powers.

14. The piles is canker below the reach of medicine given in the usual way, and must be cured by using a wash of No. 3, made strong, and by giving injections of the same, with No. 2. What is called bearing down pains in women, is from the same cause ; and must be relieved by injections made of witch-hazle or red rasp-

berry leaf tea, steeped strong, with No. 2, strained. If this does not give relief, go through a regular course of medicine.

15. Women in a state of pregnancy, ought to be carried through a regular course of the medicine, especially when near the time of delivery. When in travail, give raspberry leaf tea, with a tea-spoonful of the composition powders, or No. 2, and keep them in a perspiration. After delivery, keep up the internal heat, by giving the composition powder, or No. 2. This will prevent cold and after pains; if there should be symptoms of fever, carry them through a regular course of the medicine, which will guard against all alarming complaints, peculiar in such cases.

16. In all cases of a burn, scald, or being frozen; wrap up the part in cloths wet with cold water, often wetting them with the same, to prevent their becoming dry, and be careful to give hot medicine, such as No. 2, or the composition powders, to keep up the inward heat. Pursue this plan for twelve hours; and then, if the skin is off, apply the poultice, or salve. If there should be convulsions, or fever, a regular course of the medicine must without fail be attended to.

17. When a scald is over the whole or greatest part of the body, apply cotton cloth of several thicknesses to the whole body, wet with the tea of raspberry leaves, thoroughly wetting it with the same to prevent it from becoming dry; and give the hot medicine. When the scald is under the stocking, or any other tight garment, let it remain on, adding more cotton cloths, and wet the whole with cold water as often as the smart of the burn returns.

18. If the skin is off, or in case of an old burn, to guard against canker, apply a poultice of cracker and slippery-elm bark, made with a tea of raspberry leaves; washing it with soap suds, when the poultice is changed, and then with the same tea. When any part is frozen, the same method must be taken, as for a burn.

19. For a fresh wound, cut, or bruise, wash immediately with cold water, and bind up in cloths wet with the same; keep a hot stone at the feet, and take medicine to raise a gentle perspiration; continue this till

the inflammation is allayed, and the wound perfectly cleansed, then apply the poultice or salve, till healed. The air must be kept from all wounds or sores, as it will cause pain, and prevent them from healing.

20. In sudden and deadly attacks, such as spotted or yellow fevers, fits, drowned persons, croup, &c. the heat and activity of the patient is so much diminished, that the common administration will not give relief; the determining power to the surface, being so small, through the loss of internal heat, that it will not give the medicine operation, as its effects are resisted, and counterbalanced by the pressure of the external air. To counteract this pressure, keep the room, by aid of a good fire, about as warm as a summer heat; and more fully to rarify and lighten the air, and aid the operation of the medicine, make a free use of the steam bath; and keep the patient shielded by a blanket, at the same time give occasionally Nos. 1 and 2. This course should be unremittingly persevered in, till the patient is relieved.*

21. If the glands are dry, so that there is no moisture in the mouth, or if the patient is much pressed for breath, give a strong tea of No. 2, sweetened, and repeat it till the mouth becomes moist. No. 3, should not be used while the mouth is dry; if any is used, add a large portion of No. 2.

22. Be careful not to have the outward heat too high, by too many clothes or fire; for if this is the case, it will cause a balance of the outward and inward heat, and will prevent the medicine from operating, by stopping the circulation; and the patient will be very much distressed. When this happens, throw cold vinegar on the face and stomach, and give more hot medicine, which will let down the outward heat, and raise the inward.

---

*Keep always in mind to give the patient fresh air when steaming, and while going through a course of medicine, by making a quick fire of shavings, or very light wood, and opening a window at the same time; as this will immediately change the foul air in the room, by driving it out, and supplying its place by the fresh air from the surrounding atmosphere. This mode is essential in all disorders both in hot weather and in cold. Steaming is not essential in hot weather, except when going through a course of medicine; after which, a shower-bath is good in the morning, as it lets down the outward heat, which gives power to the inward.

23. If the patient is restless, wet the head and body with cold vinegar ; and if there are convulsions or spasms, give the nerve powder with No. 2. Injections must also be used.

24. Never make use of physic in cases where there is canker inside, for it will draw the determining powers inward, and increase the disease. I have seen so many bad effects from giving physic, that I have disapproved the use of it altogether ;. but if any is given, after the operation, be careful to keep up the inward .heat, so as to cause a free perspiration.

25. Avoid all minerals used as medicine, such as mercury, arsenic, antimony, calomel, preparations of copper or lead ; and also nitre and opium. They are all poison, and deadly enemies to health.

26. Beware of bleeding and blisters, as they can never do any good, and may be productive of much harm; they are contrary to nature, and strengthen the power of the enemy to health. Setons and issues should also be avoided, as they only tend to waste away the strength of the patient, without doing any good ; it is a much better way to remove the cause by a proper administration of medicine, which will be more certain and safe in its effects.

27. Be careful not to make use of salt-petre in any way whatever ; it is the greatest cold of any thing that can be taken into the stomach, and was never intended for any other purpose than to destroy life. It is a very bad practice to put it on meat, for it destroys all the juices, which is the nourishing part, and leaves the flesh hard and difficult to digest.

28. Never eat meat that is tainted, or any way injured, as it will engender disease ; for one ounce in the stomach is worse than the effluvia of a whole carcass. Eat salt provisions in hot weather, and fresh in cold.

29. Be careful about drinking cold water, in very hot weather, as it will tend to let down the inward heat so suddenly, as to give full power to the cold. If this should happen, its fatal effects may be prevented by giving the hot medicine, to raise the inward heat above the outward. Be careful also not to cool suddenly, after being very warm, in consequence of uncommon exercise.

30. Remember that regularity in diet is very important to preserve health; and that if more food is taken into the stomach, than is well digested, it clogs the system and causes disease. Therefore be cautious not to eat too much at a time, and have your food well cooked. This is very important to those who have weakly constitutions.

31. Ardent spirit is slow poison; it is taken to stimulate, but this effect is soon over, and much use of it destroys the tone of the stomach, injures the digestive powers, and causes disease. It is therefore much better, when the feelings require any thing of the kind, to make use of stimulating medicine, such as Nos. 2 and 6, for these will answer a far better purpose.

By a strict observance of the foregoing directions, you may save much pain and expense, and enjoy good health and long life, which is the earnest wish of the writer.

To make Milk Porridge.

Put a quart of water in a kettle, with a proper quantity of salt, and while heating, mix a gill of flour in a bowl with water, made thick, and when the water is boiling hot, drop this into it with a spoon; let it be well boiled, then add half a pint of milk. This to be eaten while under the operation of the medicine; and is also good food for the sick, at any other time, especially while the stomach is weak.

To make Chicken Broth.

Take a chicken and cut it in pieces; put the gizzard in with it, opened and cleaned, but not peeled. Boil it till the meat drops from the bone. Begin to give the broth as soon as there is any strength in it; and when boiled, eat some of the meat. Let it be well seasoned. This may be given instead of the milk porridge, and is very good for weak patients, particularly in cases of the dysentery.

When the operation of medicine is gone 'through, I have said that the patient may eat any kind of nourishing food his appetite should crave ; but the best thing is, to take a slice of salt pork boiled, or beef steak, well done, and eat it with pepper-sauce ; or take cayenne, vinegar and salt, mixed together, and eat with it, which is very good to create an appetite, and assist the digesture.

DESCRIPTION

Of several Cases of Disease, with Directions how they may be Cured.

FELONS.

This sore always comes on a joint, and is often caused by some strain or bruise, which makes a leak in the joint or muscle, and the sooner it has vent, the better. If it is brought to a head by poulticing, the skin being so thick that it will often be caused to break through the back of the hand, before it can get through the skin on the inside. The best way to give it vent, that I have ever found, is to burn a small piece of punk, the bigness of half a pea, on the place affected. If you think the flesh is dead down to the matter, you may prick the point of a needle into the dead skin, and raise it up and cut out a piece under the needle sufficient to let out the matter ; then apply poultice or salve. If painful, wrap it in cloths of several thicknesses, wet with cold water, and repeat this as often as it becomes hot or painful. Take the composition or warm medicine, to keep up an inward heat.

If the sore has been several days coming, and appears nearly ripe, apply a piece of unslacked lime to the part affected, wrap it up and wet the cloth with cold water, till the lime is slacked ; and repeat this till the skin looks of a purple colour : then open it as before directed. This method is more safe and quick in causing a cure, than laying it open with a knife, as is the practice of some doctors. By cutting the live flesh, it forms a leak and often spoils the joint ; but by searing them by either of the above modes, it secures and prevents the leak, and makes a speedy cure.

Freezes and Burns.

These two names of disorder are one and the same thing, and require the same treatment. Take a cloth wet in cold water, and wrap several thicknesses round or laid on to the part, to be kept wet as often as the pain increases. Give warm medicine inside. If the scald is dangerous, carry them through a regular course of medicine as though they had a fever, or any other acute disorder; keep the cloth or poultice on to secure it from the air, from twelve to fourteen hours, till the soreness or pain is entirely gone. If the skin is off, a poultice of flour bread wet with any of the articles composing No. 3, and keep it wet with this tea or water till the sore discharges, then wash with soap suds; when dressed, wash with the tea of No. 3, and continue the poultice or salve until a cure is effected.

A freeze is direct cold, and a burn is attracted cold; for as much as the heat opens the pores more than usual, the cold follows and closes them as much more than they were before the operation of the heat; this stops the perspiration from going through the surface, and the water collects under the grain of the skin, which is called blistering; the water applied in the cloth on the outside, opens the pores and lets the water out by perspiration, and the grain adheres to the skin; the pain ceases and the cure is completed.

Cure of My Brother's Son of a Scald.

He was about 14 years of age, and was taking off from the fire a kettle of boiling cider, the leg of the kettle caught by the log, tipped it forward, and poured the cider boiling hot, into a large bed of live embers, which covered his bare feet with this hot mass; he was obliged to hold on till the kettle was set on the floor, and then jumped into a pail of cold water, and stood there until his father procured some cloths, which he immediately wrapt his feet up in; his father laid by the fire to attend to pour on water, to keep the cloths filled, which keeps the air from the surface, and eases the pain; for as the water wastes and lets the air to the burn, the pain will increase; but by pursuing this course for about two hours, the pain abated, and the boy fell asleep. Water was poured on the cloth but two or three times during the rest of the night, and in the morning, preparation was made to dress the wound, when, to the surprise of all present, no blister had arisen, nor a particle of skin broken. He put on his stockings and shoes as usual, and went about his work, perfectly well.

Case of a Boy who was badly Scalded.

A lady took off from the fire a tea-kettle filled with boiling water, when her little son, about six years old, stepped on the bail and turned the contents on to both his feet, and falling, one hand went into the tea-kettle; both feet and one hand were very badly scalded. I happened to be present, and immediately tore up cloth sufficient to do up each part, wetting them with cold water. I then put him in bed and gave him some warm medicine, put a warm stone at his feet, and wet the cloths as often as he complained of pain. In about two hours he fell asleep, after which, two or three times wetting the cloths, kept him easy through the night. In the morning on taking off the cloths, there was no appearance of blisters, nor any skin broken; and he put on his shoes and stockings and appeared as well as before the accident happened. It had been the declared opinion of the family the night before, that the boy would not be able to go to school for a fortnight; but on finding him well in the morning, were hardly willing to believe their own senses, or that the child had been scalded.

General Remarks on Burns.

Burns are the most easily cured, if rightly managed and understood, of any wounds I ever attended; and are the most difficult and dangerous, when not understood, and wrongly treated. How often have we seen these sores continue all winter and could not be healed?

as also, burns caused by blisters made with Spanish
flies, which amount to the same thing.   By not being
treated in a proper manner in season, the canker gets in
and eats out the flesh, after which what is called proud
flesh fills up the sore.   The doctor applies his sugar of
lead, vitriol and red precipitate to eat out the dead flesh,
this affects the cords and draws them out of shape, and
many times makes a sore that they cannot cure, which
terminates in a mortifying canker sore.   My friends, if
you wish to avoid all this trouble, attend to what belongs
to your peace and comfort, before it is hidden from your
eyes; that is, to attend to the canker, which always
awaits such cases, and where the skin is off, in all cases
of burns or blisters, apply a poultice of cracker, or elm
bark wet with a tea of No. 3, until the canker is gone.
Sometimes add ginger; if the imflammation is high add a
little of No. 2, with the ginger, keeping the poultice wet
with cold water; when the sore discharges, apply salve
till a cure is effected.

I shall continue my remarks on burns, by showing the
evil consequences arising from blistering.   Not long
since I knew a case where a doctor drew a blister on a
child's breast up to the neck, for being stuffed at the
lungs.   It lingered, with this scald near its vitals, about
a week; I was then called to visit the child and found
it to be dying.   The mother asked me what I thought
was the matter with it; I took off the dressing and
showed her the mortified flesh all over the blister, and
told her that was the disorder.   She seemed much surprised; and I then asked her if the child had been
scalded and it had mortified in like manner, whether she
would have had any doubt of its being the cause of her
child's death? she said that she should not.   I gave her
my opinion, that it was exactly a similar case, and that
the child's death was caused as much by the blister as it
would have been by a scald.   The child died before morning.   I had declined doing any thing for it, as I was satisfied that I could do it no good; and if I had made the attempt, it would have been said that I killed it.

I have seen many cases where I was perfectly satisfied that the patients died in consequence of blisters,
not only on the stomach, but on the head.   In many

that I have witnessed, where a blister was drawn on the head, as soon as it began to draw, their senses were gone, and did not return till they died raving, or stupified. More than half the cases where the head was shaved and blistered, that have come within my knowledge, have died. I never could see any reason why a scald on the head or body, done on purpose, should have a tendency to effect a cure, when the person is sick, and the same thing happening to them by accident, when well, should destroy their health or cause their death. If a person should have their head or stomach so badly scalded as to take off the skin, we should consider them in the most dangerous condition; but nothing is said about it when drawn on purpose. I shall leave it to the reader to reconcile, if he can, this inconsistency. I have known most dangerous stranguaries caused by blisters on the sides and limbs, and those who applied them did not know the cause, and I have been applied to for relief.

Mortification of the Limbs.

I was called on to go on board a vessel, at Eastport, to see a young man, who had had a block fall from mast head on his foot, weighing 13½ pounds, which bruised all his toes to pieces except the little one. The accident happened on Friday, and I did not see him till the Tuesday following; during which he had neither eat nor slept. His nerves were much affected, and had spasms and convulsions through the whole system. I took off the dressing from his foot, and found it black, and the smell very offensive. The captain of the vessel appeared to be very anxious about him, asked me if I could help his foot; I told him that I must first try to save his life, for his whole body was as much disordered as his foot. He requested me to do what I thought best. I put a poultice of meal on his foot, and wet the cloth with cold water, to allay the heat; then gave him medicine the same as though he had been attacked with a nervous fever. The captain attended him through the night, and I went to see him the next morning, and found him much better. The captain said he was astonished at the operation of the medicine, for that his vomiting and sweating had carried off all the pain in his body and foot, and had also reconciled the nerves.

I unbound his foot and found that the black and yellow streaks up the leg had disappeared, and on the foot, all the flesh that was alive, seemed to receive fresh support from the body ; and the living and dead flesh appeared as though two colours were painted by the side of each other. I then made a lie of pearlash in warm water, and soaked his foot in it, which caused a slimy glaze all over his foot; this took away all the offensive smell ; and I washed it with vinegar to kill the alkali and keep it from irritating the skin. The acid cleared off all the slimy matter, so that it wiped clean. I then cut off the great toe at the middle joint, and the two next at the upper joint, and set the next, which was broken. I cut none of the flesh but what was dead, to stop in part the putrefaction. I then put on another poultice, and ordered it to be kept wet with cold water, and, a warm stone wrapped in a wet cloth, to be put to his feet to keep a steam, giving him warm medicines inside to keep up the inward heat; and by wetting the foot with cold water, it kept the determining power to the surface ; thus raising the fountain and lowering the stream. By this treatment it becomes impossible that mortification can go from the limbs to the body, any more than a log that floats over the dam, can go back again into the pond, when the fountain is kept full. The next day I dressed his foot and found that the dead flesh had digested very much ; I again soaked it in pearlash, and then washed in vinegar as before, which was of great service in allaying the bad smell. I then caused him to be carried through a regular course of medicine, which completely restored his bodily health ; his appetite was good, and all pain and soreness abated, so that he took food regularly, and lost no sleep afterwards, till he got entirely well, which was in about four weeks. The captain was a very good nurse, and was faithful in attendance on the young man till he got well ; and expressed the highest gratitude for my attention and success ; and as a proof of his confidence in the medicine, he purchased a right, for which he paid me twenty silver dollars, observing at the same time, that he never paid for any thing with more satisfaction.

Old Canker Sores on the Legs.

When I was a young man, I was much troubled through the winter, for many years, with sores on my legs. At the commencement of cold weather, if I broke the grain on my shin, it would become a bad sore, and continue through the winter; the canker would get into it and eat to the bone, and sometimes spread under the grain like a burn, and feel the same, being extremely sore, with stings and twinges like a cancer. These sores were so troublesome, that it led me to invent a cure; finding the cause to be canker, I took some of the articles composing No. 3, steeped strong, and washed the part affected, with it; if there was a bad smell, I first washed the sore with strong soap suds, taking off all the loose skin, which was blistered with cankery humour, and then washed with a tea of No. 3, to destroy the canker and harden the sore; sometimes wetting it with the drops. If the inflammation run high, and the sore spread fast, I put into it a pinch of fine No. 2; then put on a poultice of white bread and ginger, wet with the above tea, wrapping it up with several thicknesses of cloths wet with cold water; wetting them as often as dry, so as to be painful, and did not let the sore come to the air for twenty-four hours. In this time, if kept well wet and warm, it will discharge ripe matter, and the inflammation and canker will abate. When next dressed, wash first with soap suds as before, then with the tea; if the soreness is gone, you may apply the healing salve, with the wet cloths, if going to bed, to keep out the air; put occasionally a hot stone wrapped in wet cloths, to the feet to keep up a steam, and wetting the sore if painful with cold water. Take medicine to keep up the inward heat; such as composition or hot bitters, and when these do not answer the purpose, go through a course of the medicine, and repeat as occasion may require. This method, if persevered in, I seldom knew to fail of success.

9*

I was called to attend a case of this kind, not long since, where the inflammation and pain was very great, and fast spreading under the grain of the skin; there had been applied an elm and ginger poultice, made with tea of No. 3. I opened and only added a pinch of No. 2, and laid on the poultice again, putting on a wet cloth, and ordered it kept wet with cold water till next morning; when on dressing it, found the inflammation abated, the sore discharged ripe matter, and by two dressings more of the same, the cure was completed.

Case of the Bite of a Rat, supposed to be Mad.

Not long since, I was sent for to attend a man who had been bitten on one of his eyebrows by a rat, supposed to be mad. The wound healed in a few days, then turned purple round it, as though the blood had settled, and turned more black, until he was blind. He was sick at the stomach, and had a high fever. I carried him through a course of the medicine, but with little advantage. The swelling and dark colour progressed till he was about the colour of a blackberry pie. These appearances led me to suspect that the madness of the rat was caused by eating rats-bane, and communicated this poison to the man by the bite, as he appeared the same as a person I had once seen, who had been killed by taking that poison. I then washed his face with a strong tea of Nos. 1 and 2, and gave the same inward with No. 3, carried him through another course of medicine, keeping a cloth on his face wet with the tea as before, to keep out the air when under the operation of the medicine, to sweat his face and throw the poison out. I kept him in a sweat for several days, occasionally with his face secured from the air, which method had the desired effect, by bringing the poison out. By continually keeping up the perspiration, the swelling abated; but whenever this was not well attended to, so as to keep the determining powers to the surface, the spasms would increase to such a degree that his life was frequently despaired of. He was carefully attended in this manner about one month, before I could determine in my own mind, whether the disease or nature would gain the victory; after which time he began gradually to gain his health, and in about six months, he appeared to be clear of the poison. The man was sixty years of age; and the accident happening in the fall of the year, it was much more difficult to conquer this cold and deadly poison, than it would have been in warm weather. This case convinced me that the cause of mad rats and mad cats, is owing to the rats having been poisoned by ratsbane, the cats eat them and become affected by the poison, which makes them mad, and by biting the people, communicate the poison, from which many fatal consequences have frequently happened.

Bad wound in the Eye cured.

While I was at Eastport, Maine, a man was cutting turf, about twelve miles from that place, and accidentally had a pitchfork stuck into one of his eyes, by a person who was pitching the turf near him. It passed by the eyeball and stuck fast in the scull, so that it was with considerable exertion that he could draw it out. The eye swelled and closed up immediately, and the people were much frightened, and sent for me; but it so happened that I could not go. I gave directions to the man who came after me, to return and carry him through a course of medicine as soon as possible, keeping several thicknesses of cloth wet with cold water on his eye, and not open it for twelve hours; and to keep him in a perspiration the whole time. This was faithfully attended to; and on opening the wound after the above time, the swelling was all gone, the eye was open, and a large quantity of blood was in the wet cloth, which had been drawn from the eye. They continued the wet cloth, and gave him warm medicine inside, keeping him in a gentle perspiration for the next twenty-four hours, which cleared the eye of all the blood, restored the sight, and amended his health, that he was well in about a week, to the astonishment of all who saw him.

Cancer Sores.

A concise and general treatise on this violent and often fatal disease may convey some useful ideas on the subject. The cause of this sore is very little understood. In all sores of an eating nature, there is more or less canker, according to their violence. A cancer is the highest degree of canker, being the most powerful effects of cold, and consequently the greatest degree of inflammation, therefore the remedies ought to be those of a warming nature, as the greatest preventives against canker. Whenever a violent inflammation is discovered, it is supposed that heat causes the difficulty; but the fact is, it is only evidence of a war between heat and cold; for there is no inflammation where there is perfect health, because heat then bears complete rule; and no disease can take place until the cold makes an attack on the body, which causes an unnatural heat to oppose an unnatural cold; wherever the cold takes possession, the inflammation shows itself, by stopping the circulation; the effect is swelling, inflamed calous, arising from some leak, caused by the natural course being stopped. If it supperates, and discharges, it is called ulcer, bile, and the like, and the canker goes off with the putrefaction. If the leak is so slow as to calous as fast as they discharge it, it becomes a hard dead lump of flesh, and not having circulation enough to support it, it begins to rot; here the canker shows its eating nature; being seated in the dead flesh, and eating on the live flesh, which is intermixed with it, causes pain and distress, in proportion as the body is filled with coldness and canker; if this is sufficient to keep the power above the natural circulation, the patient will continue in this distressed situation, being eaten up alive, until worn out with the pain, death comes as a friend to relieve them. This is the natural termination of this dreadful malady; which is far better than to combine with it the common form of practice in using arsenic, which only helps to eat up and distress the patient.

In order to give a more correct idea of the dangerous effect of making use of arsenic in cancers, I shall make a short extract from Thatcher's Dispensatory, on the subject. "Arsenic has long been known to be the

basis of the celebrated cancer powder. It has been
sprinkled in substance on the ulcer ; but this mode of
using it is excessively painful, and extremely dangerous;
fatal effects have been produced from its absorption.
This fact I have known in several instances, where
Davidson's agents, and others have undertaken to draw
out cancers when the patient would absorb enough of
this poison, which seating on the lungs, caused them to
die with the consumption in the course of one year."
My wish in exposing this nostrum, is to benefit those
who may be ignorant of the imposition; for it may be
relied on as a truth, that there is more or less poison in
all those burning plasters, used to cure cancers; and I
would advise all to beware of them; it will be much
safer to risk the cancer than the cancer quack.

The principal object aimed at is to take out the bunch,
and in doing that by the above method, a worse evil is
inoculated, which is more fatal than the cancer. The
tumour is a mixture of live and dead flesh, and is often
under a live skin ; if it is necessary to make an incision
through the live skin in order to disolve the dead flesh,
the best way is to burn a piece of punk on the place,
and repeat it till the flesh is dead enough to suppurate.
The smart will be but two or three minutes, and not so
painful as the arsenic for the same time, which will last
for twelve hours. Where the tumour is small, the cancer balsam, will be found sufficient, by repeating the
plaster for two or three weeks, to take out the dead
flesh, and remove the canker; after this is done, apply a
ginger and elm poultice wet with a tea of No. 3. If the
system appears to be generally affected with the cancer
humour, carry them through a common course of medicine, and repeat the same while attending to the sore.

I had a cancer on my foot about the bigness of an Indian corn, which had troubled me twice, by acute dart-
ing pains and twinges. I cured it by applying a plaster of the cancer balsam; repeating it twice at each
time. Where there is dead flesh under the skin, it is
best to burn the punk first and then apply the poultice
or balsam; and it is also recommended to always give
medicine to eradicate the canker from the system, both
before and after the operation on the sore.

Three cancers on the breast have come under my care, that I could not cure. One of them was as large as a half peck measure, and grew fast to the breast bone. I carried the woman through a course of medicine several times and applied a poultice of butternut shucks, to dissolve the dead flesh, and continued this course for some months, until the bunch had more than half dissolved, and had grown off from the bone, so that it was quite loose; and I was in hopes to have effected a cure; but she was taken with a fever in my absence, and died. The other two I could relieve and keep them free from 'pain, making them comfortable as long as they lived; but nature was too far exhausted to complete a cure: I have had under my care many other cases of cancers on the breast and other parts of the body, which I had no difficulty in curing in the manner before stated.

I shall conclude this subject by a few general remarks, viz: Guard thoroughly against canker and coldness. Attend to the canker by a course of medicine, and repeat it. Use the ginger poultice if the inflammation is great, putting some No. 2, raw in the sore, then apply the poultice, keeping it wet with cold water, not forgetting the composition and No. 2 inside, at the same time. Let all poisonous drugs, burning plasters, and caustics alone. Attend faithfully to the directions here given; honour your own judgment; keep your money; and bid defiance to doctors.

PILES; how cured.

I was called to attend an elderly man in South Reading, who had been confined to the house, and much of the time to his bed, for seven weeks, with the Piles. Seven doctors attended him before I was sent for, and he had continued to grow worse. The doctors had operated on one side, and said they must on the other; it was their opinion, as well as his, that he was in a decline. The side that they had operated upon was much worse to cure than the other. I carried him through a regular course of medicine twice in three days, when he was able to go out of doors. The injection composed of No. 3, steeped, and a small quantity of No. 2, was used; warm tallow was applied freely several times in the day, sometimes washing externally with the same tea. He had been dieted very low; I restored his digestive powers, and recovered his appetite; his sores healed, his general health amended to such a degree, that he was no more confined with that complaint. A little tallow used when going to bed, prevents piles and chafes in young and old. Remember this.

Sore Heads in Children; (Scalt Heads.)

This sore often comes after having had the itch; kernels form in the neck; it is contagious, being caused by canker and putrefaction. The most effectual way to cure this disease, is to carry them through a course of medicine several times, as the case may require, previous to which the head should be oiled, and covered with cabbage leaves; or draw a bladder over the head, to keep out the cold air. The head should be covered so as to make it sweat as much as possible, in order to dissolve the hard scabs. After laying all night the smell will be offensive; wash the head in soap suds; when clean, wash it also with a tea of No. 3, after which wash with a tea of No. 1. Sometimes annoint it with the Rheumatic drops and nerve ointment—let it come to the air by degrees. Be careful to guard the stomach by giving composition, warm bitters, &c. The ointment, drops and No. 1, in powder or juice, may be occasionally used together or separate. Continue to wash with soap suds, and then with No. 3, occasionally, until a cure is effected.

Sore Breasts.

Some women suffer very much from this complaint, which is caused by cold, occasioning obstructions in the glands of the breast. When they are swelled, bathe with the rheumatic drops, or pepper vinegar; if this does not remove the swelling, and it should be necessa-

ry to bring it to a head, apply a poultice of lily root
made thick with ginger or slippery elm bark; at the
same time give the composition powder or No. 2, to
keep up the inward heat. If the woman is sick, carry
her through a regular course of the medicne, which
will remove the complaint and restore her to health in
a short time. I have cured many who were very bad,
by pursuing the above plan, and never met with difficulty. I attended a woman in Portsmouth, who had both
breasts badly swelled. She was setting by the window
with it up, and could hardly get her breath; she could
not bear to have any fire in the room, complaining that
it made her faint. I told her that if I could not make
her bear heat, I could do her no good. I gave her some
No. 2, to raise the inward heat, and caused a good fire
to be made in the room. The inward heat gained as
fast as the outward, and in one hour she could bear as
warm a fire as I could. I carried her through three regular courses of the medicine in five days, and at the
same time applied the lily poultice, which brought them
to a head without pain; and she was soon well.

To stop Bleeding.

Internal bleeding is from the stomach or lungs, and
is caused by canker, or soreness of the stomach; it often
takes place very suddenly, and creates much alarm.
The patient sometimes trembles with fright, and often
has fits of the ague, which is caused by the cold increasing in proportion to the loss of blood. In the first place
shield them from the air with a blanket, by the fire, and
give the hottest medicine you have; if nothing better
can be had, give hot water or any kind of hot tea; and
get a perspiration as soon as possible; then apply the
steam bath; giving ginger tea, or No. 2, if you have it,
if not, black pepper. As soon as there is an equilibrium
in the circulation, there will be no more pressure of the
blood to the stomach or lungs, than to the extremities,
and the bleeding will cease. It has been my practice in
cases of this kind, to give some of the rheumatic drops,
shield them from the air with a blanket, placed by the

fire; then give a dose of the composition powders, and No. 2; and if this does not answer the purpose, give a dose of No. 1, which, with the steam, I never knew fail of stopping the blood; and by giving medicine to remove the canker and restore the digestive powers, I have always been able to effect a cure. . The same application will answer for other weakening and alarming complaints in women.

External bleeding, caused by wounds in the limbs, may be stopped by placing the wound higher than the body. One of my sons cut his leg very badly; I placed him on the floor and took his foot in my lap; as soon as the wound was higher than the body, the bleeding ceased. I then poured on cold water till the wound was white; then put in a few drops of No. 6, took two or three stitches to bring the wound together, dressed it with salve, and it soon got well with very little soreness. Another case of a little girl, who cut off the main artery of the middle finger, and it bled very fast. I put my thumb above the wound and stopped the blood; then poured on cold water with my other hand, and washed the wound well; then placed her hand above her head, which prevented it from bleeding, till I could get ready to dress the wound. It bled no more, and soon got well.

Rupture.

This difficulty is caused by a hurt or strain, which makes a breach in the tough film, or membrane, that supports the bowels in their place, and the intestines come down into the cavity between this membrane and the skin; being sometimes very painful and difficult to be got back; and have to be kept from coming down by a truss. When the bowels come down and remain any length of time, they become swelled, and are very painful, causing great distress and danger; and sometimes have proved fatal, as they cannot be got up again till the swelling is removed. This may be effected by a course of the medicine without danger.

A Mr. Woodbury, of Durham, was troubled with a rupture; his bowels came down, swelled, and was very

10

painful; a doctor was sent for from Portsmouth, who applied a bag of snow, which drove the pain to the stomach and caused puking. The swelling increased, and became very hard. The case now becoming desperate, and the family being alarmed, I was sent for, and on hearing the circumstances, sent some medicine, and gave directions to sweat him as soon as possible. My directions were faithfully attended to, and as soon as he became warm, the nerves slackened, the swelling abated, all appearance of mortification disappeared, the bowels went back, and in twelve hours he was restored from a dangerous situation, to almost his usual state of health. In this case may be seen the difference between the artificial doctor, and nature's physician, which is the same as between fire and snow.

Ague in the Face.

This is caused by cold in the glands of the mouth, which keeps back the saliva till it causes swelling and soreness; the canker becomes prevalent at the same time, which causes severe pain in the face and throat. The sooner a cure is attempted the better; to effect this, take a dose of the tea of No. 3, with a tea-spoonful of No. 6, in it, for the canker; then tie a small quantity of No. 2 in a fine piece of cloth, wet with No. 6, and put it between the teeth and cheek; on the side where the pain is; set by the fire covered by a blanket, and breathe the warm air from the fire; this will prick the glands and cause the saliva to flow very freely, which will take out the soreness and relieve the pain. The face may be bathed at the same time with No. 6. If the case is of long standing, so that the system is affected, and this does not remove the complaint, give a dose of No. 1. If it is caused by decayed teeth, fill the hollow with cotton wool, wet with oil of summersavory, or spirits of turpentine, which will deaden the nerve, and stop its aching. This is good in all cases of the teeth-ache, and will generally effect a cure without extracting.

To relax the Muscles in setting a Bone.

This may be done by bathing the part with warm water, and is much better than the method that is generally practised, of extending the muscles by the strength of several persons, which weakens the part so much, that the bones are liable to get out of place again ; besides, the operation causes severe pain to the patient and much trouble to the operator, which is all obviated by my method. In cases where a joint is put out, or a bone broken, give a dose of No. 2, or the composition powder with half a tea-spoonful of nerve-powder, which will promote a perspiration, prevent fainting, and quiet the nerves; then wrap the part in cloths wet with water as hot as it can be borne, and pour on the warm water, placing a pan underneath to catch it, for 'a short time, when the muscles will become relaxed, so that the bones may be put in their place with little trouble.

I was once called to a woman who had put her elbow out of joint by a fall from her horse. It was badly out, being twisted about one quarter of the way round. I ordered some water to be made hot immediately, stripped her arm, and as soon as the water was hot, put a towel in a large tin pan and poured the hot water on it till well wet; as soon as cool enough, wrapped it round her arm from her wrist to her shoulder; then placed the pan under her arm, and poured on the water from a pitcher, as 'hot as she could bear it, for about fifteen minutes. I then took off the towel and directed one person to take hold of the arm above the elbow and another below, to steady it ; and then placed my fingers against the end of the bone on the under side, and my thumb against that on the upper side, and by a gentle pressure each way, set the joint without pain, or force on the muscles, to the astonishment of all present, who calculated that it would require the strength of several men. I then wrapped it up with the same towel, which had become cold ; this brought the muscles to their proper tone, and kept the joint firm in its place; put her arm in a sling and she walked home that night about, a mile, and the next day was well enough to knit all day.

In case a shoulder is out of joint, I relax the muscles in the same manner, and put the arm over my shoulder and lift up, which has always put the joint in its place, without any danger and with very little pain to the patient; and then by applying cold water, the muscles will become braced, so that there will be no danger of its getting out again. I knew of a case where a man had his hip turned out, and several doctors had exhausted all their skill in vain to set it; when one of my agents being present, undertook it by my plan of treatment, and after he had relaxed the muscles sufficiently, put his knee against the hip joint, and placing his hand on the inside of the knee, turned the leg out and crowded the joint into its place without any difficulty.

Poison by Ivy or Dogwood.

Many people are troubled with this difficulty every season, and I have been much afflicted with it myself in my younger days, often being poisoned in such manner as to swell and break out very badly, and knew no remedy but to let it have its course, which was almost as bad as the small pox. One of my sons was often afflicted in this way, and one season was poisoned three times, so as to be blind for several days. I long sought a remedy without success, till I found it in the emetic herb. By washing with a tincture of the green plant as is directed in the second preparation of the emetic herb, on the first appearance of the disease, is a certain remedy. If the complaint has been for any length of time, and has become bad, it will be necessary to take a dose of the powdered emetic, first preparation, to clear the system of the poison, at the same time of washing with the tincture. A tea made of the powdered leaves and pods, will do to wash with, when the tincture, or green plant cannot be had. The powdered seeds, with Nos. 2 and 6, third preparation, may also be used for the same purpose.

Measles.

This disease is very common, especially among children, and is often attended with bad consequences, when not properly treated. It is a high state of canker and putrefaction; and if the determining powers are kept to the surface, it will make its appearance on the outside, and go off of itself; but if cold overpowers the inward heat, so as to turn the determining powers inward, the disease will not make its appearance, and the patient will become much distressed, frequently producing fatal consequences, if some powerful stimulant is not administered to bring the disorder out. To give physic in, cases of this kind is very dangerous, as it strengthens the power of cold, and keeps the canker and putrefaction inside, which sometimes seats upon the lungs and causes consumption; or turns to the stomach and bowels, when they die suddenly, as has been the case with hundreds, for a few years past. I have attended a great many cases of the measles in the course of my practice, and never lost one; and never have known of any that have died of this disorder, who were attended by any of my agents. When the symptoms make their appearance, give a dose of the composition powder, or of No. 2; then give the tea of No. 3, to guard against canker, and add some No. 2, to overpower the cold; and when the second dose is given, add No. 1, to clear the stomach and promote perspiration. As soon as this takes place, the disorder will show itself on the outside. By continuing to keep the determining power to the suface, nature will take its regular course, and the disease will go off without injuring the constitution. If the bowels appear to be disordered, give an injection; and be careful to keep the patient warm.

I once had a case of a young woman who had the measles; she lingered with the symptoms four or five days, and then become very sick, turned of a dark purple colour, and had a high fever, when I was called to attend her. I gave her a strong dose of No. 3, steeped, and put in it a spoonful of the third preparation of No. 1, which caused such a violent struggle, that I had to hold her in the bed; but it was soon over, for in about ten minutes she vomited, and a perspiration took place, which was followed by the measles coming out, so that she was completely covered with the eruption. She was soon well and about her work.

10*

Small Pox.

This disease is the highest state of canker and putrefaction, which the human body is capable of receiving,
and is the most contagious, being taken in with the breath,
or may be communicated by inoculation, in which case
it is not so violent and dangerous as when taken in the
natural way. The distressing and often fatal consequences
that have happened in cases of the small pox, are more
owing to the manner in which it has been treated, than
to the disease. The fashionable mode of treatment in
this disease, has been to give physic, and reduce the
strength, by starving the patient and keeping them cold.
This is contrary to common sense, as it weakens the
friend and strengthens the enemy; and the same cause
would produce similar effects in any other disorder. All
that is necessary, is to assist nature to drive out the canker and putrefaction, which is the cause of the disease,
by keeping the determining powers to the surface, in
which case there will be no danger. The same manner
of treatment should be used in this complaint as has been
directed for the measles. The canker-rash, and all
kinds of disease that a person is not liable to have but
once, such as chicken-pox, swine-pox, &c. are from the
same cause, and must be treated in a similar manner.

Cough.

The general opinion is, that cough is an enemy to
health, and ought to be treated as such; but this idea I
hold to be altogether an error; for it is the effect, and
not the cause of disease. When the lungs are diseased,
there will be a collection of matter, which must be
thrown off; and the cough is like the pump of a ship,
which discharges the water, and prevents her from sinking; so also the cough throws off what collects on the
lungs, which, if suffered to remain, would soon putrify
and cause death. It is a common saying, that I have
a bad cough, and can get nothing to stop it; and the
doctor often says, if I could stop your cough, I should
have hopes of a cure; but this is as unreasonable as it
would be to stop the pumps of a ship, which would cause.

ker to sink the sooner. Ask a sailor what he would do, and he would say, keep the pump going till you can stop the leak, and when that is stopped, the pump will become useless, as there will be nothing to throw off. Such medicine should be given as will promote the cough, till the cause can be removed, which is cold and canker on the lungs; after this is done, there will be no more cough. If a cough is caused by a sudden cold, it may be removed by taking the composition powder on going to bed, with a hot stone wrapped in wet cloths put the feet, to produce a perspiration, and at the same time taking the cough powder, which will make the patient raise easy, and also help to remove the cause. When the cough has become seated, and the lungs are diseased, they must be carried through a regular course of the medicine, repeating the same as occasion may require, till a cure is effected, at the same time giving the cough-powder, especially on going to bed.

Whooping cough must be treated in the same manner; continue to give the cough-powders till cured.

Jaundice.

Much has been said about the bile, or gall, being an enemy in case of sickness; but this is a mistake, for it is a friend, and should be treated as such. It is the main spring to life, and the regulator of health, as without it the food could not be digested. When people have what is called the jaundice, it is the prevailing opinion that they have too much bile, and it is said they are bilious; this is a mistaken notion, for there is no such thing as being too much gall, it would be more correct to say there was not enough. The difficulty is caused by the stomach being cold and foul, so that the food is not properly digested; and the bile not being appropriated to its natural use, is diffused through the pores of the skin, which becomes of a yellow colour. The symptoms are want of appetite, costiveness, faintness, and the patient will be dull and sleepy; these are evidences of bad digesture and loss of inward heat. The only way to effect a cure is to promote perspiration, cleanse the stomach, and restore the digestive powers, which will cause the bile to be used for the purpose nature designed it.

Nature has contrived that each part of the body should perform its proper duty in maintaining health, and if there is no obstruction, there would never be disease. The gall bladder grows on the liver, and is placed between that and the stomach, so that when the latter is filled with food, the bile is discharged into the stomach to digest it.　The bile never makes disorder, for it is perfectly innocent, being nature's friend; and those appearances called bilious, show the effect of disease, and not the cause. The gall is a very bitter substance, and it is the practice of the doctors, to order bitter medicine to cure the jaundice, and this seems to be the universal opinion, which is correct; but it certainly contradicts the notion that there is too much bile, for if there be too much, why give medicine to make more? I have attended many cases of this kind, and never had any difficulty in effecting a cure.　My method is to give No. 2, or the composition powders, to raise the internal heat, and No. 1, to cleanse the stomach and promote perspiration; then give the bitters, No. 4, to regulate the bile and restore the digestive powers.　If the complaint has been of long standing, and the system is much disordered, they must be carried through a regular course of the medicine, and repeat it as occasion may require, at the same time give the bitters two or three time a day, till the appetite is good, and the digesture restored.　Any of the articles described under the head of No. 4, are good, and may be freely used for all bilious complaints.

Worms.

A great deal is said about worms causing sickness, and there is scarcely a disease that children are afflicted with, but what is attributed to worms.　The doctors talk about worm complaints, worm fevers, worm cholics, &c. and give medicine to destroy the worms; by so doing, they frequently destroy their patients.　There was never a greater absurdity than their practice, and the universal opinion about worms causing disease.　The fact is, they

are created, and exist in the stomach and bowels for a
useful purpose, and are friendly to health, instead of 'being an enemy; they are bred and supported by the cold
phlegm that collects in the stomach and bowels; this is
their element; and the more there is of it, the more
there will be of the worms; they never cause disease,
but are caused by it. Those who are in health, are never
troubled with worms, because they are then quiet, and
exist in their natural element; every one has more or
less of them; and the reason why children are more
troubled with what is called worm complaints, is because
they are more subject to be disordered in their stomach
and bowels than grown persons. When children are sick,
and their breath smells bad, it is said they have worms,
and every thing is laid to them ; but this is owing to disease caused by canker, for there is nothing in the nature
of worms that can affect the breath.   In cases of this
kind, the only thing necessary is to cleanse the stomach
by getting rid of the cold phlegm, and restoring the digestive powers, when there will be no difficulty with
the worms.

The common practice of the doctors is to give calomel and other poisons to kill the worms; this must appear to any one, who examines into the subject, to be
very wrong as well as dangerous; for the worms cannot be killed by it, without poisoning the whole contents
of the stomach.   I once knew of a case of a child who,
after eating a breakfast of bread and milk, was taken
sick ; a doctor was sent for, who said it was caused by
worms, and gave a dose of calomel to destroy them, which
caused fits; the child vomited and threw up its breakfast ; a dog that happened to be in the room eat what the
child threw up; he was soon taken sick and died; the
child got well.   The fortunate accident of the child's
throwing off its stomach what it had taken, probably
saved its life, for if there was poison enough to kill a dog,
it must have killed the child.   The absurdity of such
practice is like the story related by Dr. Franklin, of a
man who was troubled with a weasle in his barn, and to
get rid of the weasle he set fire to his barn and burnt it up.
I had the following relation from the doctor who attended
the cases; three children had what he called a worm fe-

ver; and he undertook to kill the worms. One of them died, and he requested liberty to open it to see what would destroy worms, in order to know how to cure the others; but the parents would not consent. The second died, and the parents consented to have it opened; but after searching the stomach and bowels, to their surprise, no worms could be found. The third soon after died. The fact was, their death was caused by canker on the stomach and bowels, and the medicine given increased the difficulty by drawing the determining powers inward, which aided the cold to promote the canker. Where children die by such treatment, the blame is all laid to the worms, and the doctor escapes censure.

I have had a great deal of experience in what are called worm complaints; and after having become acquainted with the real cause have had no difficulty in curing all that I have undertaken. I began with my own children. One of them was troubled with what was supposed to be worms; I employed a doctor, who gave pink root, and then physic to carry it off with the worms. It would shortly after have another turn, which would be worse; he went on in this way, and the worms kept increasing, till I became satisfied that he was working on the effect, and neglected the cause, when I dismissed him and undertook the cure myself. I firstly gave the warmest medicine I then knew of to clear off the cold phlegm; and gave bitter medicine, such as poplar bark, wormwood, tansy, and physic made of the twigs of butternut, to cleanse the stomach and to correct the bile. By pursuing this plan the child soon got well and was no more troubled with worms. A child in the neighbourhood where I lived, about six years old, was taken sick in the morning, and the doctor was sent for, who gave medicine for worms; soon after, it had fits and continued in convulsions during the day, and at night died. I was satisfied that its death was hastened if not caused by what was given. When the stomach is diseased, or when poison is taken into it, the worms try to flee from their danger, which causes distress, and they sometimes get into knots and stop the passages to the stomach. Much more might be said on this subject; but enough has been stated to put those who attend to it on their guard against the dangerous practice of giving medicine to kill worms.

My practice has been what I shall recommend to others to do, in case of what is called worm complaints, to give the composition powders, or No. 2, to warm the stomach, a tea of No. 3, to remove the canker, and the bitters or either of the articles described under No. 4, to correct the bile. If they are bad, carry them through a course of the medicine, and give the bitters. When there are nervous symptoms give the nerve powder. Injections should also be frequently given. The butternut syrup is very good. If there should be danger of mortification, make use of No. 6, both in the medicine given, and in the injections.

The tape-worm is from the same cause as other worms, and may be cured in the same manner. They are, when single, about half an inch long, and one third as wide; they join together and appear like tape, and often come away in long pieces of several yards. I was once troubled with them, and used to be faint, and have no appetite; I cured myself by taking the butternut physic, which brought away several yards at a time; and by taking the bitter medicine, to correct the bile, was never troubled with it again.

I have often heard about people having a greedy-worm; but this is a mistaken notion, for there was never any such thing. The difficulty is the stomach being cold and disordered, so that the food is not properly digested, passes off without nourishing the system, and this creates an unnatural appetite. Remove the cause by warming the stomach and correcting the digestive powers, and there will be no farther difficulty. In the year 1805, I was called to see a young woman who it was supposed had a greedy-worm. It was thought to be very large, and would frequently get into her throat and choke her, almost stopping her breath. Her mother told me that the day before, one of the neighbours was in, and told a story about a person having a monster in their stomach, which was taken in by drinking at a brook; this terrible account so frightened her daughter, that the worm rose into her throat, and choked her so bad that she had fits. I took the girl home with me, and gave her a dose of hot

bitters, with some of the nerve powder that night; the
next morning I carried her through a course of the medicine, as well as I knew at that time, which cleared the
stomach and bowels, and strengthened the nervous system. I told her there was no worm that troubled her,
and she had faith in what I said. I gave her medicine to
correct the bile and restore the digesture, and she soon
got well, being no more troubled about the worm. The
difficulty was caused by a disordered stomach, and want of
digesture, which produced spasms in the stomach and
throat.

Consumption.

This complaint is generally caused by some acute disorder not being removed, and the patient being run down
by the fashionable practice, until nature makes a com-
promise with disease, and the house becomes divided
against itself. There is a constant warfare kept up between the inward heat and cold, the flesh wastes away in
consequence of not digesting the food, the canker becomes seated on the stomach and bowels, and then takes
hold of the lungs. When they get into this situation, it
is called a seated consumption, and is pronounced by the
doctors to be incurable. I have had a great many cases
of this kind, and have in all of them, where there was
life enough left to build upon, been able to effect a cure
by my system of practice. The most important thing is
to raise the inward heat, and get a perspiration, clear the
system of canker, and restore the digestive powers, so that
food will nourish the body and keep up that heat on which
life depends. This must be done by the regular course
of medicine, as has been directed in all violent attacks of
disease, and persevering in it till the cause is removed.

This complaint is called by the doctors a hectic fever,
because they are subject to cold chills, and hot flashes on
the surface; but this is an error, for there is no fever
about it; and this is the greatest difficulty; if there were
a fever, it would have a crisis, and nature would be able
to drive out the cold and effect a cure; the only difficulty
is to raise a fever, which must be done by such medicine as will raise and hold the inward heat till nature

has the complete command. When patients are very
weak and low, they will have what is called cold sweats;
the cause of this is not understood; the water that collects on the skin does not come through the pores, but is
attracted from the air in the room, which is warmer than
the body, and condenses on the surface; the same may
be seen on the outside of a mug or tumbler, on a hot
day, when filled with cold water, which is from the same
cause. It is of more importance to attend to the preventing of this complaint, than to cure it. If people
would make use of those means which I have recommended, and cure themselves of disease, in its first stages, and avoid all poisonous drugs, there would never be
a case of consumption, or any other chronic disorder.

Fits.

These are produced by the same cause as other complaints, that is, cold and obstructions; and may be cured
by a regular course of the medicine, which overpowers
the cold, promotes perspiration, and restores the digestive powers. Poison, or any thing else, which gives the
cold power over the inward heat, will cause fits, because
the natural tone of the muscular power is thereby destroyed, which produces violent spasms on the whole system. So much has already been said on this subject,
that it is unnecessary to say more, to give a correct idea
of the manner of cure.

St. Anthony's Fire, Nettle Spring, or Surfeit.

These are all caused by overheating the system and
cooling too suddenly, which leaves the pores obstructed,
and then by taking more cold, will bring on the warfare
between cold and heat, when they break out and itch
and smart, as if stung by an insect. When the heat
gets a little the upper hand, so as to produce perspiration,
it will disappear till they get another cold. The only
way to effect a cure is to give the hot medicine, and steam
till they are brought to the same state of heat as that
which first caused the disease, and then cool by degrees.

11

This I have proved in several instances, and never had
any difficulty in entirely removing the cause in this way.
Make use of a tea of No. 3, for canker, and the bitters to
correct the bile, and a little nerve powder to quiet the
nerves, and they will soon be restored to perfect health.

Stranguary, or Gravel.

This disorder is often caused by hard labour, and ex-
posure to cold, in the early part of life; and when they
grow old their heat diminishes, the bile becomes thick,
and a sediment collects in the bladder, which obstructs
the passages; the glands through which the urine passes
are clogged and become diseased, so that there is a
difficulty in voiding the water, which causes great pain.
It is seldom that there is a cure in such cases; but relief may be obtained, by a course of the medicine, and
making free use of the poplar bark tea.   A tea of the
hemlock boughs is very good; and also I have known
great relief from using the wild lettuce and pipsisway,
the tops and roots bruised and steeped in hot water.
Many other articles that are good to promote the urine
may be used to advantage.

Dropsy.

There are two kinds of this complaint; one is caused
by losing the inward heat so as to stop the natural perspiration, which causes the water that is usually thrown
off in this way, to collect in the body and limbs.   This
may be cured by raising the internal heat and causing
a profuse perspiration, when the water will pass off in a
natural way; then make use of such medicine as will
remove canker and restore the digestive powers, when
the food being digested will keep up the natural heat
of the body and continue the perspiration.   The other
kind is caused by cold and obstruction; but instead of
the water collecting and remaining in the body and
limbs, a leak forms in the glands and lets it into the
trunk of the body, where there is no vent to let it off.

This cannot be cured without tapping, and is very seldom completely cured. I have never known but two who were in this situation to be perfectly restored. One was a girl whom I attended; I tapped her and took away seventeen pounds of water; then swathed her up close, and gave medicine to keep a perspiration; she did not fill again, and was completely cured. The other was a man, he had been tapped twice. I carried him through the course of medicine several times, and gave the juniper ashes, with molasses and gin, which carried off large quantities of water, and he entirely recovered from the disorder. I have cured a number who had the first mentioned complaint, by the common course of medicine; one woman was cured by taking the wild lettuce, bruised and steeped in hot water. Mention has been made of several cases of this disease, in my narrative, which were cured; and enough has been said to give an idea of the cause and manner of treatment.

Bilious Cholic.

The name of this complaint is erroneous; for bilious means the bile, and no one ever heard of a bile cholic, or pain caused by gall, as it is a friend to health, and never caused disease or death. This pain is caused by a disordered stomach and want of digesture; the stomach is filled with canker, which gets into the narrow passage from the stomach, when the action of the bowels ceases; after the pain subsides, those parts where it was, are very sore. To cure it, raise the inward heat, by giving the hot medicine, remove the canker with No. 3, and give the bitters to correct the bile, and repeat it, till a cure is effected. If the case is bad, carry them through a course of the medicine, and often give injections.

Pleurisy.

This is a distressing complaint, and is caused by cold, or want of inward heat; I never had any difficulty in curing it by my common practice. The only remedy made use of by the doctors, is to bleed; this only in-

creases the disease, by reducing the strength of the patient, without removing the cause. I was once called to
a soldier at Eastport, who had a violent pain in his side ;
the doctor that attended him, had bled him five times,
without removing the pain, which made him so weak, that
it was with difficulty he could be held up in the bed. I
relieved him in one hour, by a common course of medicine, and bathing his side with the rheumatic drops. It
took three weeks to get up his strength, which might
have been done in three days, if he had not been bled.
I was called to another case of the kind, of a soldier, at
the same place. He had been bled, and a large blister
put on his side to remove the pain, which caused a stranguary, and he was in great distress. I declined doing
any thing for him without the consent of the command-
ing officer, who was not present. The soldier begged of
me to tell him what to do for the latter complaint, as he
could not live so. I told him to take off the blister, which
was immediately done, and it gave instant relief. By
carrying them through a course of medicine, as has been
directed for other violent attacks, it will cure all cases of
this complaint without danger ; and it is much better than
bleeding, or blisters, which only increases the difficulty.

Relax.

This complaint is caused by indigestion, or loss of
the powers of the gall, which becomes thick, in consequence of cold, or loss of inward heat, when the stomach
will be sour. The best remedy is, to give No. 2, which
will thin the gall ; cleanse the stomach with No. 1, and
give the bitters to correct the digesture. A dose of the
composition powders, with a tea-spoonful of No. 6, in it,
will in most cases effect a cure. The bayberry and poplar bark is good, and also many other articles that have
been described as good to restore the digestive powers.

Dysentery.

This is a distressing complaint, and is very common,
especially among children ; although much has already

been said on this subject; yet its importance will justify
some further directions.　It is caused by cold, which
gets the ascendency over the inward heat, so as to draw
all the determining powers inward; the stomach is disordered, the digestive powers are lost, the bowels become coated with canker, the food is not digested so as
to afford any nourishment or heat to the system, and all
the juices flow inward, and pass off by the common
passage.　The canker makes the bowels very sore, and
when any thing passes them, it causes excruciating pain.
The best plan of treatment is, to carry the patient
through a regular course of medicine, and repeat it, if
occasion should require, every day till relief is obtained.
During the operation, give the chicken broth, and after
the disease is checked, give occasionally a little brandy
and loaf sugar burned together, and a strong tea of poplar bark.　Give the syrup, No. 5, two or three times a
day, until entirely recovered; and the bitters, No. 4,
may be given night and morning, to restore the digesture.
Care must be taken to keep up the inward heat in the
interim, by giving occasionally, No. 2 in a tea of No. 3,
sweetened.　Steaming is very important in this complaint, and injections must often be administered.

Rheumatism.

This complaint is caused by cold obstructing the natural circulation, which causes pain and swelling.　It
often affects the joints, so that they grow out of shape.
A cure is easily effected, if timely and properly attended
to, which must be done by such medicine as will cause
perspiration and remove obstructions.　In common cases,
by taking the rheumatic drops, and bathing the part
affected, with the same, will remove the complaint.
When the case is bad, carry them through a course of
the medicine, and bathe with the drops, repeating it as
occasion may require, till cured.　At the same time, give
a tea of poplar bark or hemlock boughs; and many other
articles which have been described as good for this complaint, may also be made use of to advantage.

11*

The gout is from the same-cause, and the stomach being greatly disordered, and very sour, which produces a burning sensation. I have cured several cases by the common course of medicine, and giving the bitters to restore the digestive powers.

Sore Lips.

They are common in very hot or cold weather, when there is nearly a balance of the power of outward and inward heat, or outward and inward cold, which produces canker. To cure it, take a strong dose of a tea of No. 3, with a tea-spoonful of No. 2 in it, when going to bed, and wash them with the same, then wipe them dry to take off the matter collected; then wet them again with the tea, and put on as much ginger as will stick, repeat the same again for two or three times, till the coat is sufficient to keep out the air; when this comes off, repeat the same process again, until the soreness is gone, then wash again with the tea, and wipe them dry, and apply warm tallow till a cure is completed.

Sore Eyes.

This is generally caused by being exposed to sudden changes of heat and cold, which produces canker; and where this is, there will be inflammation. There are many things good for this complaint; but the best that I have found, is white pond lily root, marshrosemary, witch hazle and red raspberry leaves; make a strong tea with all or either, and add one third as much of No. 6, with a little of No. 2; bathe the eyes several times in a day; every morning put your face in cold water, open and shut the eyes till well washed; repeat this till a cure is effected. At the same time take the tea to clear the system of canker.

Headache.

This pain proceeds from a foul stomach, the bile loses its powers, the food clogs, by not being digested, and the effect is felt in the head, which is the fountain of sense.

Sometimes there is sickness at the stomach; when this happens, it is called sick headache, and when they vomit, the head is relieved. This proves that the cause is in the stomach. It must be cured by cleansing the stomach and restoring the digestive powers. A dose of composition powders, sitting by the fire wrapped in a blanket, will generally give relief; but if it should not, take a dose of No. 1, in a tea of No. 3, and take the bitters to correct the bile; No. 2 should also be taken, to warm the stomach, and if it is sour, take the pearlash water. It is very fashionable with the doctors, to tell about dropsy in the head, but in this I have no belief; for there is no disease in the head but what proceeds from the stomach, except from external injury. If they understood the real cause, and would give the proper medicine to remove it, there would be no difficulty in the head; but when a child is sick, they give calomel and other poisons, which increases the disease; and if they die, it is laid to the dropsy in the head, and this is satisfactory, because the doctor says so.

Corns.

These come on the joints of the toes, and are very troublesome. They may be cured by soaking the foot in warm water till the corn is soft, shave it thin; take a strip of bladder or skin of suet, eight or ten inches long, and half an inch wide, rub it till soft; then supple it well in rattle-snake's oil, or the nerve ointment; wrap it round the toe, and keep it on till worn out; if this does not cure, repeat the same till the corn is removed. I have seldom known this to fail of a cure.

Venereal.

This disease, that is called by this name, is more common in seaports than in the country, because there is a more promiscuous and illicit intercourse of the sexes, than in other places. It is a very high state of canker and putrefaction, which takes hold of the glands of those parts that are first affected with it; and if not checked,

the whole system will become diseased by the venereal
taint. It is more common among sea-faring men, because of their being long absent at sea, and on coming
on shore, they give free scope to their passions, without
being very scrupulous about the manner of their indulgence. It originates, probably, with those common
women, who have connection with many different men,
and going beyond the impulse of nature; this impure
connection causes uncleanness, which produces the disease, and when seated, is contagious.

The reason why this disease causes so much fright
and alarm, is owing to two causes; the first is the disgrace that is attached to the dishonesty in getting it; and
the other is the manner in which it has generally been
treated, in giving mercury to cure it; the remedy becomes worse than the disease. That this disorder cannot
be cured by any other means, is altogether an error; for
I have cured a number of cases by very simple means.
The first symptoms felt, is a scalding sensation and pain
when voiding the urine; and within twenty-four hours
after this is experienced, it may be cured in that time, by
applying cold water, and making use of the rheumatic
drops; if there is much soreness, make use of the tea of
No. 3, with the drops in it; which must be taken, as well
as applied to the parts. If the disease has been of long
standing, and the whole system has become affected,
they must be carried through a course of the medicine.
Where there has been mercury made use of, and there is
all the attendant consequences of such treatment, it is
much more difficult to effect a cure; and is only done by
a full course of the medicine, and repeating it for a number of times; raising the heat by steam, each time as
high as they can bear, to throw out the mercury and remove the canker, at the same time applying the poultice;
then give the bitters to correct the bile.

I had a case of a woman, who was brought to me on
a bed, fifteen miles. She was in a very putrid state, and
as bad as she could well be, with all the consequences
that are caused by being filled with mercury. Different
doctors had attended her for eleven months, and she had
constantly been growing worse. She had been kept
ignorant of her disease, till a few days before brought to

me, on account of her husband. I carried her through
five courses of the medicine in two weeks, and applied a
poultice of white bread and ginger made with a tea of
No. 3. This completely broke up the disorder, and by
giving medicine to correct the bile and restore the digesture, she was cured, and returned home in three weeks
after coming to me. By taking things to restore her
strength, has enjoyed good health ever since. Another
woman was cured in the same manner, who had been in
this way for six years, and unable to do any business. I
attended her three weeks, when she was restored to
health, and returned home. In less than a year after,
she had two children at a birth, and has enjoyed good
health to this day.

This disease may be produced by other means than
what have been described. It may be taken in with the
breath by being much exposed in attending on those
who are in a very putrid stage of the complaint; or may
be communicated to parts where the skin is broken, and
in many other ways; when they will have many of the
symptoms the same as when taken in the common way.
Children will sometimes be affected with the venereal
taint, whose parents have had the disease. A disease
similar in appearance, with much the same symptoms,
may be brought on by overdoing and being exposed to
the cold. I once had the case of a young married man,
who, by straining himself from loading mill logs and being exposed to wet and cold, caused a weakness in the
back and loins, and he had what is called a gleet, and an
inflammation, with all the symptoms common in the venereal. His wife became affected in the same manner,
and they continued in this situation three months, when
I was called to attend them; and by making use of such
things as I then had a knowledge of, to strengthen the
loins and remove the canker, was able to cure both in a
short time. The man had all the symptoms that appear
in the venereal except hard bunches in the groins, called
buboes. These I am satisfied are caused by mercury,
for I never knew any to have them except they had taken
mercury. By syringing with mercury and sugar of lead,
it dries the glands and contracts the passage, and stops the
discharge, when the putrid matter instead of going off,

collects in the groin and forms hard tumours, which remain a long time and have to be brought to a head to let off the putrid matter.   Bunches of a similar kind often come on different parts of the body caused by mercury.

Much more might be written on this subject, but it is difficult to find proper terms to convey all the directions that may be necessary in all cases.   Enough has been said to give to those who are so unfortunate as to have the disease, a general knowledge of the nature of the complaint and the best manner of effecting a cure ; and to those who are fortunate enough to escape it, any thing further will be unnecessary.   If the disease be of recent standing, let it be considered merely a case of local canker, and treated as such ; but if the whole system has become tainted, and especially if mercury has been given, the disease is more difficult to remove, and must be treated accordingly.

MIDWIFERY.

This is a very difficult subject to write upon, as I know of no words, that would be proper to make use of, to convey the necessary information to enable a person to attempt the practice with safety.   The great importance of the subject, however, induces me not to be silent ; and I shall endeavour to make known to the public such thoughts and conclusions as long experience and much solicitude has enabled me to form, concerning those who are suffering and are constantly liable to suffer from the erroneous and most unnatural practice of the present day.   The practice of midwifery at this time, appears to be altogether a matter of speculation with the medical faculty, by their exorbitant price for attendance.   The tax on the poor classes is very heavy ; and this is not the greatest grievance that they have to bear, for they are often deprived of their wives and children, by such ignorant and unnatural practice as is very common in all parts of the country.

Thirty years ago the practice of midwifery was principally in the hands of experienced women, who had no difficulty ; and there was scarce an instance known in those days of a woman dying in child-bed, and it was very uncommon for them to lose the child; but at the present time these things are so common that it is hardly talked about. There must be some cause for this difference, and I can account for, it in no other way than the unskilful treatment they experience from the doctors, who have now got most of the practice into their own hands. In the country where I was born, and where I brought up a family of children, there was no such thing thought of as calling the assistance of a doctor; a midwife was all that was thought necessary, and the instances were very rare that they were not successful, for they used no art, but afforded such assistance as nature required; gave herb tea to keep them in a perspiration and to quiet the nerves. Their price was one dollar; when the doctors began to practise midwifery in the country, their price was three dollars, but they soon after raised it to five; and now they charge from twelve to twenty dollars. If they go on in this ratio, it will soon take all the people can earn, to pay for their children.

All the valuable instruction I ever received, was from a woman, in the town where I lived, who had practised as a midwife, for twenty years; in an interview of about twenty minutes, she gave me more useful instruction, than all I ever gained from any other source. I have practised considerably in this line, and have always had very good success. It is very important to keep up the strength of women in a state of pregnancy, so that at the time of delivery, they may be in possession of all their natural powers; they should be carried through a course of the medicine several times, particularly a little before delivery, and keep them in a perspiration during and after delivery, which will prevent after pains, and other complaints common in such cases. Beware of bleeding, opium, and cold baths; invigorate all the faculties of the body and mind, to exert the most laborious efforts that nature is called upon to perform, instead of stupifying, and substituting art for nature. I will relate a case that I was knowing to, which will give a pretty fair view of the practice of the doctors. A woman was taken in travail, and the midwife could not come; a doctor was sent for; when he came, the prospect was, that she would not be delivered in two hours; he gave her some medicine, which caused vomiting, and turned the pains to the stomach; she continued in this situation for twelve hours, when her strength was nearly gone; he then bled her, and to stop the puking, gave so much opium, as to cause such a stupor, that it required all the exertions of the women to keep the breath of life in her, through the night; in the morning, she remained very weak, and continued so till afternoon, when she was delivered with instruments. The child was dead, and the woman came very near dying, and it was six months before she got her strength again. Many more cases might be given of the bad success of bleeding and giving opium to stupify, and making use of art, instead of assisting nature to do her own work.

I have given instruction to several who have bought the right, and their practice has been attended with complete success. Many men that I have given the information to, have since attended their own wives, and I have never known an instance of any bad consequences; and if young married men would adopt the same course, it would be much more proper and safe, than to trust their wives in the hands of young inexperienced doctors, who have little knowledge, except what they get from books, and their practice is to try experiments; their cruel and harsh treatment, in many instances, would induce the husband to throw them out at the window, if permitted to be present; but this is not allowed, for the very same reason.

The following cases, and the mode of treatment, each of which presents something new, and difficult, will present to view all that will be further necessary on this subject. These will be added by way of supplement.

SUPPLEMENT

TO THE THIRD EDITION.

INTRODUCTION.

"The Hebrew women are lively, and are delivered ere the midwives come in unto them." Exodus, i. 19.

As an introduction to what I have further to say on the subject of midwifery, the above may answer as a text; from which, I have only to observe, that, had this important branch been preserved in its simplicity, attended only by women, as it seems to have been in the days of the ancient Egyptians, when the Hebrews were slaves under Pharaoh, who ordered the midwives to kill all the Hebrew male children at their birth, women might still have been delivered with as little trouble to the midwives, and as little pain to themselves, as from the account, it appears that they were then. For, as a cover to their humanity, and to escape punishment from the king, the midwives excused themselves for not killing the male children on account of the liveliness of the Hebrew women. If those women had had the doctors of the present day, with their pincers, Pharaoh would have had less cause to have issued his decree to kill the male children, as many might have been killed with impunity before it was known whether they were male or female. Has the nature of women altered, which makes the mode of having children so much more difficult and mysterious now than it was then? or is it the speculation of the doctors, for the sake of robbing the people of *twenty dollars*, the regular tribute here, for each child born? And should the child be born, fortunately for the mother and child both, before the arrival of the doctor, he even then, instead of the price of a common visit, considers himself entitled to a half fee; that is, ten dol-

12

lars.   In all this, you may see the mystery of iniquity.
Then dismiss the doctor; restore the business into the
hands of women, where it belongs; and save your wife
from much unnecessary pain, your children, perhaps,
from death, and at all events, your *money*, for better purposes.   Then will your children be born naturally, as
fruit falls from the tree, when ripe, of itself.

From this source, the doctors and their pincers, may
be traced the miserable health of women, unable to stand
on their feet for weeks and months, and never finally
recover; all caused by those horrid instruments of steel,
to extend the passage not only for the child, but for the
instruments also.   In this harsh and unnatural operation,
they often not only crush the head of the child, but also
the neck of the bladder.   After this, there is an invol-
untary discharge of the urine, bearing-down pains, &c.
insomuch that life becomes an intolerable burden without
remedy.   Can any one believe there was ever an instance of this kind among the Hebrew women, where
midwives only were known, or where nature only was
the midwife?   I think not.   Is there any such thing
known among the natives of this country, where nature
is their only dependence?   History gives us an account
of their squaws' having a pappoos at night, and wade
several rivers the next day, when driven by *Christians*
in warfare; and by the simple use of taking the unicorn
root, they would prevent themselves from taking cold.
If all these views of the subject, what has been stated
in the body of this work, and what is here to follow,
be not satisfactory, neither would people be persuaded
though one should arise from the dead.

Further Remarks on Midwifery.

As I am often called upon for verbal information on
this important subject, I shall endeavour in this supplement to give some further instructions, by relating several important cases, and their mode of treatment, which
have occurred since my last edition was published.

In addition to the bad practice of the doctors, as before related, I will state another case of which I was an

eye-witness. My brother's wife, about thirty years old, was in travail with her first child. The midwife called on me for advice, on account of a violent flooding, which I immediately relieved by the hot medicine; at the same time, some people present, privately sent for a doctor. When he came, I told him there was no difficulty, and all that was wanting was time. After examination, he said the woman had been well treated. He then took the command, and very soon began to use too much exertion. He was cautioned by the midwife; but he showed temper, and said, " Why did you send for me, if you know best." I told him he was not sent for by our request; we found no need of any other help. The doctor persisted in this harsh treatment for about seven hours, occasionally trying to put on his instruments of torture. This painful attempt caused the woman to shrink from her pains, and the child drew back. After making several unsuccessful attempts, got himself tired out; he asked me to examine her situation. I did so, and told him that the child was not so far advanced as when he came. He asked me to attend her. I refused the offer; and told him that he pronounced the woman well treated when he came; but she had not been so treated since, and I was not liable to bear the blame. He then sent for another doctor, and let her alone till the other doctor came, in which time nature had done much in advancing her labour. The doctors were astonished at her strength, in its thus holding out; and 1 now firmly believe that with the use of the medicine which had been given her, and which ought to have been continued, nature would have completed her delivery. The second doctor did but little more than to say, the instruments could now be put on; which shows how far nature had completed her work. The first doctor put on the instruments of death, and delivered her by force; using strength enough to have drawn a hundred weight! Thus the child was, as I should call it, murdered; the head crushed, and the doctor put it in a tub of cold water twice; an application, one would have supposed, sufficient to kill it, had it been well ! !

The woman flooded, like the running of water, so as to be heard by all in the room. The doctor called for

cold water to put on as soon as possible. I told the
doctor that he need not trouble himself any further about
the woman, I would take the care of her. I gave her a
spoonful of fine bayberry, cayenne and drops; got her
into bed as soon as possible; the alarming situation soon
abated; but her senses were gone, and her nerves all in
a state of confusion. I repeated the dose with the addition of nerve powder. I put a hot stone, wrapped in
cloths wet with vinegar, at her feet, and also at her back
and bowels, until she got warm. Then her nerves became more composed. When the doctor left her, he
said there was a doubt whether she lived over twelve
hours. At that time she was so swollen as to stop all
evacuations, besides other injuries she had received by
the use of force instead of aid. The midwife used her
best endeavours to promote a natural discharge, but in
vain. But, when all other sources fail, then comes my
turn. I succeeded, and saved her from mortification.
The second day, I carried her through a course of medicine; steaming her in bed; for she was as *helpless* as
though all her bones had been broken. All the way she
could be turned was to draw her on the under sheet, and
so turn her that way. After the second course, she began to help herself a little. I was with her most of the
time for five days and nights. I then left her, with medicines and directions, and she gained her health in about
two months. I gave them directions how to proceed in
case she should ever be in the like situation again. She
had another child in about two years; the *child lived*,
and both did well, by keeping away the doctor, as I am
satisfied would have been the case the first time, had
this scourge of humanity been kept away.

I have been more particular in relating this case, than
I otherwise should have been, had I not been an eye-
witness to all the proceedings, and of course to all the
facts which I have stated, which I could not have believed had I not seen them; and had it been at my own
house, I think I should not have waited for a door, but
have pitched the monster out at the window. Yet I
have reason to believe that this is only a sample of the
general practice where nature moves slowly. The argot
or rye spur, which is a very improper medicine, was

also frequently given in this case; but it ought to be particularly guarded against, in all cases.

———

Another instance happened in the country, very recently, only about six weeks since, where the doctor was with a young woman in travail, who had fits. The doctor bled her, and took away her child dead by force. The woman is yet in a poor state of health. What could we expect otherwise, where learned men forbid the laws of nature to take their course, take the blood, " which is the life," to enable women to go through with the most laborious task which nature is called on to perform? Consider of these things, my friends, and govern yourselves accordingly.

———

Now let me exhibit the other side of the picture. I was called upon to attend a young woman in child-bed, about four weeks ago, eighty miles in the country. I attended. She had been sick, and sent for help, before I arrived, and had got about again. About one week after, she was taken again, with every appearance that she would be delivered soon. In about six hours the pains all flatted away; she grew pale and dull in spirits, and the motion of the child had nearly ceased. She had laboured hard and got cold, and had a bad cough; and the moisture of the glands was so thickened, that she could not spit clear of her mouth. I saw that there was no use in any further delay. On Thursday I carried her through a thorough course of medicine, and steamed her twice in the course of the day, and then let her rest. About the same time she was taken the night before, to wit, about eleven o'clock, her pains were regular, her animation and vigour returned, a fine son was born about three o'clock, she walked from the fire to the bed, a portion of coffee and cayenne was administered, and a steaming stone put to her feet. As soon as her perspiration was free, all after-pains ceased, and there were none of those alarming symptoms common to learned ignorance. The second day she showed symptoms of a child-bed fever and broken breasts. I carried her

12*

through another course of medicine and steam.   The
fifth day she took breakfast and dinner below with the
family, and carried her child up stairs.   The eighth day
she rode out two miles, paid a visit and come back.   On
the ninth day, I carried her through another course of
medicine, and got her so far cleared, that she could spit
clear of her mouth for the first time after I saw her.   On
the tenth day, she rode the same distance; and I have
no doubt that, had she been-attended in the common
way, she would have had the child-bed fever, broken
breasts, and a poor health afterwards.

This case caused much conversation.. Why so? It
was the different mode of treatment, reversing every
mode commonly attended to.   What shall we do? say
the people, we shall never dare to employ a doctor again.
I answer.   Call the doctor and obtain his advice; and
then reverse every prescription given by him in a case of
child-bed.   If he tells you to have a doctor, have a midwife.   If he says, "be bled," keep your blood for other
uses.   If he says, "keep yourself cold," Sweat yourself.   If he says, "put cold water on your bowels,"
take hot medicine inside, and a steaming stone at your
feet.   If he says, "take physic," use warm injections.
If he says, "starve yourself," eat what your appetite
craves.   By strict observance of the foregoing anti-di-
rections, you may enjoy your health, and save the heavy
bill for the many visits of the doctor, besides saving him
from the trouble of keeping you sick.   This is the mode
of having patent babies, so highly recommended by Dr.
Robinson in his 12th lecture, who says, "Even in child-
bed delivery, a matter never to be forgotten, this practice has very nearly removed the pain and punishment
from the daughters of Eve, threatened to our progeni-
tor and entailed upon her offspring.   A lady of good
sense, and without the least colouring of imagination,
said it was easier to have five children under the operation and influence of this new practice, than one by the
other management and medicine.   And she had had experience in both cases, and has been supported in the
evidence by every one who has followed her example."

This extract speaks volumes in favour of the treatment
in the last named case.

The following case of midwifery I shall mention, with the mode of treatment, for the purpose of giving instruction to others.

I was called to visit a woman in Greenfield, Saratoga Co. N. Y. who had been in travail ten days, and her life despaired of. I think there was not less than ten men and women present, and the seal of despair was set upon each one's countenance. The woman in a low voice said, "I cannot see what can be the use of a woman's undergoing the distress I have for ten days, and die after all, as two sisters of mine have done in a similar case but a short time ago." I replied, that pain and distress were the common lot of all mankind, and the duty of every one is to alleviate the miseries of others as far as it is in our power. She asked me if I thought I could help her. I assured her that I would do every thing I could for that purpose. There were several persons present who owned the right. I took out my medicine, and put in a tea-cup a large spoonful of composition, one tea-spoonful of cayenne, one of nerve powder, and one spoonful of sugar, filled the cup with boiling water, stirred them well together, and set it down. While settling, I took a large tea-spoonful of brown emetic, and having poured off the tea into another cup, stirred in the powder, and handed it to the woman, who swallowed it, apparently with all possible faith that it would help her. I called for assistance, to regulate the bed and other things, which were in disorder about the room, as soon as possible. Every attention was paid, the medicine roused the efforts of nature, so that the woman was in readiness before we were. This called all to her assistance; the desired object was obtained in less than fifteen minutes after taking this friend of nature; a fine son was born alive, and the woman comfortable and able with steadying, to walk from the fire to the bed, to the great joy of all present. The gloomy veil of despair was raised from the countenance of all, and they heartily partook of the joy and thankfulness of the woman and family; insomuch that some of the women present, declared that they would never have any other children but patent ones hereafter.

One of my agents, Joseph Michell, went with me; and we returned in the space of two hours, in a violent snow storm. He declared that that expedition was worth one hundred dollars to the society. The next day, the husband came, and purchased the right, with instruction on the branch of midwifery; and has attended his wife twice since, with unusual success. One of my agents says he has frequently heard the woman relate the foregoing case; but never without shedding tears.

Case of Midwifery in Columbus, Ohio.

This woman I agreed to be with when confined, which was expected in about three weeks. I went to see my son, about 130 miles. While there, I fell and broke two of my ribs. I had a violent cough, and almost lost my life. I did not return short of about six weeks, and then in a very poor state of health. I arrived at the house about eleven o'clock at night. The woman was then in travail. She said she had waited for me three weeks. The midwife said the waters had been discharged three days, and the woman was in a low and lingering state, often wishing for me. I went to bed that night, but did not sleep much, on account of the distress of the woman, and noise of the moving in the house. I was solicited about noon the next day, by the husband and wife, her father and mother, my agent and his wife, with an earnest desire to attend the woman, as her mind was set on my attention. I reluctantly consented, as I was weak in body and mind, and hardly able to undergo the anxiety and responsibility of so difficult a case. I however agreed to do the best I could. I prepared a dose similar to that mentioned in the foregoing case. It was given. It soon had the desired effect, by rousing the system to action. I delivered her in about half an hour. But the child was apparently dead. I took the placenta or after-birth, with the child; the grandmother being seated in the corner, she placed the after-birth on a bed of embers, while rubbing the child; and as soon as the substance on the coals had gained warmth enough to fill the umbilical cord with warmth and moisture, it was stripped towards the body of the child, and so continued until a sufficient degree of warmth through this medium was conveyed into the body of the child, as to expand the lungs, which was effected in about fifteen or twenty minutes; then the string was separated in usual form.

I relate this case for the information of those who may not have studied the principle of heat's giving life, as is manifest in the present case. There was no other possible way of communicating heat to the vitals, except through that channel or stem which had supported the growth of the child to that time, the same as any vegetable fruit is supported from the vine or tree by the stem. If the vine be cut off, or pulled up, the fruit will wither and die. Now what was the cause of the death of this child? Recollect the fore part of this statement. The water had been discharged three days. All that time the child had been starving, the same as the fruit loses its support when the vine is cut. But by raising artificial heat, through the placenta and umbilical cord, by putting the former on the embers, and conveying the heat to the body of the child through the medium of the latter, it gave the child one more meal, which roused it into action, and which was to last till the next means nature has provided, can be obtained. Before the child is born, it is supported by this stem from the mother internally; after birth, from the breast of the mother externally. This food supports the child, till he can eat more solid food, and thus no longer need the breast.

> Now the attention of the mother,
> May be employ'd to have another;
> And so go on with all the rest,
> Your house be fill'd with children bless'd.

Case of a False Conception.

About two years ago, I was called on by one of my agents, at Eastport, Me. who appeared to be much alarmed, and requested me to go with him to visit a woman with whom he had been all night, and could give her no relief. She had flowed so much, that she lay fainted away, more than half the time, and then, the rest part

of the time, she was puking.   I asked him if she was
in a pregnant state.   He thought not.   I answered, I
thought it must be-the case.   I went with him; and, on
the way, asked him if he had given her an emetic?   He
had not.   If he had used an. injection?   No, he did not
think it would answer.   Not answer!   What is your
medicine good for, if it is not a friend in the most alarming case?   When entering the house, the man said, "My
wife has been fainted away more than half the time,
since you left, and the rest of the time she has been
puking."   I directed my agent to go after his syringe.
The first thing I could find warm was some wormwood
tea.   I took some in a cup, and added some cayenne,
nerve powder, and emetic herb, sweetened, as heretofore directed.   She took it.   I then steeped one pint of
coffee, and had time to give her about one glass, with a
requisite portion of the same articles as before, when the
syringe arrived.   I then prepared about a gill of this
liquid, and added the same proportion of the articles
taken, and charged the syringe with it, and ordered the
nurse to administer it.   I, with my agent, left the room
for the space of about ten minutes, when we were called
in, and found the nurse much surprised at the discharge.
The like was never seen by any one present.   The appearance was like a hog's heart secured in a membrane.
The people were at a loss what to call it.   My agent
was of opinion that there was some human shape in it.
I said, no.   To satisfy himself, he opened it with his
knive, and found it solid flesh.   I told them it was a
false conception, and void of human shape.   I then repeated the dose as before given, and repeated the injection in usual form, which cleared her of all disorder, and
set nature at liberty.   All flowing, puking, and fainting,
ceased from the first application I made.   The woman
soon got well, and in less than one year, had a fine son,
and her health remains good.   Many thanks were given
me by the family, believing, as they said, that what I
administered to the woman, together with what I prescribed, had saved her life.

   I shall close this subject with a few brief remarks.
   The foregoing cases I have described for the purpose
of showing the difference between forcing nature, and

aiding and assisting her. They are two theories, directly opposed to each other, and can never harmonize together. As soon as learned ignorance begins to use force to extend the passage, the child ceases from its natural progression and draws back; as nature shrinks from all such operations, and force must then do the whole; and if the child should be caught by such force, as the dog catches his game, it will be likely to share the same fate, as in the case first mentioned. I shall not follow up the simile, by comparing the doctor to a dog, though it might be made a very striking one. Is not this the cause of many women lingering out a miserable existence in pain and torment, and are often heard to say, " I have never been well since my last child was born. I was in the hands of the doctor three days, and at last was delivered with instruments. I did not stand on my feet for six weeks, and have never regained my health." Yet the doctor is looked upon as her benefactor, and is thanked for saving her life. Query. Were these evil consequences ever known where nature did her own work, and the child born before the doctor could get there ? In all my practice, I never knew an instance where the woman could not bear her weight upon her feet the same day. Nor have I ever heard of a single instance where nature had been assisted according to my practice by others, where the patient was not able to bear her weight on her feet the same day of her delivery. As to the cause of the difference between those attended according to nature, and those attended *secundum artem*, according to art, I shall leave the reader to decide for himself.

Another evil in this branch, which I shall mention here, and of which women have generally either felt or heard, is that of taking the after-birth by force. The doctor says, " It has grown fast to the side;" and tares it off, so as to be heard by those present. Alarming, if not fatal consequences are the result. The question is, what other way can be done ? Answer. The same as in taking the child. Assist nature, instead of forcing it. The only rule given by me, to those who wish to attend their own wives, or others, is simply this. After the string is separated from the child, be careful not to lose it, by letting it draw back, as this is the only sure guide to the placenta. Take the string between the thumb and finger of the left hand, drawing it straight, while having the same between the thumb and finger of the right hand, slipping it forward until you find the solid part to which the string is attached. Take a steady pull when the pain is on. After a few seconds, it will begin to give way, turning inside out as turning the lining to the sleeve of a coat. But if it stick fast, take care not to break the string, as if you do, you lose your guide. Keep the woman well fed with hot medicine, to prevent flooding. Then carry her through a course of medicine; and when the system is slackened, it will often come of itself. I would prefer having it remain till it discharges itself, according to nature, as it certainly will in time, than to be taken away by force, as I have seen done. The danger is far less. But I never knew a case of the kind where the woman had been sufficiently cleared by the medicine near the time of her delivery. I knew one instance, where the woman had been treated by force in this way, that she had been so injured that all her urine run away as fast as it collected. The doctors had so injured her, that they declared she would never live to have another child. But they were mistaken. The next one she was attended by my direction, and carried through, I think, thirteen courses of medicine before delivery. I attended her. She was sick but about two hours; was delivered and cleared without any difficulty, and both she and her child did well.

There are as great errors committed in using force for the after-birth, as for the child. The inflammation caused by using force in taking the child, causes the obstruction in taking the after-birth. When learned ignorant pretenders, who know nothing about following the umbilical cord for their guide, proceed inward, where they have no business, they often commit irreparable injury, and instead of taking the after-birth, they injure the womb, sometimes by turning it wrong side out, which causes distressing bearing-down pains, and thus the woman must linger out a miserable existence until death comes as a welcome friend to relieve her.

Thus, kind reader, I have given you the most important particulars I now think of, and as to any further general directions, I can do no better than to refer you to the *General Directions,* as laid down in this book; and it is my opinion that you are better off with your own judgment and this book, than with all the scientific ignorance, called knowledge, as taught in the schools, without it. Hence my advice to you is, dismiss all doctors of law, physic and divinity. Pray for your own soul, if you know what it is, doctor your own body, and make your own will. By so doing, you will save your share of the greatest tax ever imposed on mankind.

Outlines of Treatment in the hour of Travail.

To point out a regular rule or form for every woman, would be out of my power, as they are restless, shifting their position in every form and manner, to find a place of rest, which is as difficult as that of Noah's dove. When they become so far advanced that they cannot satisfy themselves any longer in their own way, then you may assist them in the best manner to help themselves, and to enable others to help them, by assisting nature to do her own work.

The seat is prepared in different ways, according to their fancy. Those who have had children ought to be the best judge how to aid and assist them in this particular. I shall only give advice how to proceed in some alarming and difficult cases, to be handed down for the benefit of generations yet unborn, as none can be obtained from the progress of the learned, for four thousand years. And if any beneficial information shall now be obtained, it must be from the illiterate, who have studied nature rather than books. I have no authors, dictionaries or concordance, to assist my feeble efforts in acquiring a correct judgment. Necessity and experience are the only sources of my knowledge, from which I draw all my lessons.

Among the most desperate cases, is the flowing of females; pregnant or not, the treatment is the same. If it happens before delivery, give a portion of composition

13

with more cayenne, and hot water sweetened; or some drops, cayenne and snuff, or fine bayberry, as substitutes. If after delivery, the same. When the woman grows weary and worn out, and pains begin to die away, give a portion of the third preparation, in some composition and nerve powder. This will compose the system so as to rest or reinforce nature, and hasten delivery. It is of great service, when the pains are. lingering, at the time of giving the above named medicine, to use an injection, in common form, made of the same compound. This will hasten or delay delivery, as nature requires.

Remark......About the time of delivery apply a cloth of several thicknesses wet with hot water, to slack the muscles; repeat it occasionally, and keep it hot till nature is ready to perform her work.

I attended one woman in this city, with her first child. Her strength failed; her pains slacked; I gave her a table-spoonful of the liquid of the third preparation; wrapped her warm, which caused her to vomit once, and raised a perspiration; she fell asleep, and in this situation rested four hours, when the head of the child was so far advanced, as to have been visible. She awoke, her travail re-commenced with reinforced vigour. She was delivered rather in a cold state; she flowed badly; I gave her some No. 2, and drops, with a little fine bayberry, which had the desired effect. She walked from the fire to the bed, and did well.

There is another distressing complaint incident to females, worse than having children; and often no relief from the doctors. I have seen women in as great agony with false pains, as at the delivery of a child. A strong tea of witch-hazle leaves and nerve powder, and a little cayenne, strained, used by injection either way, or both, I have seen relieve, like throwing water on the fire. The disorder is canker, and must be met with its antidote where it is.

These few remarks, together with the foregoing cases, will be sufficient information on this subject. In conclusion, I would ask, can we attach sufficient value on a medicine that will give rest to a weary patient in travail, and restore the nerves and muscles to a giant-like strength, as refreshed by wine, and continue the strength until delivery is completed ; and at the same time guard against all those alarming complaints which too often follow afterwards ? A medicine to which you may resort with perfect confidence, in times of the greatest peril, that, if any thing can, it will save your wife and child, and the *fee* of twenty dollars from the doctor. This is the regular *fce* in cities, though it is less in the country.

Supplement to the Venereal.....See page 130.

There are four diseases, or rather four names of disease, which are often made fatal, in consequence of the name. 1. Venereal. 2. Hydrophobia. 3. Smallpox. 4. Erysipelas. As the remedy is laid down in the Medical Pocket Book, the name is doctored instead of the disease. If a child has a sore ear, and it runs a yellow water, it will spread like fire, as often seen on a pot ; and it will inoculate where it touches. While on the child's ear, women call it a canker sore; and there is nothing alarming under this name. Any old woman can cure it. But take the same infection from the ear, and inoculate with it, in that part of the body where venereal is seated, and call it venereal, the consequence is the same ; and by the same mercurial treatment, there would be all the alarming consequences as though the disorder was generated in any other way. Yea, if the patient was well, with the same administration of mercury, in the same way, and to the same extent, the buboes and shankers would often make their appearance in the same manner without the supposed disease as with. They doctor the name instead of the disorder. The patient, therefore, as often loses his life by the mercury, as by the supposed disease.

Equally so in hydrophobia, by taking mercury, the remedy becomes worse than the disease.

In either of the above cases, the disorder is far easier cured by a regular course of medicine, than the poison given for it; as the mercury is harder to eradicate from the system, than all the natural disease incident to mankind.

Since my last edition was published, the smallpox has been thoroughly attended to, and the general rule, as there laid down, found to answer every purpose, and produce the desired effect. To bring out the smallpox, as in the measles and other similar disorders, be careful not to have too much outward heat while the pock is filling. I visited a family in Cincinnati, last winter, who had the smallpox, and who had had the kinepox previous. The appearance of the pustules were more like poison or measles than those of the smallpox. When it turned, it began to flat, instead of drying off; and when it had flatted down to the vitals, it turned in, and one died, and the other, it left in a miserable state of health; the pits hard and blue, like other poison sores; and I am of an opinion that more people die in consequence of having the kinepox, than it would to let the smallpox have its natural run. Because the nature of the smallpox, when taken the natural way, is to clear the system from every other putrefaction, which, on the turn, scabs off with it. Not so in the kinepox. The infection partakes of every disorder of the persons of which it was taken; itch, venereal, cancer humours, or worse than all the rest, mercurial taint given by the doctor. When part, or all of these diseases are inoculated into a healthy person, and has no way to discharge itself from the system, it creates worse disease than the smallpox. I knew a man in Portsmouth, N. H. who was inoculated with the kinepox, the infection taken from a man who had a cancer humour. He was a healthy man when inoculated. I saw him within two years, and it was judged that he had more than half a peck of cancers on different parts of the body and limbs. He imputed it entirely to this inoculation; and highly disapproved of the kinepox. He died in the most distressed condition.

The learned have added nothing to the healing art; but they have done much in taking the knowledge of the simple remedies from the people. They have substituted the poisonous minerals which have multiplied the forms of disease, and thereby added to our bills of mortality. They have taken midwifery from the tender hands of women, and substituted the torturing instruments of steel, whereby not only children, but even women have been scarified. In relation to such practice, Robinson says. Lec. viii. p. 103. "It is, in truth, like running the gauntlet among armed Indians, or red hot plough-shares, to escape from the poisons or medical practice."

Why do old people die more in a warm and rainy winter than in a severe cold one?

The answer to the above question is at hand. Old people are like the old house which they built in their younger days. The house decays about as fast as its builder, and becomes racked with wind and storms which have beaten upon it until the cracks open, the shingles blow off, and the house grows leaky and cold. So is the man in his old age. He becomes racked with the storms and hardships of life; his heat goes out, the fire-place decays, his food digests poorly, and gives but little nourishment or heat to warm the body and expand the lungs. For the inward heat rarifies the air in the lungs, and causes them to expand, by lightening the air within, and the heft of the surrounding atmosphere, being higher charged with oxygen or water, puts out the fire faster than dry cold air; and as the heat decays inward, the weight of the air crowds heavily on the lungs, and causes great difficulty in breathing; the lungs labour like the wheel of a mill in back water, the fountain almost level with the stream, until the heat in the lungs becomes insufficient to expand them any longer; the heft of the air comes to an equilibrium of heft inside, and all motion ceases. The water in the air has put out the fire. This is the cause why those people who have but little fire in the body, and such a heft of damp air outside, the heat is so soon extinguished inside; like a person falling into the water; the cause of death is, the water has put out the fire; and when the air is full of water, it puts out the fire in the same proportion. Thus I think I have given a satisfactory cause of death upon natural principles. The cause and effect are in themselves.

In this case, I would ask the Christian, of every denomination, what God, here, either gave or took away life? Was there any God in the case abstract from the cause here given? Or what soul or spirit went out at death, except the heat, or nature, which caused life and breath?

How Doctors shorten the lives of their Patients.

That the practice of the regular doctors, as they are termed, shortens the lives of their patients, is a truth of

13*

which I have not the shadow of a doubt; and the cause, to me, is obvious. The cold poisons which they administer, have the effect of chilling the stomach and killing the digestive organs; so that the food does not raise more than half the heat it did in a natural state, before those poisons had been administered. Then the bleeding and blistering lessens the remainder so as to reduce the heat to the capacity of old age. It is the same thing, no matter what age, from one hour old to an hundred years. When the heat is so far exhausted that the air is not sufficiently lightened by the heat as to expand the adjoining air, the pressure becomes equalled, external and internal, the same as in the case of a drowned person. There is no difference, as to age, sect, or denomination, so far as the practice is concerned; and so far as that goes to lessen the heat by bleeding, by fever powders, or by poison; all tend to lessen inward heat, and to diminish life in the same proportion; and when it is entirely extinguished, death follows, as a natural consequence; and from the same cause; *loss of heat*, whatever it may be that puts out the fire. The putting out of the fire, or extinguishing inward or vital heat, is the cause of death.

All practitioners, therefore, may by this rule either condemn or justify themselves by looking back on their former practice, and asking themselves the question. "Have I cultivated the heat of my patients, to prolong their lives; or have I extinguished their heat, and thereby killed or destroyed them?" Is not this question fully answered? See how the lives of human beings are daily sacrificed, at all ages, from birth to death! Who, I would ask, is authorized to say, in such a case, "The Lord gives, and the Lord taketh away, and blessed be the name of the Lord," when they are destroyed in this manner?

In every thing that breathes, the breathing is from the same cause. Without heat, their is no breathing. But when heat is continually generated or evolved in a confined room, excepting at one avenue, as in the lungs, there must be breathing, or what is the same, an inhaling of cold air, and an exhaling of oxygen or vapour from it. Every animal body has its lamp, in proportion to its bigness; and its continuing to burn, is much owing to the one who trims or takes care of the lamp. If it be replenished with water, instead of oil, and with an icicle for a wick, it is like the method in which the doctors trim the lamps of their patients. Taking out the blood, is like pouring out the oil; and the cold poison, is as the icicle for a wick. The effect soon follows, which is cold and darkness. Can we doubt this being the fact at the present time? Do we not often see the head of a family suddenly made cold by his lamp being put out; and three or four children taken from one house, all having their lamps blown out? Can any one suppose that had their lamps been trimmed with good oil, and good wicks, but that they would have continued burning as long as the body of the lamp remained whole? But if we continue not our own guards and sentinels, but employ artificial and learned fools to watch over us, and save our oil for their own use, and trim our lamps with water and ice, we cannot wonder at seeing our wives and children " dashed in pieces like the potter's vessel." When we employ seamen to drive our coach of life, instead of horsemen; and as long as custom, superstition, error and bigotry, are the ruling principles of the world, we never can expect to live-while all the oil in our lamps are consumed; but to be blown out by the breath of ignorance, if nothing worse, as mankind have been. in all ages where the poisonous breath of the Bohon Upas overtakes them.

> The Priest and Doctor claiming the control,
> One of the flesh, the other of the soul;
> Hell and the pit, from which they dig their stuff,
> Are never filled, yea, never cry enough.

The effect of religious meetings, where women chiefly attend, in the absence of their husbands.

If women are allowed to attend day and night meetings, for the purpose of having the priest pray for their souls and pardon their sins, while their husbands and children are left at home, how long will it be before the sandals of the priest will be left at the door, as in some other countries, as a token that the husband must not enter, lest he should see and learn how the priest pardons his wife's sins?

The doctor also, who comes in for a full share in these secret privileges, if he be allowed to examine secretly our wives and daughters for the purpose of finding some secret complaint, which is indecent for the husband or father to witness, or to know, as was the case of R****'s wife and Dr. A****, of this city, but a few years since, who is to be responsible for the mode of examination.

If men will allow their wives to be thus privately examined by these crafts, for the purpose of pardoning their sins, and removing their indecent disorders, will they not soon claim all the indecent jobs in their families? If it be indecent for a man to be present at the birth of his child, why not equally indecent to be present at its generation? And so we must let the priest and the doctor generate, as well as bring into the world, all our children! The priest could still baptize them in the name of the Father, Son and Holy Ghost; in whose name, also, he might pardon the sins of their mother! In this way, these two crafts might liberate the affectionate husband from all the toils of his family, excepting that of their maintenance! ! !

Arouse, husbands, from your lethargy. Gird on every man his sword by his side. The sword of truth, I mean. Go in and out of your camp, and whenever you please, till you have driven all such miscreants from your borders. Take the protection of your wives and daughters into your own hands; keep them at home at all proper times, and when they go to meeting, go with them; when they are so sick as to need a doctor, which, if properly treated, would seldom be the case, be present at the examination; if they need prayers, pray for them yourselves; if they want children, be sure to be their real father, and take a fatherly care of them in bringing into the world, as well as afterwards; nourish them with due attention, instruct them in all that is good; but save them, by all means, from the pincers of learned doctors, or the fears of missionary *mules*.

☞ All people who have been attended by Patent Doctors, are cautioned against putting themselves under regular doctors, as the cases have generally proved fatal to the patient, and the blame palmed on the Patent Doctor; some after two weeks in their care.

SEAMEN'S DIRECTIONS.

After purchasing the right, and having a sample of Medicine numbered, these Directions are the first lessons learned, as it gives a short and concise view of the system and practice. In the first stages of disease, one gill of No. 3, may be used simple, with or without sugar. In more violent attacks, use from half to a teaspoonful of No. 2; let the patient be covered with a blanket, by the fire or in bed; apply a hot stone at the feet; if this does not relieve them, add the emetic, No. 1, and nerve powder, and go through a course of medicine. In all cases where the glands are dry, and much fever, the emetic should be used without spirit; the bitters also are best taken in hot water sweetened than with spirit. The objection to physic and bleeding, is given in these directions hereafter. The complement of medicine given as a family stock, is more to show the simplicity of the articles, than the requisite quantity required. Give children drink often, sick or well.

☞The public are cautioned against employing any one who shall pretend to use his own improvements with my System of Practice, as I will not be accountable for any mal-practice of his.

Th' Emetic number ONE's design'd
A gen'ral med'cine for mankind,
Of every country, clime, or place,
Wide as the circle of our race.

In every case, and state, and stage,
Whatever malady may rage;
For male or female, young or old,
Nor can its value half be told.

To use this med'cine do not cease,
Till you are helped of your disease;
For NATURE'S FRIEND, this sure will be,
When you are taken sick at sea.

Let number TWO be used bold,
To clear the stomach of the cold;
Next steep the coffee, number THREE,
And keep as warm as you can be.

A hot stone at the feet now keep,
As well as inward warmth repeat,
The fountain 'bove the stream keep clear,
And perspiration will appear.

When sweat enough as you suppose,
In spirit wash, and change your clothes;
Again to bed, both clean and white,
And sleep in comfort all the night.

Should the disorder reinforce,
Then follow up the former course;
The second time I think will do,
The third to fail I seldom knew.

Now take your bitters by the way,
Two, three, or four times in a day;
Your appetite if it be good,
You may eat any kind of food.

Physic, I would by no means choose
To have you first or last to use;
For if you take it much in course,
It will disorder reinforce.

If any one should be much bruis'd,
Where bleeding frequently is us'd,
A lively sweat upon that day,
Will start the blood a better way.

Let names of all disorders be
Like to the limbs, join'd on a tree;
Work on the root, and that subdue,
Then all the limbs will bow to you.

So as the body is the tree,
The limbs are cholic, pleurisy,
Worms and gravel, gout and stone,
Remove the cause and they are gone.

My system's founded on this truth,
Man's Air and Water, Fire and Earth,
And death is cold, and life is heat,
These temper'd well your health's complete.

INDEX

To the New Guide to Health.

CPSIA information can be obtained
at www.ICGtesting.com
Printed in the USA
LVHW051343200423
744765LV00004B/35